CONCISE GUIDE to
Neuropsychiatry and Behavioral Neurology

THIRD EDITION

Edited by

John J. Barry, M.D.

Sepideh N. Bajestan, M.D., Ph.D.

Jeffrey L. Cummings, M.D., Sc.D.

Michael R. Trimble, M.D., FRCP, FRCPsych

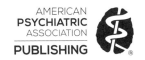

AMERICAN
PSYCHIATRIC
ASSOCIATION
PUBLISHING ®

Copyright © 2023 American Psychiatric Association Publishing

ALL RIGHTS RESERVED

Third Edition

Manufactured in the United States of America on acid-free paper
26 25 24 23 22   5 4 3 2 1

American Psychiatric Association Publishing
800 Maine Avenue SW, Suite 900, Washington, DC 20024-2812
www.appi.org

Library of Congress Cataloging-in-Publication Data
Names: Barry, John J., editor. | Bajestan, Sepideh, editor. | Cummings, Jeffrey L., 1948- editor. | Trimble, Michael R., author. | Cummings, Jeffrey L., 1948- Concise guide to neuropsychiatry and behavioral neurology. | American Psychiatric Association, publisher.
Title: Concise guide to neuropsychiatry and behavioral neurology / John J. Barry, Sepideh Bajestan, Jeffrey L. Cummings, Michael R. Trimble.
Description: Third edition. | Washington, DC : American Psychiatric Association Publishing, [2023] | Preceded by Concise guide to neuropsychiatry and behavioral neurology / Jeffrey L. Cummings, Michael R. Trimble. 2nd ed. c2002. | Includes bibliographical references and index.
Identifiers: LCCN 2022003982 (print) | LCCN 2022003983 (ebook) | ISBN 9781615374090 (paperback : alk. paper) | ISBN 9781615374106 (ebook)
Subjects: MESH: Brain Diseases--physiopathology | Mental Disorders—diagnosis | Mental Disorders—therapy | Neuropsychology—methods | Handbook
Classification: LCC RC386 (print) | LCC RC386 (ebook) | NLM WL 39 | DDC 616.8—dc23/eng/20220214
LC record available at https://lccn.loc.gov/2022003982
LC ebook record available at https://lccn.loc.gov/2022003983

British Library Cataloguing in Publication Data
A CIP record is available from the British Library.

CONTENTS

Lauren Drag, Ph.D.
Juliana Lockman, M.D.
Michael Zeineh, M.D.
Michel Medina, M.D.

Kieran C.R. Fox, Ph.D.

Sheldon Benjamin, M.D.
Delia Bakeman, D.O.

Sepideh N. Bajestan, M.D., Ph.D.
Gaston Baslet, M.D.

Simon Ducharme, M.D.
Lisa Koski, Ph.D.

Jeffrey L. Cummings, M.D., Sc.D.
Michael R. Trimble, M.D., FRCP, FRCPsych

LIST OF FIGURES

LIST OF TABLES

CONTRIBUTORS

Jesse Adams, M.D.
Director of Child and Adolescent Psychiatry, Seattle Neuropsychiatric Treatment Center, Seattle, Washington

Gregory W. Albers, M.D.
Professor, Department of Neurology, Stanford University, Stanford, California

Sepideh N. Bajestan, M.D., Ph.D.
Chief, Neuropsychiatry Services; Associate Director, Neuropsychiatry and Behavioral Neurology Fellowship; Co-Director, Individual Psychotherapy Clinic; and Clinical Associate Professor, Department of Psychiatry and Behavioral Sciences, School of Medicine, Stanford University, Stanford, California

Delia Bakeman, D.O.
Assistant Professor, Department of Neurology, University of Colorado Anschutz Medical Campus, Denver, Colorado

John J. Barry, M.D.
Fellowship Director, Neuropsychiatry and Behavioral Neurology; Director, Neuropsychiatry Clinic; Co-Director, Individual Psychiatry Clinic; Professor of Psychiatry and Behavioral Sciences, Department of Psychiatry and Behavioral Sciences; School of Medicine, Stanford University Hospital, Stanford, California

Gaston Baslet, M.D.
Director, Division of Neuropsychiatry; Co-Director, Center for Brain/Mind Medicine and Neuropsychiatry and Behavioral Neurology Fellowship Program; and Director, Medical Student Education in Psychiatry, Brigham and Women's Hospital; Assistant Professor of Psychiatry, Harvard Medical School, Boston, Massachusetts

Ori-Michael Benhamou, M.D.
Clinical Assistant Professor, Department of Psychiatry and Behavioral Sciences, School of Medicine, Stanford University, Stanford, California

Sheldon Benjamin, M.D.
Professor of Psychiatry and Neurology, University of Massachusetts T.H. Chan School of Medicine, Worcester, Massachusetts

Mahendra T. Bhati, M.D.
Clinical Professor, Chief of Interventional Psychiatry, Director of Electroconvulsive Therapy, Departments of Psychiatry and Be-

havioral Sciences and Neurosurgery, Stanford University, Stanford, California

John P. Coetzee, Ph.D.
Advanced Health Fellow, Polytrauma Division, VA Palo Alto Health Care System, Palo Alto; Postdoctoral Scholar, Department of Psychiatry and Behavioral Sciences, Stanford University, Stanford, California

Jeffrey L. Cummings, M.D., Sc.D.
Chambers-Grundy Center for Transformative Neuroscience, Department of Brain Health, School of Integrated Health Sciences, University of Nevada Las Vegas, Las Vegas, Nevada

Les Dorfman, M.D.
Professor Emeritus, active, Department of Neurology and Neurological Sciences, School of Medicine, Stanford University, Stanford, California

Lauren Drag, Ph.D.
Clinical Assistant Professor (Affiliated), Department of Neurology and Neurological Sciences, School of Medicine, Stanford University, Stanford, California

Simon Ducharme, M.D.
Douglas Mental Health University Institute, Montreal, Quebec, Canada

Alex Eischeid, M.D.
Neurologist, Department of Neurology and Neurological Sciences, Stanford University, Stanford, California; Ruan Neurology and Research Center, MercyOne, Des Moines, Iowa

Aryandokht Fotros, M.D.
Department of Psychiatry and Human Behavior, Brown University, Providence, Rhode Island

Kieran C.R. Fox, Ph.D.
School of Medicine, Stanford University, Stanford, California

Manal Khan, M.D.
University of California, Los Angeles, Los Angeles, California

Lisa Koski, Ph.D.
Scientist, Brain Repair and Integrative Neuroscience Program, Research Institute of McGill University Health Centre; Associate Professor, Departments of Neurology and Neurosurgery and Psychology, McGill University, Montreal, Quebec, Canada

Ian H. Kratter, M.D., Ph.D.
Clinical Assistant Professor, Department of Psychiatry and Behavioral Sciences, Stanford University, Stanford, California

Scheherazade Le, M.D.
Clinical Associate Professor, Department of Neurology and Neurological Sciences, Stanford Comprehensive Epilepsy Center, Palo Alto, California

Juliana Lockman, M.D.
Clinical Associate Professor, Department of Psychiatry and Behavioral Sciences, Stanford University, Stanford, California

Peter H. Marcus, Psy.D.
Department of Psychiatry, Harvard Medical School, Boston, Massachusetts

Lawrence M. McGlynn, M.D., M.S.
Clinical Professor, Department of Psychiatry and Behavioral Sciences, School of Medicine, Stanford University, Stanford, California

Michel Medina, M.D.
Department of Psychiatry and Neurology, Kaiser Permanente Northern California, Sacramento, California

Hokuto Morita, M.D.
Assistant Professor, Department of Neurology and Neurological Sciences, Stanford University, Stanford, California; Department of Neurology, The University of North Carolina at Chapel Hill, Chapel Hill, North Carolina

Jagan Pillai, M.D., Ph.D.
Lou Ruvo Center for Brain Health, Cleveland Clinic, Case Western Reserve University, Cleveland, Ohio

Kathleen L. Poston, M.D., M.S.
Professor, Department of Neurology and Neurological Sciences, and (by courtesy) Neurosurgery, Stanford University, Stanford, California

Amer Raheemullah, M.D.
Clinical Assistant Professor of Addiction Medicine, Department of Psychiatry and Behavioral Sciences, School of Medicine, Stanford University, Stanford, California

Yelizaveta Sher, M.D.
Clinical Associate Professor of Psychiatry, School of Medicine, Stanford University, Stanford, California

Reena P. Thomas, M.D., Ph.D
Clinical Associate Professor, Division of Neuro-Oncology; Vice Chair of Diversity and Inclusion, Department of Neurology; and Associate Dean, Office of Diversity in Medical Education, School of Medicine, Stanford University, Stanford, California

Michael R. Trimble, M.D., FRCP, FRCPsych
Emeritus Professor in Behavioural Neurology, Faculty of Brain Sciences, Queen Square Institute of Neurology, University College London, London, United Kingdom

Katherine E. Williams, M.D.
Clinical Professor of Psychiatry, and Director, Women's Wellness Clinic, School of Medicine, Stanford University, Stanford, California

Nolan Williams, M.D.
Assistant Professor; Director, Interventional Psychiatry Clinical Research; and Director, Brain Stimulation Laboratory, Department of Psychiatry and Behavioral Sciences, Stanford University, Stanford, California

Michael Zeineh, M.D.
Associate Professor or Radiology (Neuroimaging and Neurointervention), Department of Radiology, The Richard M. Lucas Center for Imaging, Stanford University, Stanford, California

Disclosures

Sheldon Benjamin, M.D.

Owner: Brain Educators, LLC; *Author:* The Brain Card; *Boards:* American Board of Psychiatry and Neurology (Psychiatry Board); Academic Psychiatry (Governance Board); Journal of Neuropsychiatry and Clinical Neuroscience (Editorial Board).

Jeffrey L. Cummings, M.D., Sc.D.

Consultant: Acadia, Actinogen, Acumen, Alector, Alkahest, Alzheon, AriBio, Avanir, Axsome, Behren Therapeutics, Biogen, Cassava, Cerecin, Cerevel, Cortexyme, Cytox, EIP Pharma, Eisai, Foresight, GemVax, Genentech, Green Valley, Grifols, Janssen, Karuna, Merck, Novo Nordisk, Otsuka, ReMYND, Resverlogix, Roche, Samumed, Samus, Signant Health, Sunovion, Suven, United Neuroscience. *Stock Options:* ADAMAS, AnnovisBio, MedAvante, BiOasis. *Copyright:* Neuropsychiatric Inventory. *Grants:* National Institute of General Medical Sciences P20GM109025, National Institute of Neurological Disorders and Stroke U01NS093334, National Institute on Aging R01AG053798 and P20AG068053.

PREFACE

The *Concise Guide to Neuropsychiatry and Behavioral Neurology* was first published in 1995 and has since helped hundreds of clinicians provide excellent care to thousands of patients with neuropsychiatric and neurobehavioral syndromes. The book originated from our shared passion for clinical phenomenology, neurological and psychiatric diagnoses, excellence in patient care, and teaching of these related disciplines to students at all levels of learning. The complexity of the brain is reflected in the diagnostic conundrums that patients present to clinicians. Substantial expertise in understanding how to examine an individual experiencing delusions, hallucinations or aphasia combined with a deep understanding of brain structure and function in health and disorder is required of the neuropsychiatrist/behavioral neurologist. Our goal in the *Concise Guide* was to distill this information into a brief format and to produce a volume that would fit in a pocket virtually or physically and be available when needed to assist in diagnosis and treatment of patients with neuropsychiatric and neurobehavioral disorders. The enduring popularity of this volume suggests that we succeeded.

There has been tremendous progress in neuropsychiatry and behavioral neurology since the *Concise Guide* was last published. The development of new techniques of brain imaging with amyloid and tau PET; the advances in MRI allowing examination of brain structure, function, composition, and perfusion; the improvement in electrophysiological methods to better detect and characterize epilepsy and sleep disorders; and the evolution of an ever-growing list of blood and spinal fluid biomarkers have revolutionized the diagnostic capability of the neuropsychiatrist/behavioral neurologist. Treatment alternatives have advanced markedly since the last edition. Improved therapies for psychosis, depression, mania, OCD, anxiety, and sleep disorders have materialized from innovative programs, as have treatments for epilepsy, movement disorders, stroke, multiple sclerosis, brain tumors and degenerative brain disorders. Awareness of these advances is necessary to provide neuropsychiatrists and behavioral neurologists with skills not only to achieve accurate diagnoses but also to manage patients with complex neuropsychiatric and neurobehavioral disorders once the well-prepared clinician has examined the patient thoroughly, with insight and kindness. We have endeavored to preserve this precious vision of patient care while integrating the many advances that have enriched the field.

We are very grateful to John Barry and Sepideh Bajestan for their willingness and enthusiasm in reviving the *Concise Guide*. They have done a terrific job of preserving much of the original content and intent while integrating the new approaches, technologies, and therapies. Additional chapters have been added addressing autism, substance use, endocrine and HIV neurocognitive disorders, limbic encephalities, and interventional neuropsychiatry. We are pleased to know that more generations of neuropsychiatrists and behavioral neurologists will have this companion in their pocket. Our goals remain teaching, excellent patient care, growth of individual expertise, and expansion of our understanding of mind/brain relationships. This new edition of the *Concise Guide* captures these ideals.

Jeffrey Cummings, M.D., Sc.D.
Michael Trimble, M.D., FRCPsych, FRCP

ACKNOWLEDGMENT

We offer since gratitude to Dr. Cummings and Dr. Trimble for the privilege and opportunity to update this third edition of the *Concise Guide to Neuropsychiatry and Behavioral Neurology*. We hope that this new edition will be as clinically useful as its predecessors.

John J. Barry, M.D.
Sepideh N. Bajestan, M.D., Ph.D.

NEUROPSYCHIATRIC ASSESSMENT

Lauren Drag, Ph.D.
Juliana Lockman, M.D.
Michael Zeineh, M.D.
Michel Medina, M.D.

Neuropsychiatry and behavioral neurology are specialties devoted to understanding and treating behavioral disturbances associated with neurological dysfunction. The detection and characterization of brain and behavior disorders require careful behavioral observation, formal clinical assessment, and the application of selected neurodiagnostic procedures. In this chapter, we discuss the clinical examination as well as neuropsychological testing, laboratory tests, electrophysiological techniques, and brain imaging. The symptoms of brain dysfunction are presented in more detail in Chapter 3, "Neuropsychiatric Symptoms and Syndromes," and the symptoms of each specific disease or condition are presented in the relevant chapters of the book.

■ DEFINITIONS

Symptoms are the patient's self-reported subjective complaints. *Signs* are the objective observations of the physician, the patient, or the patient's friends and family and indicate the presence of abnormal functioning of one or more body systems.

A *syndrome* is a recognizable constellation of the signs and symptoms that tend to co-occur and represent the clinical expression of an underlying, unifying disease process. A syndrome may or may not be pathognomonic for a specific etiology. The presentation of an illness depends on many factors, including environmental and personality variables.

■ CLINICAL AND LABORATORY EXAMINATION

Initial Observations

The clinician should first observe; note the patient's appearance, awareness, viscosity, and attitude; and then listen. The patient's dress may reveal the eccentricity of hysteria or the flamboyance of mania or may hint at the dishevelment of schizophrenia or dementia. Is eye contact maintained? Is there evidence of irritability, agitation, or pressured speech? Or conversely blunted affect and terse responses? Is there an excessive focus and perseveration on symptoms or perhaps an indifference and a lack of insight into a condition that is otherwise obvious to the examiner? These types of behavioral observations are invaluable to the clinical examination and case conceptualization and can be elicited even with casual conversation.

Disturbances of motor activity can aid diagnosis. In *catatonia,* muscle tone is high, leading to resistance, and in *catalepsy,* limb rigidity and postures can be maintained for hours at a time. *Gegenhalten* refers to an involuntary resistance to passive movements of the extremities.

A patient's gait may suggest an extrapyramidal disorder, with smaller steps and poverty of accessory movements indicative of parkinsonism. *Akinesia,* or poverty of movement, can be seen in parkinsonism or can reflect a side effect of neuroleptic treatment. A patient with *akathisia* may not be able to sit longer than a few minutes. A patient with agitation will pace around. *Mannerisms* (exaggerated components of the usual behavioral repertoire), *stereotypies* (repeated complex sequences of purposeless movement), and *choreoathetoid* writhing may be noted. Mannerisms and stereotypies are common in schizophrenia; choreoathetoid writhing may suggest any number of extrapyramidal problems. *Tics* (frequent stereotyped repetitive movements of small groups of muscles) may suggest Gilles de la Tourette's syndrome. Vocal tics and excessive sniffing or clearing of the throat are also characteristic of this disorder. Tics can also be commonly associated with other developmental disorders, such as ADHD or autism spectrum disorder (see Chapter 18, "Autism Spectrum Disorder").

There may be involuntary movements of the mouth, such as repetitive tongue movements or chewing motions indicative of *tardive dyskinesia,* or more sustained abnormal postures as in *dystonia.*

The hands may tremble in cases of anxiety or extrapyramidal disease. Is there any evidence of muscle wasting (loss of muscle bulk generally or in specific areas)? Observation of the fingers may reveal nicotine addiction, anxiety-related behaviors (e.g., bitten nails), or poor hygiene. When shaking the patient's hand, the clinician may detect the clammy sweat of anxiety or an underlying extrapyramidal tremor. A handshake also gives the opportunity to test grasp reflex. Left-handedness can provide insights into cerebral lateralization.

The patient's speech should be studied for form and content. The slowing of depression contrasts with the pressured overactivity of mania. *Dysarthria,* due to impairment of the neuromuscular mechanisms of speech, may hint at intoxication or cerebral or cerebellar damage. *Hypophonia* can be indicative of parkinsonism. *Prosody* of speech refers to rhythm and intonation, which can be impacted in schizophrenia or right-hemisphere lesions. A stammer may suggest anxiety; *paraphasias* and *neologisms* indicate aphasia or schizophrenia.

The patient's attention and concentration and ability to maintain a stream of thought and a reciprocal conversation should be noted. Overfamiliarity, inappropriate or impulsive comments, or perseverative tendencies during conversation can be indicative of frontal-based dysfunction. *Confabulation* can be an indicator of underlying memory loss. *Circumstantiality* refers to a persistent tendency to wander slowly over the irrelevant details of a subject before reaching a final conclusion, making it difficult to elicit an efficient history during interview.

Evaluation of speech disturbances is discussed in Chapter 6, "Aphasia and Related Syndromes."

Formal thought disorder, which refers to disorganization, incoherence, and concretization of thought processes, suggests either schizophrenia or a neurological disease. Slowing of the train of thought is seen with the psychomotor slowing of depression and with the bradyphrenia of many neurological disorders, such as traumatic brain injury, Parkinson's disease, epilepsy, and multiple sclerosis. *Viscosity* describes the "sticky thinking" of some such patients, although this term is also used to explain a clingy interpersonal style associated with temporal lobe epilepsy.

Delusions are unshakable, fixed false beliefs that are manifestly incorrect, even when cultural considerations are taken into account. They can accompany both psychiatric and neurological disorders. *Autochthonous delusions* arise suddenly, spontaneously, and fully formed. They are bizarre and nearly always signify schizophrenia. *Hallucinations* are perceptions without objects, and *illusions* are abnormal perceptions of sensory stimuli. Impaired judgment can be seen in dementia and focal frontal injuries. *Anosognosia* is the lack of awareness of deficit; it can accompany a range of conditions, including parietal lobe, subcortical, or frontal involvement; Alzheimer's disease; traumatic brain injury; and serious mental illness. In contrast, hyperawareness and concern about symptoms can accompany anxiety and depression.

Hyperesthesia, especially for sounds, is not uncommon in anxious patients, although it can also accompany neurological conditions such as traumatic brain injury. *Hypoesthesia* is common in depression. Anesthesia, in the sense of reporting *anesthetic patches* or *hemianesthesia,* may be seen in patients with hysteria (conversion disorder).

Alterations in the perceived size of objects, such as in micropsia and macropsia, may suggest ophthalmological disease or temporal lobe dysfunction. *Derealization* and *depersonalization,* in which the world and the patient him- or herself, respectively, feel different, unreal, empty, or two-dimensional, are noted in various conditions but especially in anxiety and as an aura in temporal lobe epilepsy. In *déjà vu* experiences, patients believe that everything they are experiencing they have seen before. *Jamais vu* is the opposite, an abnormal feeling of unfamiliarity.

Careful attention should be paid to patients' mood and to whether delusions are congruent or incongruent with the mood state. Incongruent delusions immediately hint at schizophrenia. *Apathy* is common after cerebral damage but is seen in a wide range of neuropsychiatric disorders. *Abulia* is related to apathy and akinetic mutism and is defined as lack of will. *Emotional lability* is noted when patients are unable to control their emotional flow, laughing at the hint of a joke or crying at the hint of sadness. *Pseudobulbar palsy* is a common cause of emotional lability associated with involvement of corticobulbar tracts. It is contrasted with the empty euphoria of patients with multiple sclerosis and meaningless playful *Witzelsucht* of frontal lobe dysfunction. Inappropriate affect is more characteristic of schizophrenia.

Neuropsychological Testing

Comprehensive cognitive testing should be completed by a neuropsychologist, often in clinic but sometimes at bedside. Nevertheless, a briefer mental status screen can be very valuable and in many patients is an essential part of the initial screening. Aspects of a cognitive screen to consider are outlined in Table 1–1. These

TABLE 1–1.   **Bedside mental state testing**

Level of consciousness
  Orientation for time, place, and person
  Name, age, marital status
  Day, date, month, season, year
  Name of president
  Current event in the news
  Estimate of the current time (without looking at a clock)
  Name of city, county, state, and hospital/clinic
  Address, phone number
Attention and vigilance
  Digit or sentence repetition
  Serial 7 subtraction
  Digits reversed, spelling reversed
  Days or months in reverse order
  Mental calculations
  Letter tapping
Expressive language
  Rate, rhythm, syntax, and semantics
  Speech errors (e.g., agrammatism, word-finding difficulties, word
    substitutions)
  Naming of objects, body parts, and colors
  Ability to describe what is happening in a picture or a scene
Receptive language
  Ability to point to objects in the environment named by the
    examiner
  Ability to perform single and multistep commands
  Ability to read a passage of text (e.g., from a newspaper) and answer
    questions
Memory ability
  Repetition of a story
  Repetition of five words
  General knowledge for recent events
  Knowledge for remote events
  Ability to recall the location of an object that was hidden in the room
Constructional ability
  Copy of a circle, cross, and cube; drawing a clock

TABLE 1–1.	Bedside mental state testing *(continued)*

Ideomotor and ideational apraxia

  Ability to perform tasks on command: complete a complex sequence of actions (e.g., hammering a nail, lighting a match)

Executive function

  Verbal fluency: number of animals named in 1 minute or number of words that begin with a certain letter in 1 minute

  Perseveration: fist-palm-side test, copy repeating sequences (e.g., ramparts design)

  Understanding of similarities (e.g., How are a train and a bus alike?)

  Proverb interpretation (e.g., a bird in hand is worth two in the bush)

  Cognitive estimation (e.g., How fast does a racehorse run? What is the largest piece of furniture in the house?)

  Ability to follow repeating motor sequences (e.g., fist, edge, palm)

  Right-left disorientation

  Follow commands using right and left extremities

  Paper and pencil calculations

tests should be done routinely, but any suspicion of cognitive dysfunction should lead to a request for more comprehensive cognitive evaluation. When referring for a neuropsychological evaluation, the clinician should specify possible differential diagnoses and areas to focus on—for example, asking that emphasis be placed on tests of executive functioning—so that the neuropsychological test battery and report can be tailored to optimize differential diagnosis and directly address the referral question.

Patients with confusional states cannot be reliably tested, but the degree, content, and variability of their mental state must be noted. Patients with typical *delirium* (see Chapter 10, "Delirium") seem confused and are disoriented for time and possibly also for place. Simple attention span and mental arithmetic are abnormal, and memory is unreliable. Hallucinations are predominantly visual, complex, and silent. Delusions are often paranoid. Typically, the severity of the symptoms fluctuates with time.

Attention span can be tested by repetition of digits or sentences. More complex attention, such as working memory, can be tested using the serial 7s subtraction test (or other mental arithmetic tasks) or having the patient sequence strings of numbers or days/months in backward order. Longer periods of attention (*vigilance*) are tested by reading a series of letters aloud and asking the patient to tap every time a certain letter is called out.

Memory is tested by having the patient recall previously pre-sented words or stories, current events in the news, or the loca-tion of an object that he or she watched being hidden in the room. Items of general knowledge should be tested that are relevant to the patient's cultural and intellectual background. Tests of general knowledge about news items, famous people, or events should be given. The ability to accurately recall events from the more distant past (remote memory) should also be tested.

Expressive and receptive language should be assessed, both formally and qualitatively. Attention should be paid to the rate, prosody, volume, and grammar of speech output. Expressive speech can be elicited by asking the patient to describe a visual scene or to name common objects. Receptive language can be as-sessed by having the patient follow both simple and multistep commands or read a passage and answer questions.

Testing for *aphasia* and *apraxia* is discussed in Chapter 6.

Anosognosia is a deficit of awareness of a disability associ-ated with a medical condition. It often consists of lack of insight and impairs the ability to perceive a deficit and to seek treat-ment. It also may be associated with a refusal of medication and is one of the most significant reasons for lack of adherence to medication regimens in patients with psychiatric diseases. Ano-sognosia may result in a denial of hemiparesis and most com-monly accompanies right-hemisphere disease. *Finger agnosia* is the inability to recognize different fingers, either the patient's own or those of the examiner. *Autotopagnosia* is the same as finger agnosia, except that it applies to any body part. Finger agnosia and right/left disorientation usually indicate a left-hemisphere lesion.

Tests of constructional ability require the patient to draw a familiar object, such as a clock or a house, or to copy line drawings (e.g., a cube). *Neglect* of one-half of the drawing is seen with contralateral-hemisphere lesions. Neglect is more common and more severe with right-hemisphere lesions.

Tests of *frontal lobe* or *executive function* are often indicated in neuropsychiatric patients. These are described in detail in Chapter 5, "Frontal Lobe Syndromes" (see Table 5–1).

If possible, another person who knows the patient should be interviewed to confirm the accuracy of the patient's account of his or her illness. Family history should always be sought, and any potential genetic diseases should be noted. Question-ing about early history can elicit behavior problems relevant to the clinical presentation, including a history of sleepwalking, enuresis, stammering, tics, phobias, or hyperactivity. Developmental delay, especially for motor development, speaking, and language, should be inquired about. *ADHD, learning disorders, conduct disorder, oppositional defiant disorder,* and *autistic behavior* should be noted.

Neurological Examination

All patients should receive a neurological examination. A screening examination for neurological disease is shown in Table 1–2. This brief examination takes 10 minutes; if abnormalities are revealed, more detailed testing is needed. In addition to the items listed in the table, the screening neurological examination includes aspects of the mental status assessment detailed in Table 1–1. These include, but are not limited to, level of consciousness, orientation, language, memory, and general fund of knowledge.

Neurological "soft signs" may be subtle, not readily localizing, and do not always correlate with a well-defined neurological syndrome. They are thought to represent a connectivity abnormality among cortical and subcortical structures. They are classified as clusters of signs with presumed localization. Categories include integrative sensory function, motor coordination, sequencing of complex motor acts, and primitive reflexes (as detailed in Table 1–2). Soft signs are best described in schizophrenia but can also be seen in conditions such as OCD and the dementias. Their presence can aid in the differential diagnosis and prognosis of neuropsychiatric conditions.

Formal Tests of Neuropsychological Function

Formal tests of neuropsychological function are listed in Table 1–3 and in Chapter 5, Table 5–1.

Metabolic and Biochemical Investigations

The following tests are done for all patients:

- Hemoglobin, red blood cell count, and related indices (hematocrit, mean corpuscular volume, and mean corpuscular hemoglobin concentration)
- White cell and platelet count
- Sedimentation rate
- Serum electrolytes (sodium and potassium chloride)
- Tests of liver function (alanine aminotransferase [ALT], alkaline phosphatase, aspartate aminotransferase [AST])

TABLE 1–2.	Brief neurological screening examination

Cranial nerves*

Assess olfaction (identification of the presence of odor) (I)

Check visual fields (confrontation testing in each quadrant) (II)

Examine fundus (perform an ophthalmoscopic exam) (II)

Test visual pursuit (follow the examiner's finger in horizontal and vertical directions) (III, IV, VI)

Assess bulk of temporalis and masseter muscles (opening jaw against force; muscle bulk on tight bite) (V)

Observe facial symmetry (ask patient to raise eyebrows and smile) (VII)

Assess hearing (rub finger and thumb an inch from the patient's ears) (VIII)

Observe palate (ask patient to say "ah") (IX, X)

Test sternocleidomastoids and trapezius (push chin against the examiner's hand, test muscle bulk, shrug shoulders) (XI)

Observe tongue for abnormal movements or deviation on protrusion (XII)

Motor system

Observe for adventitious movements (e.g., tremor, dystonia, chorea, fasciculations) or limited movement suggesting paresis

Check tone in each limb (ask patient to relax limb to allow passive flexion and extension by the examiner, assessing for flaccidity, spasticity, rigidity, paratonia, and "giveway")

Assess power (test pronator drift, test the force of each limb against resistance applied proximally and distally)

Reflexes

Test muscle stretch (biceps, triceps, supinator, knee, ankle); pathological (plantar "Babinski sign")

Coordination

Finger-nose test

Rapid movements (quickly tap the back of one hand with the palm of the other)

Heel to shin testing

Sensory testing

Stroke skin on representative parts of the body, especially the distal extremities

TABLE 1–2.	Brief neurological screening examination *(continued)*

Stance and gait

  Observe walking and turning

  Balance with feet together and eyes closed (Romberg's test)

Primitive reflexes (when seen are called "Frontal Release Signs")

  Palmomental (stroke the palm from the thenar eminence and watch for a reflex contraction of the ipsilateral mentalis muscle)

  Grasp (stroke the patient's palm firmly moving outward and watch for hand closing in)

  Jaw jerk (examiner places index finger on jaw and taps with reflex hammer)

  Snout and pout reflexes (tap lips and watch for puckering)

*Numerals in parentheses refer to the cranial nerve tested.

- Tests of renal function (blood urea nitrogen, creatinine)
- Blood glucose (if abnormal, order an extended glucose tolerance test)
- Blood A1c

The following tests are done for selected patients:

- Vitamin B_{12} and folic acid
- Iron and total iron-binding capacity
- Creatinine clearance test
- Calcium and phosphorus estimations
- Thyroid-stimulating hormone, triiodo-thyronine, and thyroxine
- Drug screen (for illicit drugs)
- Dexamethasone suppression test (see Chapter 19, "Evaluation and Treatment of Endocrine Disorders With Neuropsychiatric Symptoms")
- Syphilis serology (Venereal Disease Research Laboratory, fluorescent treponemal antibody absorption)
- HIV serology, CD4 lymphocyte cell count, and CD4 percentage (see Chapter 21, "HIV Neurocognitive Disorders")
- Prolactin (increased by neuroleptics and transiently by seizures, especially generalized seizures)
- Cholesterol and fatty acids
- Heavy metals screening
- Ammonia (for encephalopathy)

TABLE 1-3. Examples of common neuropsychological tests

Boston Diagnostic Aphasia Examination	Comprehensive measure of expressive and receptive language
California Verbal Learning Test	Measure of learning and delayed memory of a word list
Continuous Performance Test	Computerized measure of sustained attention, vigilance, and inhibition
Delis-Kaplan Executive Functioning System	Battery of subtests measuring multiple aspects of executive functioning
Judgment of Line Orientation	Assessment of spatial judgment requiring the matching of angles and orientations of lines in space
Rey-Osterrieth Complex Figure	Measure of constructional ability and delayed memory for a complex visual figure
Stroop Color-Word Interference Test	Measure of executive function requiring the patient to inhibit and override a prepotent response
Test of Premorbid Functioning	Word-reading test used to determine premorbid IQ
Trail Making Test	Speeded test requiring sequencing of numbers and alternating numbers and letters to assess processing speed and rapid set-shifting
Verbal Fluency	Test of speeded word generation in response to both letter and category cues
Wechsler Adult Intelligence Scale	A comprehensive measure of IQ including assessment of verbal abilities, visuospatial abilities, processing speed, and working memory
Wechsler Memory Scale	Battery of visual and verbal learning and memory tasks
Wisconsin Card Sorting Test	Measure of reasoning assessing the patient's ability to utilize feedback to identify reinforced rules and set-shift

- Lactate and pyruvate (for mitochondrial disorders)
- Genetic tests (chromosome analysis, specific gene tests, human leukocyte antigen genotypes)

The following tests are done in association with specific diagnoses:

- Alcoholism: red-cell transketolase, serum γ-glutamyl transferase, ALT, and AST
- Systemic lupus erythematosus (lupus): lupus erythematosus cells and serum antinuclear or anti-double stranded DNA antibodies, antiphospholipid antibodies
- Fatigue: infectious mononucleosis monospot and heterophile antibody test
- Polydipsia: plasma and urine osmolality
- Porphyria: urinary or fecal porphyrins
- Dexamethasone suppression test (see Chapter 19, "Evaluation and Treatment of Endocrine Disorders With Neuropsychiatric Symptoms (Thyroid and Adrenal")
- Dementia: see Chapter 11 ("Dementia")
- Movement disorders: serum copper and ceruloplasmin, serum creatine phosphokinase (CPK), acanthocytes in blood; see Chapter 12 ("Movement Disorders")

The following tests are done for patients taking specific drugs:

- Lithium: routine lithium level
- Anticonvulsants: see Chapter 22, "Treatments in Neuropsychiatry"
- Antidepressants: levels are determined to check compliance or to detect unusual metabolism (e.g., patient complains of side effects on low doses)

Lumbar puncture is done to look for CNS infections (e.g., cerebral syphilis), to help in the differential diagnosis of dementia, and for the diagnosis of multiple sclerosis (oligoclonal bands). For workup for limbic encephalitis, see Chapter 20 ("Limbic Encephalitis").

Electroencephalography

The electroencephalogram (EEG) was discovered by psychiatrist Hans Berger in 1924. The electroencephalographic signal is created by the average of electrical currents from the surface dendrites of neurons.

The usual 10–20 system of electrode placement covers only 20% of the cortical surface. In general, abnormal electrical activity must span at least a few square centimeters to be detected on scalp EEG. Additional electrodes, in the following placements, may improve the detection of abnormalities:

- Sphenoidal—in the region of the foramen ovale
- Nasopharyngeal—in the nasopharynx at the base of the skull
- Intracranial—subdural or intracerebral

Activation procedures facilitate detection of abnormal rhythms. These procedures include hyperventilation, photic stimulation, sleep induction or deprivation, and occasionally drugs (e.g., pentylene-tetrazol).

Waveforms

The four main types of waveforms seen on scalp EEG are

- Alpha: 8–13 Hz or cycles per second (cps), maximal occipitally, blocked by eye opening
- Beta: 13–30 Hz or cps, increased by many psychotropic drugs, especially sedatives and hypnotics
- Delta: 0.5–4 Hz or cps, in the alert state often a sign of pathology
- Theta: 4–7 Hz or cps (Figure 1–1)

Faster (e.g., gamma >30 Hz) and infraslow waveforms (0.5 Hz and lower) can be seen on subdural or intracerebral recordings. These waveforms are influenced by genetics, age, sleep, drugs, and disease. Anticonvulsants such as valproic acid are notable for the potential to normalize interictal abnormalities in the EEG. Waveforms do not correlate well with intelligence. Theta and delta waves predominate EEGs in the very young. Adult EEGs feature mainly alpha and beta waveforms in wakefulness.

During the night, there are usually six periods of rapid eye movement (REM) sleep lasting up to 30 minutes, approximately 90 minutes apart—around 20%–25% of total sleep time. The first REM onset is after about 90 minutes (REM latency). This period may be altered in disease states; for example, patients with de-

14

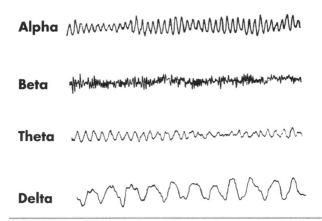

Alpha

Beta

Theta

Delta

FIGURE 1–1. Typical electroencephalogram waveforms.
Source. Reprinted from Scott D: *Understanding EEG*. London, Duckworth, 1976, p. 24. Copyright 1976. Used with permission.

pression have a short REM latency. Dreaming typically occurs during REM sleep.

The EEG is an important test in patients who present with paroxysmal behavioral disorders and in the workup of patients with epilepsy. Recordings during the period of the change or the ictus are of most value. The EEG is helpful in diagnosing epileptic states such as nonconvulsive status epilepticus, some types of dementia, infectious encephalitis, and toxic/metabolic encephalopathy (see Chapters 9 and 10).

Evoked Potentials

The technique of evoked potentials allows the very small potentials generated by a stimulus to be exaggerated and studied. The results of many similar stimuli are averaged, and the signal-to-noise ratio is thus enhanced. The waveform is derived from computer analysis of the data; a series of positive and negative waves is detected, and the latency (time from stimulus) of these waves is one index used to detect pathology. Visual, auditory, or somatosensory evoked potentials are usually recorded.

Several potentials can be evoked by endogenous events. These include the contingent negative variation (CNV, or expectancy wave), the P300 wave, and premotor potentials such as the *Bereitschaftpotential*. The CNV arises from anticipation of an expected response. It is a slow negative shift at the vertex and frontal regions. The P300 wave is thought to relate to a process of cognitive appraisal of a stimulus.

Other Electroencephalographic Techniques

Ambulatory monitoring involves placing electrodes on the head (or heart), signals from which are continuously recorded onto a small recording device that patients attach to themselves. Patients can walk around wearing this recorder, and recordings over days can be made, for example, in the home. With *video telemetry*, a picture of the patient's behavior is recorded simultaneously with the EEG, and both are replayed side by side on a screen. The behavior and the EEG can be directly compared.

Computerized electroencephalographic mapping produces topographical images of the brain's electrical activity by means of computerized analysis of the various EEG components.

Magnetoencephalography

Magnetoencephalography, which detects magnetic source fields in the brain, complements electroencephalography. However, because the skull does not interfere with magnetic signals, magnetoencephalography provides better spatial resolution and detects fields beneath the surface.

Brain Imaging

Brain imaging is typically divided into two categories: structural and functional neuroimaging. Structural imaging evaluates the physical appearance and integrity of brain tissue. In routine clinical practice, *computed tomography* (CT) and *magnetic resonance imaging* (MRI) are the key imaging modalities. Functional imaging produces images that measure the physiological changes (blood flow, glucose, oxygen utilization) that indirectly reflect brain activity; clinically, the most frequently utilized functional brain imaging technologies include *single-photon emission computed tomography* (SPECT) and *positron emission tomography* (PET). Others (e.g., functional MRI) are primarily research tools with limited clinical utility at this time.

Although CT/MRI are the most common imaging modalities in clinical practice, there are no clear guidelines for when a physician should or should not order structural brain imaging for a psychiatric presentation. Studies investigating this question have identified the presence of focal neurological signs, cognitive decline, advanced age at symptom onset (>50 years),

TABLE 1–4. Clinical indications for structural brain imaging in psychiatric patients

Atypical psychiatric symptoms

Catatonia

Cognitive decline or dementia

Delirium

Eating disorder

First-episode psychosis

Focal neurological signs

New-onset personality changes

New-onset psychiatric symptoms after age 50 years

Pre-electroconvulsive therapy workup

Refractory to treatment

Seizure history

Traumatic brain injury

and atypical symptoms as being clinical features suggestive of a psychiatric presentation masquerading as a general medical condition. From our perspective, neuroimaging should be considered in any clinical situation in which neuroimaging data may assist with differential diagnosis, modify the treatment plan, provide prognostic value, or provide insight into atypical psychiatric manifestations. Table 1–4 includes a broad list derived from clinical experience of psychiatric presentations that may warrant further investigation with structural imaging.

Computed Tomography

Like a conventional radiograph, CT measures the differential absorption of X-rays. X-rays are projected through the brain in many directions around the patient's head, and the number detected depends on the density of the particular tissue. This gives rise to relative attenuation values, which are measured in Hounsfield units. Bone will appear white (higher density; almost complete absorption of the X-rays or higher attenuation), air will appear black (very low attenuation), and brain tissue will appear gray (intermediate density). For brain matter, the shades of gray are influenced by the tissue composition; for example, white matter, which has higher lipid content (from myelin), appears darker on CT than gray matter.

Magnetic Resonance Imaging

Based on the technical foundations of *nuclear magnetic resonance*, MRI uses the magnetic properties of the atomic constituents of biological matter (hydrogen atoms, a major component of water in soft tissue) to construct a visual representation of tissue. Patients are placed at the center of a large magnet (the strength of magnet is measured in teslas [T]), and their hydrogen atoms are exposed to a carefully calculated series of radiofrequency pulses while they are within the scanner's magnetic field. Brain images are obtained by measuring the proton (hydrogen atoms) spin relaxation parameters (T1, T2) after excitation by these radiofrequency pulses.

T1-weighted images are best for displaying anatomy and resemble anatomical brain sections (gray matter appears medium gray, white matter appears very light gray, cerebrospinal fluid [CSF] appears black). *T2 weighted images* resemble film negatives and are best for detecting pathological changes (appear bright or hyperintense). A variant of the T2-weighted scan is called the *fluid-attenuated inversion recovery* (or FLAIR) image, which subtracts the CSF signal (CSF appears black) and improves visualization near CSF-filled spaces, allowing identification of subtle lesions. The *gradient echo* sequence, also sometimes called susceptibility weighted, is also commonly used to detect any type of hemorrhage (or blood breakdown products), such as from amyloid angiopathy. Another important MRI sequence is *diffusion weighted imaging* (DWI), which measures the diffusion of water protons in brain tissue, making it ideal for detecting cellular changes associated with acute ischemic strokes (DWI is often combined with imaging of the *apparent diffusion coefficient* to improve specificity). Various additional specialized MRI pulse sequences and techniques exist that are primarily research tools and are beyond the scope of this chapter (e.g., diffusion tensor imaging, functional MRI, magnetic resonance spectroscopy).

Structural Imaging: CT and MRI

The choice of imaging modality should be based on the anatomy or pathology that one wants to view. CT and MRI each are preferable in certain situations (Table 1–5); however, for clinical neuropsychiatry, MRI is the preferred modality in most cases. Structural imaging for psychiatric purposes may be indicated in several clinical situations (see Table 1–4).

TABLE 1–5. Comparison of CT and MRI

Characteristic	CT	MRI
Availability	Universal both in terms of location and time	Less accessible (available in most hospitals but access may be limited outside of regular hours)
Cost	Relatively inexpensive	More expensive
Resolution, *mm*	1.0	1.0
Sensitivity	Good	Superior
Acquisition time, *min*	3–4	~30
Parameter measured	Tissue density	Many properties of tissue (T1 and T2 relaxation times, spin density, magnetic susceptibility, water diffusion, blood flow)
Clinical conditions for which it is preferred (within neuropsychiatry)	Acute setting or medically unstable patient Status postacute head trauma Suspect: acute hemorrhage, bone injury/ fracture, lytic lesions, mass effect, herniation, calcified lesions	Subacute or chronic setting Superior sensitivity for acute ischemic injury All subcortical lesions Demyelinating disorders or in evaluating extent of white matter disease Superior anatomical detail is needed; e.g., temporal lobe or cerebellum

TABLE 1–5. Comparison of CT and MRI (*continued*)

Characteristic	CT	MRI
Plane of section	Axial (although coronal or sagittal reformatted images can be quickly constructed with newer scanners)	Any plane of section
Contraindications	No absolute contraindications for a noncontrast CT	Any magnetic metal in the body (e.g., sutures, surgical clips)
	If using contrast-enhanced CT, concern for history of anaphylaxis, elevated creatinine, or metformin administration on day of scan	Implanted electrical, mechanical, or magnetic devices (e.g., pacemakers, nerve stimulators)
		History of welding (requires skull films before MRI)
		Claustrophobia (open-design magnets may be an option)
		Pregnancy (legal contraindication)

The use of contrast media significantly improves the ability to visualize vascular structures and lesions that compromise or disrupt the blood-brain barrier (e.g., aneurysms, dissections, arteriovenous malformations, inflammatory or infectious processes, tumors). For brain CT, the contrast agents contain iodine (iodinated and appear white on the scan). Without a companion noncontrast CT scan, preexisting dense areas (calcified or hemorrhagic) might be mistaken for contrast-enhanced lesions. In MRI, the contrast agents contain gadolinium, which changes the T1 and T2 properties of hydrogen atoms in nearby tissues, resulting in increased signal better visualized in T1-weighted images (seen as white, or brighter).

Functional Neuroimaging: SPECT and PET

In contrast to the imaging methods just described (which, apart from the newer MRI techniques, assess brain structure), SPECT and PET measure numerous aspects of brain function that have growing clinical indications in neuropsychiatry. Both PET and SPECT are based on imaging the distribution of a radiotracer that is injected intravenously. As the radiotracer decays, it emits photons (or positrons in PET) that are detected and provide an indirect measure of neural activity; for example, the distribution of the radiotracer may indicate regional blood flow or cellular metabolism.

In SPECT, two tracers for cerebral blood flow (perfusion) are approved for clinical use in the United States: technetium hexamethylene-propyleneamine oxime ($[^{99m}Tc]$-HMPAO; Ceretec) and technetium ethyl cysteinate dimer ($[^{99m}Tc]$-ECD; Neurolite). A SPECT tracer for imaging the dopamine transporter (ioflupane $[^{123}I]$; DaTscan) has also been approved for the evaluation of neurodegenerative movement disorders. These tracers are taken up by tissue and then temporarily trapped, decaying and emitting a photon in the process. Radiation is detected by rotating gamma cameras, and an image of blood flow is obtained via a process of tomographic reconstruction. SPECT is generally less expensive and more widely available than PET.

The most commonly used PET tracer is 18-fluoro-2-deoxyglucose ($[^{18}F]$FDG), and there are three tracers for β-amyloid imaging (amyloid PET). The tracer is taken up by the cells, similar to glucose, and undergoes metabolism, which provides a measure of cerebral metabolic activity. These are detected by a scanner, and, via computerized reconstruction of the data, an image is created that shows the distribution of the radiotracer, with areas of high concentration appearing as "hot spots" or resembling a map of glucose metabolism. PET has the advantage of higher spatial resolution and true attenuation correction.

Clinical neuropsychiatric applications of SPECT and PET include aiding in differential diagnosis, treatment planning, and prognostic information. Currently, their primary use is for the evaluation of neurodegenerative disease (e.g., distinguishing Alzheimer's disease from frontotemporal dementia or utilizing SPECT dopamine transporter imaging for diagnostic evaluation for early Parkinson's disease) and in the preoperative evaluation of patients with medically refractory epilepsy (e.g., ictal perfusion SPECT).

■ REFERENCES

Arciniegas D, Anderson C, Filley C (eds): Behavioral Neurology and Neuropsychiatry. Cambridge, UK, Cambridge University Press, 2013

Arnold DL, Matthews PM: Practical aspects of clinical applications of MRS in the brain, in MR Spectroscopy: Clinical Applications and Techniques. Edited by Young IR, Charles HC. London, Martin Dunitz, 1996, pp 139–159

Dougherty DD, Rauch SL, Rosenbaum JF (eds): Essentials of Neuroimaging for Clinical Practice. Washington, DC, American Psychiatric Publishing, 2004

Erhart SM, Young AS, Marder SR, Mintz J: Clinical utility of magnetic resonance imaging radiographs for suspected organic syndromes in adult psychiatry. J Clin Psychiatry 66(8):968–973, 2005 16086610

Grant I, Adams KM: Neuropsychological Assessment of Neuropsychiatric Disorders, 3rd Edition. New York, Oxford University Press, 2009

Hales RE, Yudofsky SC: Clinical Manual of Neuropsychiatry. Washington, DC, American Psychiatric Association Publishing, 2012

Hurley RA, Patel SS, Taber K: Neuroimaging in neuropsychiatry, in Textbook of Neuropsychiatry and Clinical Neurosciences, 6th Edition. Edited by Arciniegas DB, Yudofsky SC, Hales RE. Washington, DC, American Psychiatric Association Publishing, 2018, pp 117–138

Lezak M, Howelson DB, Bigler ED, Tranel D: Neuropsychological Assessment, 5th Edition. New York, Oxford University Press, 2012

Malhi GS, Lagopoulos J: Making sense of neuroimaging in psychiatry. Acta Psychiatr Scand 117(2):100–117, 2008 18028255

Moore DP: Textbook of Clinical Psychiatry. London, Arnold, 2001

Schnider A: Neuropsychological testing: bedside approaches. Handb Clin Neurol 88:137–154, 2008 18631689

Strub RL, Black FW: The Mental Status Examination in Neurology, 4th Edition. Philadelphia, PA, FA Davis, 2000

Trimble MR: Clinical presentations in neuropsychiatry. Semin Clin Neuropsychiatry 7(1):11–17, 2002 11782887

Uher R, Treasure J: Brain lesions and eating disorder. J Neurol Neurosurg Psychiatry 76(6):852–857, 2005 15897510

2

BEHAVIORAL NEUROBIOLOGY

Kieran C.R. Fox, Ph.D.

■ NEUROANATOMY, NEUROPHYSIOLOGY, AND NEUROCHEMISTRY

To understand the biological underpinnings of neuropsychiatric illness, it is necessary to know basic neuroanatomical, neurophysiological, and neurochemical principles. Many of these principles were discovered in other species and then assumed to apply to the human brain. The advent of noninvasive neuroimaging modalities, however, combined with a resourceful use of invasive methods, has led to enormous advances in our understanding of the human brain in recent decades.

The brain is composed of *neurons* and *glial cells*. The main link between neurons is the synapse. The *synaptic cleft* is around 20 nm wide. *Neurotransmitters* are released from the *presynaptic* terminals and diffuse across the synapse to bind to specific receptors on the *postsynaptic* membrane. Calcium is essential for neurotransmitter release.

There are four main ions in cells: sodium, potassium, chloride, and organic anions. A negative *resting potential* is maintained by the action of the sodium-potassium pump, which uses energy in the form of adenosine triphosphate (ATP) to maintain an electrochemical voltage difference across the neuron's membrane. Known as Na^+/K^+-ATPase, this pump forces sodium ions out and draws potassium ions into the cell. This is the energy store of the cell. The *action potential* is generated by the influx of sodium and the loss of potassium during synaptic transmission, and the resulting current is propagated along the cell membrane.

Postsynaptic potentials are either inhibitory or excitatory, and these summate to determine the ultimate excitability of the postsynaptic cell.

Receptors are proteins to which neurotransmitters and other *ligands* bind. Many of the receptors in the CNS have been cloned and their molecular structures identified. Once a transmitter has interacted with a receptor, either ion exchange occurs with alteration of the neuron's membrane potential or there is stimulation of a *second messenger*, which may then alter intracellular metabolism and gene expression. Adenylate cyclase, generating cyclic adenosine monophosphate, is one common second messenger pathway. Genes such as c-Fos may be switched on.

Many receptors have been described, but the main ones of relevance are shown in Table 2–1.

Neurons have a soma (cell body), a single axon (output), many dendrites (inputs), and thousands of synapses connecting them to other neurons. Tubulin, a protein in the axon, acts in the transport of molecules down the axon. Larger axons are surrounded by a fatty sheath of *myelin* that increases the speed of conduction by electrically insulating the cell.

There are five types of glial cells: astrocytes, oligodendrocytes, microglia, Schwann cells, and ependymal cells. These cells provide structural, phagocytic, and metabolic support for neurons and manufacture myelin.

The main *neurotransmitters* are shown in Table 2–2. Many others are known to exist, but their function is poorly understood. These include peptides such as the enkephalins, substance P, and cholecystokinin. In individual neurons, two or more neurotransmitters may coexist.

Dopamine is related to the control of movement and to psychosis, *γ-aminobutyric acid* (GABA) to inhibitory postsynaptic potentials and seizure activity, *serotonin* to impulse control and mood, and *acetylcholine* to memory.

■ ESSENTIAL NEUROANATOMY

Limbic System

The limbic system is involved in the experience of emotion, and its integrity is essential for emotional well-being. Alteration of the structure or function of the limbic system is found in many neuropsychiatric illnesses.

The main nuclei and pathways of the limbic system are shown in Table 2–3. The cortex of the limbic system proper (archicortex, allocortex) is three layered, as opposed to the six layers of the neocortex. Intermediate is the mesocortex.

Nearly all limbic structures are strongly interconnected with the hypothalamus, amygdala, and hippocampus. The connections between the midbrain nuclei, which are the origin of neu-

TABLE 2–1. Neuroreceptors of clinical relevance

Receptor	Subtypes	Comments
Acetylcholine	Nicotinic, muscarinic	Linked to memory and cognition; five types of muscarinic receptors now identified
Dopamine	5	D_2 is related to movement disorder; all neuroleptics bind to it; antipsychotic effect of typical neuroleptics is related to intensity of binding; abundant in striatum
		D_1 has relevance in psychosis
		D_4: clozapine has good affinity
		Grouped into those receptors that are similar to D_1 (D_1 and D_5) or D_2 (D_2, D_3, and D_4)
Endocannabinoid	CB_1, CB_2	Related to appetite, mood, and pain
GABA	A, B	Linked to the benzodiazepine receptor; on activation, chloride channels open; inhibitory; abundant all over brain; type A linked to seizures and anxiety
Glutamate	NMDA, AMPA Kainic acid	Related to seizures
Norepinephrine	α, β	Predominant in cortex, limbic system, and striatum
		α_2 linked to depression
		All subtypes are metabotropic and diffuse in CNS
Opioid	μ, δ, κ	Related to pain
Peptide	Many	Various functions, many still poorly understood
Serotonin (5-hydroxytryp-tamine [5-HT])	At least 11, with 7 subtypes	5-HT_{1a} linked to anxiety and depression
		5-HT_{1d} linked to migraine
		5-HT_2 linked to depression, sexual function, and sleep
		5-HT_3 linked to memory

Note. Many of these receptors have subtypes not noted here.
AMPA=α-amino-3-hydroxy-5-methyl-4-isoxazole propionic acid; NMDA= N-methyl-D-aspartate.

TABLE 2–2. Some neurotransmitters

Neurotransmitter	Synthesized from	Metabolite	Main location
Acetylcholine (slow activation and inhibition)	Choline	Acetyl-CoA	Cortex
			Spinal cord
			Caudate
			Hippocampus
			Nucleus basalis of Meynert
Dopamine (slow inhibitory activation)	Tyrosine	Homovanillic acid	Substantia nigra Ventral tegmental area
			Basal ganglia
			Limbic system
GABA (inhibitory) and glutamate (excitatory)	Glutamate	Glutamic acid	Ubiquitous
			Cortical/ Subcortical
Norepinephrine	Tyrosine	MHPG	Locus coeruleus
			Limbic system
			Cortex
Serotonin (5-HT)	Tryptophan	5-HIAA	Raphe nucleus
			Limbic system
			Cortex

5-HIAA=5-hydroxyindoleacetic acid; 5-HT=5-hydroxytryptamine; MHPG= 3-methoxy-4-hydroxyphenylglycol.

rotransmitters so relevant to the regulation of behavior, to the forebrain structures such as the nucleus accumbens, are referred to as the *mesolimbic system*. The orbitofrontal cortex (OFC) is also typically included as part of the limbic circuitry.

Figure 2–1 outlines the most important structures of the limbic system. The amygdala plays a role in many emotional processes, including the control of aggression, affective tone of incoming sensations, anxiety, learning associations between stimuli and reinforcement, laying down emotional memory, and possibly psychosis.

The *hippocampus* plays a major role in episodic memory.

The *parahippocampal gyrus* (part of which is referred to as the *entorhinal cortex*) is a meeting point where sensory informa-

TABLE 2–3.	Limbic system	
Main nuclei	**Principal target**	**Main pathways**
Amygdala	Cingulate, medial temporal, thalamus, hypothalamus, dorsal and ventral striatum, orbital frontal cortex	Stria terminalis, ventral amygdalofugal pathway, uncinate fasciculus
Anterior and mediodorsal thalamic	Cingulate and dorsolateral frontal lobes	Thalamocortical tracts
Hippocampus	Parahippocampus, hypothalamus, limbic cortex	Fornix, medial forebrain bundle
Hypothalamus	Pituitary, limbic cortex	Tuberoinfundibular pathway, medial forebrain bundle
Locus coeruleus	Diverse cortical regions	Ascending pathways
Mammillary bodies	Anterior thalamus	Mammillothalamic tract
Nucleus accumbens	Globus pallidus	Frontal-subcortical circuits
Raphe	Diverse cortical regions	Ascending pathways
Ventral tegmental area	Ventral striatum, orbital frontal cortex	Tegmental-cortical pathways

tion from the outside world is integrated with data from inside the organism. Thus, sensory information first reaches the cortex at *unimodal primary sensory areas*. It is then projected to *secondary sensory areas* and to the *multimodal association cortex*. These cortical regions project to the parahippocampal gyrus, providing integrated sensory information. This information is further projected to hippocampal structures and the amygdala. The latter two, in turn, influence and are influenced by information on the internal state of the organism derived from hypothalamus and other subcortical limbic structures. The hypothalamus has extensive connections with the visceral nuclei in the brain stem.

The *cingulate gyrus* is an extensive cortical gyrus that is part of the so-called *Papez circuit*. The Papez circuit is *hippocampus–mamillary bodies–anterior thalamic nucleus–cingulate gyrus–hippocampus*. The cingulate gyrus is involved in some highly complex mammalian activities, such as maternal behavior, play,

28

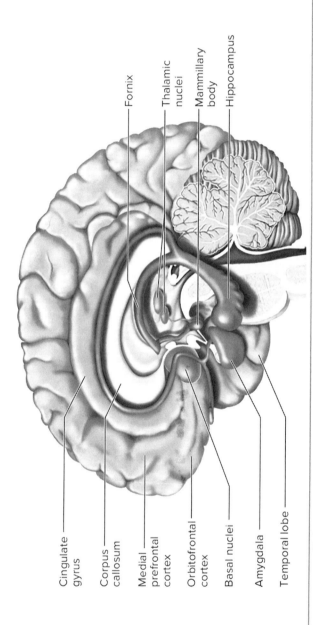

Cingulate gyrus

Corpus callosum

Medial prefrontal cortex

Orbitofrontal cortex

Basal nuclei

Amygdala

Temporal lobe

Fornix

Thalamic nuclei

Mammillary body

Hippocampus

FIGURE 2–1. **Major limbic system structures in medial view.**

pain, and attention. It is sometimes lesioned in neurosurgical procedures to treat OCD, pain, and depression.

The term *extended amygdala* refers to the amygdala (mainly the centromedial nuclei) and a connecting group of cells and fibers that extend medially under the basal ganglia to the bed nucleus of the stria terminalis and also posteriorly, looping anteriorly, like the fornix (see Figure 2–1) in the stria terminalis. The extended amygdala thus can be conceptualized as a group of interconnected structures that receive rich monoamine input from ascending midbrain afferents; through its efferents, it broadly influences hypothalamic, autonomic, and somatomotor functions.

Basal Ganglia

The *basal ganglia* typically encompasses the *caudate nucleus, putamen,* and *globus pallidus*. The *striatum* refers to the caudate and the putamen, the former being a large C-shaped nucleus that adheres throughout its length to the lateral ventricles and is continuous anteriorly with the putamen.

Medially within the head of the caudate nucleus is the *nucleus accumbens*. The nucleus accumbens and some adjacent dopamine-rich nuclei are sometimes referred to as the *ventral* or *limbic striatum*. The extended amygdala outputs to the ventral striatum and thus influences emotional motor behavior.

The basal ganglia are members of brain circuits that mediate cognitive and motor processes. Five frontal-subcortical circuits have been described that link specific frontal regions with the basal ganglia and thalamus. The five loops originate in the supplementary motor cortex, the frontal eye fields, the dorsolateral prefrontal cortex (PFC), the OFC, and the anterior cingulate cortex. The three behaviorally relevant circuits are shown in Figure 2–2. Each circuit has sequential connections between the frontal lobes, caudate or putamen, globus pallidus and substantia nigra, and thalamus, as well as an indirect pathway (not shown) that interposes connections between the subthalamic nucleus, globus pallidus externa, and globus pallidus interna before rejoining the direct pathway. Thus, the main outflow from the caudate and putamen occurs via the globus pallidus, which then connects to the thalamus. The ventral striatum flows to the *ventral pallidum* and then to the *thalamus*. The ventral pallidum is sometimes called the *substantia innominata*, an area rich in acetylcholine and associated with the *nucleus basalis of Meynert*.

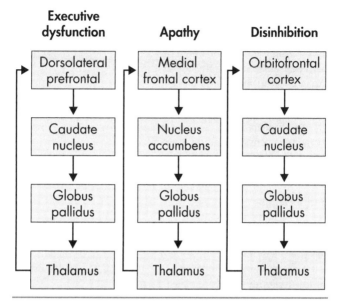

Executive dysfunction

Dorsolateral prefrontal → Caudate nucleus → Globus pallidus → Thalamus

Apathy

Medial frontal cortex → Nucleus accumbens → Globus pallidus → Thalamus

Disinhibition

Orbitofrontal cortex → Caudate nucleus → Globus pallidus → Thalamus

FIGURE 2–2.   Frontal-subcortical circuits.

The three circuits relevant to behavior are shown. Injury to the dorsolateral prefrontal circuit produces executive dysfunction, damage to the orbitofrontal circuit causes disinhibition, and dysfunction of the medial frontal circuit produces apathy.

MD=medial dorsal nucleus; VA=ventral anterior nucleus.

Source.   Reprinted from Cummings JL: "Frontal-Subcortical Circuits and Human Behavior." *Archives of Neurology* 50:873–880, 1993 (Figure 2, p. 875). Copyright © 1993, American Medical Association. Used with permission.

The most important loops for emotional behavior involve the ventral striatum, which has limbic connections. The substantia nigra–caudate pathway is involved in Parkinson's disease. These frontal-subcortical circuits provide an explanation for the similarities between the behavioral abnormalities that accompany frontal lobe dysfunction and those that occur with basal ganglia and thalamic injury.

Of great importance for neuropsychiatry is the influence of the limbic system on the basal ganglia. The ventral striatum is one of the crossroads where emotional and motoric information come together and can influence each other. Taken together, the basal forebrain structures are involved in a wide variety of functions related to many basic social behaviors; they integrate somatomotor and emotional motor activity.

Reticular Activating System

The *reticular activating system* (RAS) is a large collection of fibers and nuclei throughout the brain stem that include the main monoamine nuclei, extending from the medulla oblongata to the thalamus. Structures within the RAS modulate arousal, sleep-wake cycles, and conscious activity.

Cerebral Cortex

The *cerebral cortex* is traditionally numbered after the scheme devised by the famous neurologist Korbinian Brodmann, who identified several dozen regions distinguishable by their histological characteristics (*cytoarchitecture*). The four lobes—frontal, parietal, occipital, and temporal—are defined solely on the basis of surface markings (Figure 2–3). The cortex has a large number of association fibers that link areas of the same hemisphere and commissural fibers that link homotopic areas of the two hemispheres. The largest commissural fiber bundle is the *corpus callosum*, the primary pathway connecting the two hemispheres. The *arcuate fasciculus* is a bundle of association fibers that connects many parts of the cortex on the lateral surface of the hemisphere.

The two main fissures of the cortex are the *Sylvian fissure*, which separates the temporal lobe from the frontal and parietal lobes, at the bottom of which is found the *insular cortex*, and the *Rolandic fissure* (or *central sulcus*), which runs obliquely across the dorsolateral surface of each hemisphere, separating the frontal from the parietal lobe.

Sensory information from the receptive organs is relayed through the thalamus to the *primary sensory areas* of the cortex. The *primary motor cortex*, where brain control of musculature originates, is in the precentral gyrus, immediately anterior to the central sulcus. The primary somatosensory cortex—where body sensations are processed—is located posterior to the central sulcus along the postcentral gyrus. More posteriorly are the somatosensory association areas. The primary auditory cortical areas are in the superior temporal gyrus, and the primary visual areas are in the striate cortex of the occipital lobe.

The *frontal lobes* are represented anatomically by those areas anterior to the central sulcus. The motor strip is Brodmann area 4 (BA4); the premotor area is in front of the motor strip (BA6, BA44, and BA45). The frontal eye field is BA8. The supplementary motor area is BA6, on the medial aspect of the hemisphere.

32

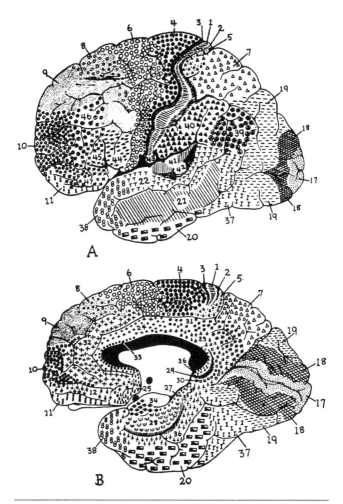

FIGURE 2–3. **Anatomical areas as depicted by Brodmann.**
Main anatomic areas to note are the 1, 2, and 3=primary somatosensory
areas; 4=primary motor cortex; 6=premotor area; 8, 9, 10, 11, 12, 45, 46, and
47=prefrontal granular cortex; 17=visual cortex; 22=superior temporal gyrus; 23, 24, 31, and 33=cingulate gyrus; 27, 28, and 34=parahippocampal
gyrus; 38=temporal pole; 39 and 40=inferior parietal lobule; and 41 and 42=
auditory cortex (Heschl's gyri).
Source. Reprinted from Carpenter MB: *Core Text of Neuroanatomy*, 4th Edition. Baltimore, MD, Williams and Wilkins, 1991, p. 399. Copyright © 1991,
Lippincott Williams and Wilkins. Used with permission.

The *prefrontal cortex* designates the more anterior (mostly nonmotor) parts of the frontal lobe. It is divided into the dorsolateral PFC (BA9, BA10, and BA46), the medial frontal cortex (BA24 and BA32; anterior cingulate cortex), and the OFC (BA11 and BA12).

The frontal lobes are the six-layered neocortex, and the motor and premotor areas are the agranular cortex. Layers III and V contain the long projection fibers that descend from these areas to the brain stem and spinal cord and are enlarged compared with other cortical regions. The PFC is the granular cortex: layers II and IV are larger and layers III and V are smaller than the cortex of the motor and premotor areas. The caudal orbitofrontal cortex and cingulate cortex of the frontal lobes are the paralimbic regions, composed of the mesocortex and transitional between the archicortex (three layered) and the neocortex (six layered).

The frontal lobes receive afferent association fibers from other cortical areas and projections from subcortical structures. In addition, each frontal lobe receives inputs via commissural fibers from the contralateral frontal areas. The PFC receives fibers from the unimodal association cortex (visual, auditory, somatosensory) and posterior heteromodal cortex of the inferior parietal lobule. These projections are reciprocal and are distributed in the *arcuate fasciculus*. Fibers from the amygdala and medial temporal cortex enter the prefrontal regions through the *uncinate fasciculus*. The principal subcortical projections to the PFC originate in the *medial dorsal nucleus of the thalamus*. Afferent connections from the hypothalamus are also present. Thus, the PFC receives sensory information from the posterior cortical regions and limbic input from temporal, thalamic, and hypothalamic structures, creating the opportunity for integrating environmental, emotional, and interoceptive information.

The efferent connections of the frontal lobes include reciprocal connections with the sources of afferent input from other cortical and subcortical regions. These connections create the opportunity for the frontal lobes to modulate and modify their own input. In addition, the frontal cortex has unidirectional projections to the head of the caudate nucleus, nucleus accumbens, and putamen (see Figure 2–3). Connections to the hypothalamus are largely efferent in nature. The final output of the nervous system is mediated by frontobulbar connections and frontospinal connections descending to the brain stem and spinal cord nuclei through the pyramidal tract. It is via this tract that humans effect environmental change, through speech and movement.

The frontal-subcortical projections use glutamate as their principal transmitter. However, afferents to the frontal cortex include extensive dopaminergic, noradrenergic, and serotonergic neurons from the midbrain and pons. The nucleus basalis also provides cholinergic input. GABA, an inhibitory transmitter, is present in high concentrations throughout the cerebral cortex.

Functional neuroimaging methods, such as functional MRI and PET, can provide dynamic pictures of brain function and metabolism. In particular, functional MRI (fMRI) has become the workhorse of human cognitive and clinical neuroscience because it is safe and noninvasive, but the limitations of these methods should be kept in mind. For instance, fMRI provides only a very indirect measure of brain function, measuring the brain's metabolic demands (i.e., blood oxygenation levels) as a proxy for real neuroelectrical activity.

Despite these limitations, neuroimaging has revealed that even distant regions of the cerebral cortex are linked together into cooperative *functional-anatomical networks* (Figure 2–4). Some of these brain networks have clear functions, such as the visual network (largely coextensive with the occipital lobe). Other networks, such as the frontoparietal network, are distributed throughout the brain in nonintuitive ways, serving complex and still controversial functions. Intrinsic networks are not static structures but are dynamic patterns of interconnectivity shaped by development, learning, and disease. Just as healthy acquisition of new knowledge and skills leads to changes in network activity and connectivity, so too can pathological disease processes and mental illness.

The *default network* plays an essential role in self-referential thinking, mind-wandering, and rumination and is therefore thought to be of great relevance for many neuropsychiatric diseases. The default network is overactive or abnormally coupled with other networks in a wide variety of conditions, including depression, anxiety, ADHD, and schizophrenia. Abnormal default network functioning is also implicated in neurodevelopmental and neurodegenerative conditions, such as Alzheimer's disease and autism spectrum disorder. Other important networks include the central executive and salience networks.

The network organization of the brain has potentially profound implications for understanding the consequences of brain injury. Network architecture helps explain the well-known ef-

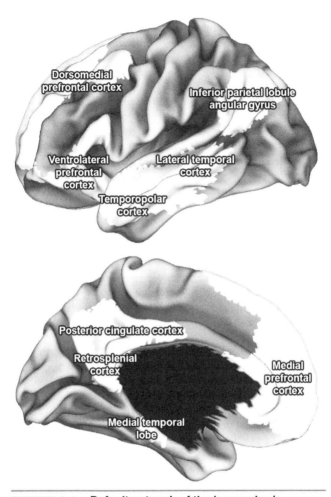

FIGURE 2–4. **Default network of the human brain.**

The cerebral cortex can be parcellated in functional-anatomical networks that show cooperative, correlated activity at rest, during tasks, and even in deep sleep when consciousness is absent. The default network (shown in *white*) consists of many regions distributed throughout the brain. The major nodes of the network are labeled. Abnormal activity and connectivity of the default network plays an important role in various neuropsychiatric diseases.

fect of *diaschisis*, in which damage to a given brain region results in deleterious effects on the function of distant, ostensibly uninjured brain areas. Because brain networks function as integrated wholes, damage to a single node can have a negative effect on the entire network. This is especially true for network *hubs*—crucial connectors that facilitate communication among the various nodes of a network. For instance, although the default network contains approximately nine regional nodes, only two or three of these are considered hubs. Hubs therefore represent high-risk loci in brain disease and injury, and damage to hubs is likely to result in negative consequences out of proportion to the extent of the lesion.

The brain's network architecture also has potential upsides, however, in terms of treating neuropsychiatric disease. Many noninvasive *neuromodulation* methodologies have emerged in recent decades, such as *transcranial magnetic stimulation* and *transcranial direct current stimulation*. Although still experimental, these methods aim to safely modulate brain activity to improve the symptoms of various neuropsychiatric conditions. However, the signals emitted by these methods generally are not able to penetrate more than a few centimeters through the skull and brain tissue. Many highly desirable targets of neuromodulation located deeper in the brain are therefore inaccessible, including many default network regions and limbic and subcortical regions crucial to emotion, such as the amygdala and hippocampus. The brain's network organization presents the possibility of modulating these otherwise inaccessible regions by targeting the more superficial brain areas on the cortical surface with which deeper regions are reciprocally connected. Such an approach is already being tried for treating refractory depression. Likewise, when using invasive neuromodulation methods such as *deep brain stimulation*, a single electrode well-placed within a crucial network hub can be expected to have widespread effects throughout the brain.

Cerebellum

The *cerebellum* lies posterior to the brain stem. Its cortex is divided into the central vermis and the cerebellar hemispheres. The cerebellum plays an important role in maintaining balance, posture, and fine control over voluntary muscle movements. Recently, direct links between this structure and the limbic system have been found. Some important associations between neuroanatomical sites and behavior are listed in Table 2–4.

TABLE 2–4. Some brain-behavior associations

Structure	Behavior
Amygdala	Fear, anxiety, aggression, sexual behavior, psychosis, mood
Cingulate gyrus	Maternal behavior, play, vocalization, attention, pain, motivation
Entorhinal cortex	Memory, sensory integration
Hippocampus	Memory, anxiety
Hypothalamus	Eating, drinking, sex, aggression, hormonal regulation
Reticular activating system	Arousal, sleep-wake cycle
Septum	Pleasure, addiction
Ventral striatum	Motivation

■ BRAIN-BEHAVIOR RELATIONSHIPS

Theories of *localization* argue that specific mental functions are subserved by specific brain regions. *Lateralization of function* implies that some functions are predominantly mediated by one hemisphere or the other; a classic example is the left-hemisphere dominance of language in most people. *Theories of equipotentiality* deny such localization, whereas the concept of *parallel distributed processing* (PDP) seeks an intermediate ground. PDP implies the existence of integrated neuronal circuits that are widely distributed in the brain and have the capacity to change their response bias with learning. Any point in the circuit may interconnect with other circuits; hence, a single lesion may have multiple potential effects. Likewise, similar effects could emerge from lesions in different parts of the same circuit.

Classical lesion studies provide strong evidence for localization of certain functions. For instance, lesions of BA44/45 in the left hemisphere—known as Broca's area—commonly result in a deficit in the production of language (*Broca's aphasia*). Bilateral lesions to the hippocampus yield *anterograde amnesia*, a profound inability to form new memories. Most functions cannot be so strictly localized, however, and evidently involve the cooperation of many regions distributed throughout the brain.

In the early twentieth century, the increasing prevalence of neurosurgery to treat epilepsy and brain tumors provided an unprecedented opportunity to explore human brain function via direct electrical stimulation of neural tissue: awake surgical pa-

38

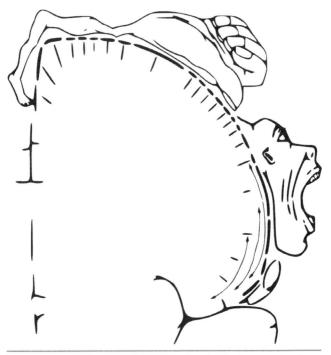

FIGURE 2–5. Sensory homunculus in the human brain.
The postcentral gyrus of the parietal lobe contains the primary sensory cortex, where body sensations are first processed in the cerebral cortex. Directly applying electrical stimulation to the cortical surface in neurosurgical patients revealed that larger areas of cortex are dedicated to processing information from the most sensitive parts of the body, such as the face, hands, and fingers.
Source. Based on Penfield and Jasper 1954. This file is licensed under the Creative Commons Attribution-Share Alike 4.0 International license.

tients were able to provide detailed reports of the wide variety of effects elicited on their minds and bodies. Direct electrical stimulation led to classic discoveries, such as the topographical organization of body maps in primary sensory and motor regions (the so-called homunculus; Figure 2–5). Recent work has revealed that the effects of direct electrical stimulation are not determined merely by local function but are also influenced by the brain's hierarchical network architecture. Taken together, the findings of the past century suggest that both local and global properties contribute to the functionality of specific brain regions. The phenomenon of diaschisis may be operative here, in which an injury at one brain location, because of interconnecting networks, may affect a distant anatomical and functional site.

The realization that injecting electrical current into human brain tissue could have profound effects on perception, mood, and memory led to the development of chronically implanted neuromodulation devices, commonly referred to as deep brain stimulation. These devices are increasingly being used as interventions for neuropsychiatric disorders that have proven refractory to pharmaceutical treatment.

■ REFERENCES

Aggleton JP (ed): The Amygdala: A Functional Analysis, 2nd Edition. New York, Oxford University Press, 2000

Alhourani A, McDowell MM, Randazzo MJ, et al: Network effects of deep brain stimulation. J Neurophysiol 114(4):2105–2117, 2015 26269552

Borchers S, Himmelbach M, Logothetis N, Karnath HO: Direct electrical stimulation of human cortex: the gold standard for mapping brain functions? Nat Rev Neurosci 13(1):63–70, 2011 22127300

Buckner RL, Andrews-Hanna JR, Schacter DL: The brain's default network: anatomy, function, and relevance to disease. Ann N Y Acad Sci 1124:1–38, 2008 18400922

Catani M: The anatomy of the human frontal lobe. Handb Clin Neurol 163:95–122, 2019

Cole EJ, Stimpson KH, Bentzley BS, et al: Stanford accelerated intelligent neuromodulation therapy for treatment-resistant depression. Am J Psychiatry 177(8):716–726, 2020 32252538

Cummings JL: Frontal-subcortical circuits and human behavior. Arch Neurol 50(8):873–880, 1993 8352676

Fox KCR, Shi L, Baek S, et al: Intrinsic network architecture predicts the effects elicited by intracranial electrical stimulation of the human brain. Nat Hum Behav 4(10):1039–1052, 2020 32632334

Fuster JM: The Prefrontal Cortex: Anatomy, Physiology, and Neuropsychology of the Frontal Lobe, 3rd Edition. Philadelphia, PA, Lippincott-Raven, 1997

Harmsen IE, Elias GJB, Beyn ME, et al: Clinical trials for deep brain stimulation: current state of affairs. Brain Stimul 13(2):378–385, 2020 31786180

Holtzheimer PE, Mayberg HS: Deep brain stimulation for psychiatric disorders. Annu Rev Neurosci 34:289–307, 2011 21692660

Huntenburg JM, Bazin PL, Margulies DS: Large-scale gradients in human cortical organization. Trends Cogn Sci 22(1):21–31, 2018 29203085

Mak LE, Minuzzi L, MacQueen G, et al: The default network in healthy individuals: a systematic review and meta-anaysis. Brain Connect 7(1):25–33, 2017 27917679

McGinty JF (ed): Advancing from the ventral striatum to the extended amygdala: implications for neuropsychiatry and drug abuse. Ann N Y Acad Sci 877 (entire volume), 1999

McIntyre CC, Hahn PJ: Network perspectives on the mechanisms of deep brain stimulation. Neurobiol Dis 38(3):329–337, 2010 19804831

Menon V: Large-scale brain networks and psychopathology: a unifying triple network model. Trends Cogn Sci 15(10):483–506, 2011 21908230

Mesulam M-M: Patterns in behavioral anatomy: association areas, the limbic system, and hemispheric specialization, in Principles of Behavioral Neurology, 2nd Edition. Edited by Mesulam M-M. New York, Oxford University Press, 2000, pp 1–70

Penfield W, Jasper H: Epilepsy and the Functional Anatomy of the Human Brain. Oxford, England, Little, Brown & Co., 1954

Whitfield-Gabrieli S, Ford JM: Default mode network activity and connectivity in psychopathology. Annu Rev Clin Psychol 8:49–76, 2012 22224834

Yeo BTT, Krienen FM, Sepulcre J, et al: The organization of the human cerebral cortex estimated by intrinsic functional connectivity. J Neurophysiol 106(3):1125–1165, 2011 21653723

3

NEUROPSYCHIATRIC SYMPTOMS AND SYNDROMES

Sheldon Benjamin, M.D.
Delia Bakeman, D.O.

Neuropsychiatric diagnosis is based on the elicitation of clinical symptoms, careful examination, construction of a differential diagnosis, use of laboratory tests and neuroimaging to support or exclude specific diagnoses, and identification of the most likely etiology of the behavioral disturbance. In some cases, longitudinal assessment and careful monitoring of treatment responses may be necessary to clarify the diagnosis. Treatment depends on accurate diagnosis.

This chapter addresses neuropsychiatric symptoms and syndromes and their differential diagnosis. The syndromes described include depression, mania, mood and affective lability, delusions, hallucinations, anxiety, OCD and other repetitive behaviors, personality changes indicative of brain dysfunction, dissociative disorders, altered sexual behavior, and aggressive behavior. Neuropsychiatric syndromes associated with frontal lobe disorders are described in more detail in Chapter 5, "Frontal Lobe Syndromes," and symptoms and syndromes indicative of epilepsy and limbic system dysfunction are described more extensively in Chapter 9, "Epilepsy and Limbic System Disorders." Treatment of neuropsychiatric disorders is discussed in the relevant disease-oriented chapters (Chapters 8–21) and is summarized in Chapter 22, "Treatments in Neuropsychiatry."

■ DISORDERS OF MOOD AND AFFECT

Depression

Depression has mood, affective, motivational, cognitive, motor, neurovegetative, immunological, inflammatory, and endocrine dimensions. DSM-5 specifies that patients with major depressive episodes must have five or more of the symptoms described in this section during the same 2-week period, with one of those symptoms being anhedonia or depressed mood. A patient meets criteria for persistent depressive disorder if these symptoms are consistently present for a period of 2 years. *Mood* changes in depression include sadness and loss of ability to experience pleasure (anhedonia). Anxiety is common in depression, and irritability may be present. *Affect* refers to the outward expression of one's internal mood state reflected in posture, facial expression, prosody, and gesture. Depressed affect may include cataleptic posture; restricted, flat, sad, or tearful facial expressions; monotonous speech; and absence of spontaneous gestures. *Motivational alterations* characteristic of depression include the loss of motivation with apathy and diminished initiative. *Cognitive characteristics* include thoughts of worthlessness, hopelessness, helplessness, guilty or somatic preoccupation, and decreased concentration. Recurrent thoughts of death or suicide may be present. Patients with depression may develop the dementia syndrome of depression (previously known as pseudodementia), which includes withdrawn avoidant behavior, executive dysfunction, diminished cognitive processing speed, and impaired memory retrieval. The risk for dementia of any etiology has been shown to be increased ≤70% in patients with late-life depressive symptoms. Some patients display mood-congruent hallucinations (e.g., the smell of feces or of rotting substances) and delusions (e.g., belief that they are dying or are guilty of serious offenses). In addition to *cataleptic posture*, *motor symptoms* of depression may include hypophonic, monotonous speech; decreased eye contact; and psychomotor slowing or agitation. *Neurovegetative features* of depression include altered sleep patterns (i.e., early morning awakening, multiple nocturnal awakenings, difficulty falling asleep, hypersomnia, decreased rapid eye movement latency), appetite alterations (decreased or increased), excessive fatigue, and diminished libido. *Endocrine abnormalities* in depression may include changes in the hypothalamic-pituitary-adrenal axis or the hypothalamic-pituitary-thyroid axis.

Secretion of excess cortisol, hyperstimulation of corticotropin-releasing hormone, and failure to suppress cortisol response to dexamethasone in the dexamethasone suppression test have all been found in major depression. In addition, patients with depression show abnormal responses to thyroid-stimulating hormone (TSH) and thyrotropin-releasing hormone, elevated thyrotropin-releasing hormone concentrations in cerebrospinal fluid, and increased prevalence of antithyroid antibodies (see Chapter 19, "Evaluation and Treatment of Endocrine Disorders With Neuropsychiatric Symptoms [Thyroid and Adrenal]"). Variation in sex hormone levels during characteristic periods of puberty, peri- and postpartum, and menopause have also been linked to depression risk. *Inflammatory abnormalities*, such as elevated levels of proinflammatory cytokines and increased blood-brain barrier permeability, have been found in depression, and higher rates of depression are present in patients with autoimmune diseases compared with the general population.

Depression occurs in a wide variety of brain diseases in which it exacerbates cognitive impairment and functional disability (Table 3–1) and adds to the overall cost of treatment. The diagnosis of depression, which involves symptoms expressed verbally, experienced cognitively, or involving neurovegetative features, may be complicated by the presence of damage to brain structures subtending these functions and may be facilitated by obtaining collateral information from someone close to the patient. Onset at a later age, onset in proximity to the diagnosis of a medical condition, absence of family history, and presence of atypical features are indications that depression may be due to a medical condition. The treatable nature of depression makes it imperative that depression be sought and actively treated in patients with brain disorders.

Review of the disorders listed in Table 3–1 reveals that depression may be linked to dysfunction in specific brain regions. Disorders affecting the frontal lobes, temporal lobes, and basal ganglia (especially the caudate nuclei) are particularly likely to be accompanied by depressive symptoms. Involvement of the left frontal lobe or left caudate nucleus is more likely than right-sided dysfunction to precipitate depression, and depression is more severe and more frequent the closer the left frontal lesion is to the frontal pole. Patients with late-onset depression often have evidence of ischemic white matter injury when they are studied with MRI. Serotonergic, noradrenergic, and dopaminergic transmitter systems are implicated in the pathogenesis of depression, and abnormalities of motivation, stress response, and behavioral programming mediated by frontal-subcortical circuits are involved in many symptoms.

Depression can be treated with psychotherapy, pharmacotherapy, and neuromodulation with electroconvulsive therapy or transcranial magnetic stimulation. Pharmacological agents

44

TABLE 3–1. Frequency of depression in neurological disorders

Neurological condition	Frequency of depressive syndromes, %*
Brain tumor	40–50
Frontotemporal dementia	40–50
Parkinson's disease	40–50
Stroke	30–60
Huntington's disease	30–40
Vascular dementia	25–60
Multiple sclerosis	25–50
Traumatic brain injury	25–50
Migraine	20–30
Alzheimer's disease	16–44
Epilepsy	10–50

*Depressive disorders include both major depressive episodes and less severe symptomatic depression syndromes.

used to treat depression include selective serotonin reuptake inhibitors (SSRIs), noradrenergic reuptake inhibitors, serotonin-norepinephrine reuptake inhibitors (SNRIs), tricyclic antidepressants (TCAs), monoamine oxidase inhibitors, and NMDA blockers (ketamine/esketamine). Evidence-based psychotherapies for depression include cognitive-behavioral, interpersonal, and psychodynamic psychotherapies.

Mania

The manic syndrome includes abnormalities of mood, affect, cognition, motor activity, and neurovegetative functions. *Mood changes* may include euphoria, lability, and irritability. Depressive symptoms may be mixed with the expansive, elevated mood state of mania to create a mixed mood disorder. *Affective alterations* are characterized by excessive laughter, smiling, and animation. *Cognitive changes* include disorganization, distractibility, impaired concentration, and tangentiality. Impaired judgment may result in increased risk-taking behaviors such as substance use, hypersexuality, impulsive business endeavors, or speeding. Inflated self-esteem, mood-congruent delusions (e.g., grandiose delusions of having special powers or abilities), hallucinations, flight of ideas related by clang associations, rhyming, echolalia, or incoherence may be present. *Motor symptoms* of mania include hyperactivity, increased gesturing, restlessness, and logorrhea. Speech may be loud, pressured, and excessively fast (tachyphemic). The patient may be intrusive, domineering, demanding, or threatening in social interactions. *Neurovegetative features* include insomnia, decreased need for sleep, and increased appetite, libido, and energy. Hypomania has many of the same features as mania, but psychosis is not present; symptoms are less severe and typically do not cause impaired social or occupational function. The DSM-5 criteria for manic episode require a distinct period of mood, energy, and behavioral disturbance in addition to three or more of the symptoms just described lasting at least 1 week.

Mania and hypomania have been associated with various neurological conditions (Table 3–2). Nearly all of the focal lesions that produce mania are located in the right hemisphere and involve the orbitofrontal cortex, caudate nuclei, thalamus or perithalamic regions, or basotemporal area. Mood modulation, hypothalamic control of neurovegetative functions, and limbic system activities are disrupted in mania.

Mania and hypomania are treated with mood-stabilizing agents, including lithium, antiepileptics, and antipsychotics (see Chapter 22). Temporary medication to aid with sleep may be required during the acute manic phase. Establishment of a long-term therapeutic relationship promotes medication compliance and early detection of hypomanic symptoms.

■ MOOD AND AFFECT LABILITY

Lability of mood refers to the rapid shift from one mood state to another. Patients may alternate among happiness, anger, and irritability within short periods of time, as may be seen in orbitofrontal dysfunction. *Lability of affect* refers to sudden changes in emotional expression. Although they are typically linked, affect may not reflect mood in some neurological disorders. Neurological causes of affective and mood lability are listed in Table 3–3. Pathological affect regulation, which is also known as pathological laughing and crying or pseudobulbar affect and has more recently been called involuntary emotional expression disorder, is one component of pseudobulbar palsy. Patients with pseudobulbar affect overreact to the presence of what would ordinarily be a mild emotional cue. Pseudobulbar palsy, an upper motor neuron disorder caused by bilateral corticobulbar lesions, includes pseudobulbar affect, dysarthria, dysphagia, facial and

TABLE 3–2.	Neurological disorders associated with mania or hypomania

Autoimmune
  Autoimmune limbic encephalitis
  Multiple sclerosis
  Systemic lupus
Degenerative
  Basal ganglia calcification
  Creutzfeldt-Jakob disease
  Frontotemporal dementia
  Huntington's disease
  Leukodystrophies
  Parkinson's disease with dopaminergic therapy
Epilepsy
  Post temporal lobectomy for epilepsy
  Temporal lobe epilepsy with interictal psychosis
Functional neurosurgery
  Deep brain stimulation of subthalamic nucleus for Parkinson's disease
  Deep brain stimulation of ventral striatum/ventral capsule for OCD
Infectious
  Cryptococcal meningitis
  Herpes encephalitis
  HIV encephalitis
  Infectious mononucleosis
  Influenza A
  Lyme disease
  Neurosyphilis
Stroke (especially right frontal lobe and right basal ganglia)
Traumatic brain injury

Note. Many toxic (medications, metals) and metabolic causes of secondary mania should be considered in any differential.

tongue weakness, and extensor plantar reflexes. Some common causes of pseudobulbar palsy are listed in Table 3–4.

Epileptic seizures may also cause abnormalities of affect. Gelastic seizures, consisting of brief spells of mirthless laughter, and dacrystic seizures, consisting of brief tearful outbursts, are often associated with hypothalamic hamartoma. Sudden fear, sadness, or elation may occur during partial seizures of tempor-

TABLE 3–3.	Neurological disorders associated with mood and affective lability

Angelman syndrome

Anterior communicating artery aneurysm

Behavioral variant frontotemporal dementia

Herpes encephalitis

Huntington's disease

Idiopathic basal ganglia calcification (Fahr's disease)

Pseudobulbar palsy

Orbitofrontal meningioma

Seizure disorders

  Dacrystic epilepsy

  Frontal lobe epilepsy

  Gelastic epilepsy

  Temporal limbic epilepsy

Traumatic brain injury

TABLE 3–4.	Causes of pseudobulbar palsy

Amyotrophic lateral sclerosis

Bilateral vascular lesions (including lacunar state, Binswanger disease)

Demyelinating disease

Metabolic abnormalities

Neoplasm

Parkinson's disease

Progressive supranuclear palsy

Traumatic brain injury

olimbic origin. Angelman syndrome typically includes laughter and drooling in the setting of puppet-like jerky movements and dysmorphic features. Right (greater than left) bifrontal lesions may cause *Witzelsucht* (constant joking) or *moria* (inappropriately cheerful affect) without pathological affect regulation.

■ PSYCHOTIC SYMPTOMS

The manifestations of *psychosis* include positive symptoms (delusions, hallucinations, formal thought disorder [tangentiality, illogicality, incoherence, derailment], bizarre or disorganized behavior) and negative symptoms (avolition/apathy, poverty of speech or alogia, affective flattening, anhedonia/asociality).

▪ DELUSIONS

Delusions are fixed false beliefs unsupported by facts, inconsistent with cultural background, and from which a person cannot be dissuaded. Types of delusions are shown in Table 3–5.

Delusions may be mood congruent, with grandiose beliefs of personal power or wealth in mania and beliefs of personal inadequacy, guilt, disease, or death in depression.

Delusions in primary psychiatric disorders are not known to have neuroanatomical correlates. However, delusional misidentification syndromes can occur in the setting of right frontal dysfunction, and delusions in neurological disorders are more likely to occur following right than left hemisphere damage. Delusions are more likely to be related to neurological insult if they are monothematic and not preceded by evidence of paranoia or persecutory delusions. Table 3–6 lists neuropsychiatric conditions reported to be associated with delusion formation.

Delusions are treated with neuroleptics (see Chapter 22). Anticonvulsants ameliorate delusions when they occur as part of an ictal event. A combination of antidepressant and antipsychotic treatment is often used to treat depressive delusions, and combined mood stabilizer and antipsychotic therapy is used to treat delusions in mania.

▪ HALLUCINATIONS AND ILLUSIONS

Hallucinations are sensory experiences that occur without stimulation of the relevant sensory organ. In primary psychotic disorders, they are experienced as real, whereas in psychosis due to neurological disorders hallucinations are recognized as false perceptions. *Illusions* are misperceptions or incorrectly perceived sensory stimuli and commonly occur in the same disorders as hallucinations. Hallucinations may involve any sensory modality: visual, auditory, gustatory, olfactory, or tactile. They may be complex (formed, recognizable; e.g., visual hallucinations of people or animals; auditory hallucinations of voices) or simple and unformed (e.g., visual hallucinations consisting of spots, lights, or colors; auditory hallucinations of machine-like noises).

Visual hallucinations occur with lesions of the eyes, optic nerves, geniculocalcarine tracts, occipital cortex, or temporal

TABLE 3–5. Types of delusions

Delusion	Definition/Examples
Delusional misidentification syndromes	Belief that people, objects, or places have been replaced by a lookalike. Examples include
	Capgras, delusion that a person close to the patient has been replaced by a double
	Cotard's, delusion that one does not exist, is dead, or that one's organs or body parts are missing, lost, or have been replaced
	Doppelganger, conviction that one has a double;
	Fregoli, delusion that one's persecutor has disguised her- or himself to look like a familiar person
	Heautoscopy (*autoscopy*), seeing an image of one's own self at a distance
	Intermetamorphosis, delusion that one's close contacts look like one's enemies
	Lycanthropy, delusion that person has or can turn into an animal
	Mirror agnosia, delusion that one's reflection is actually a stranger
	Reduplicative paramnesia, delusion that a person, place, or object has been relocated or duplicated
Erotomanic (de Clerambault syndrome)	Belief that another person, often of higher status, is in love with the individual; *incubus syndrome*, delusion one was approached during the night by an unseen lover.
Folie à deux	DEelusion shared by two people.
Delusional jealousy (Othello syndrome)	Belief that one's sexual partner is unfaithful.
Grandiose	Sense of inflated self-worth, power, knowledge, fame, or having a relationship with someone famous or powerful; religious delusions of being God or chosen by God.

TABLE 3–5.	Types of delusions *(continued)*
Delusion	**Definition/Examples**
Persecutory	Delusions of being attacked, followed, poisoned, monitored, harassed, or conspired against; *delusions of reference* describes belief that others are talking or thinking about the person.
Somatic	Delusions involving bodily functions or sensations. Examples include
	Anosognosia, denial of deficit
	Anton's syndrome, denial that one is blind in cases of cortical blindness
	Asomatagnosia, denial that a body part is one's own
	Bromosis, delusion one has terrible body odor
	Delusions of control, conviction that one's body or thoughts are under the control of another/others
	Delusional parasitosis (Ekbom's syndrome, Morgellon's disease)
	Koro, delusion that one's penis is retracting into the abdomen
	Pseudocyesis
	Somatoparaphrenia, belief that one's own body part belongs to someone else
	Thought broadcasting, belief that others can hear one's thoughts
	Thought insertion/withdrawal, belief that an external entity is inserting or withdrawing one's thoughts

lobes (Table 3–7). Blindness due to cataracts, retinal disease, or macular disease may be associated with formed or unformed hallucinations. *Charles Bonnet syndrome* is characterized by ocular disease and hallucinosis in elderly persons. Hallucinations may occur with destructive lesions of the hemispheres (*"release" hallucinations*) or as ictal events in the course of focal epileptic seizures. *Ictal hallucinations* are usually brief and stereotyped and are associated with other seizure manifestations (e.g., head and eye turning, interruption of consciousness), whereas the hallucinations that occur with destructive lesions are typically

TABLE 3–6.	Neuropsychiatric disorders associated with delusions

Adrenoleukodystrophy

Alzheimer's disease

Autoimmune limbic encephalitis

Brain tumors (especially right hemisphere)

Creutzfeldt-Jakob disease

Delusional disorder

Dementia with Lewy bodies

Depression with psychotic features

Epilepsy (especially temporal limbic epilepsy)

Frontotemporal dementia

GM2 gangliosidosis

Huntington's disease

Idiopathic basal ganglia calcification

Mania with psychosis

Metachromatic leukodystrophy

Mitochondrial encephalopathy

Multiple sclerosis

Neuronal ceroid lipofuscinosis

Parkinson's disease with dopaminergic treatment

Posttraumatic encephalopathy

Schizophrenia

Stroke (with Wernicke aphasia or right hemisphere lesion)

Vascular dementia

Viral encephalitis (especially herpes encephalitis)

Vitamin B_{12} deficiency

more prolonged and variable and occur within a visual field defect. Cortical irritability in the primary visual cortex (Brodmann area 17) causes simple elementary visual hallucinations such as geometric structures (phosphenes) and flashes of light (photopsias). Irritability in the visual association cortices (Brodmann areas 18 and 19) causes more complex visual hallucinations such as lifelike images, scenes, or people. Lilliputian or Brobdingnagian hallucinations can also occur in which the person perceives miniature or giant people engaged in fantastical activities. Formed hallucinations occurring in temporal lobe seizures may be based on visual memories.

TABLE 3–7.	Neurological disorders associated with visual hallucinations

Alzheimer's disease

Dementia with Lewy bodies

Depression or mania with hallucinations

Drug intoxication or withdrawal

Geniculocalcarine radiation lesions ("release" hallucinations)

   Multiple sclerosis

   Stroke

   Tumors

Inborn errors of metabolism

Metabolic encephalopathies

Midbrain lesions (peduncular hallucinosis)

   Stroke

   Tumors

Migraine

Narcolepsy (hypnagogic and hypnopompic hallucinations)

Occipital or temporal cortex

   Stroke

   Tumors

Ocular disorders (Charles Bonnet syndrome)

   Cataracts

   Enucleation

   Macular degeneration

Optic nerve and tract disorders

   Compression

   Ischemia

   Multiple sclerosis

Parkinson's disease after dopaminergic treatment

Posterior cortical atrophy

Schizophrenia

Peduncular hallucinosis is a unique hallucinatory syndrome occurring with midbrain lesions and consisting of sleep disturbance and well-formed, often Lilliputian, hallucinations that occur in the evening and have an amusing quality. *Migraine* headaches may be preceded by the classic scintillating scotoma (teichopsia) or fortification spectra or by metamorphopsia, micropsia, or macropsia, in which objects or body parts appear to change shape or size, sometimes referred to as *Alice in Wonderland* syndrome. *Narcolepsy* is a brain stem dysregulation syndrome manifested by the tetrad of visual hallucinations, sleep attacks, cataplexy, and sleep paralysis. Hallucinations in narcolepsy occur on falling asleep (hypnagogic) or on awakening (hypnopompic). Visual hallucinations may also occur with degenerative brain disease and are particularly common in dementia with Lewy bodies and in Parkinson's disease after initiation of dopaminergic treatment.

Auditory hallucinations occur with acquired deafness or inner ear disease, brain stem lesions, temporal lobe seizures, PTSD, borderline personality disorder, dementia subtypes, or any psychotic disorder. When attempting to categorize auditory hallucinations, evaluate accompanying symptoms because a minority of healthy individuals experience auditory hallucinations without underlying organic disease. Hallucinations may vary from voices that are speaking complete sentences to muffled speech sounds, tones with varying pitches, sounds of music, tapping, or noises made by animals. *Musical hallucinations* are common in elderly individuals with partial deafness. *Auditory illusions* such as hypoacusis or hyperacusis often occur in migraine.

Gustatory hallucinations are most common with seizures affecting the medial temporal (uncus) region and involve tastes that are not secondary to a physical stimulus.

Olfactory hallucinations (phantosmia) may be of pleasant or disturbing odors. Neuropsychiatric conditions associated with olfactory hallucinations include epilepsy, vascular dementia, Alzheimer's disease, medial temporal lobe tumors, and delusional bromosis.

Tactile or *haptic hallucinations* refer to false perceptions of touch or surface sensations. The feeling of insects crawling under the skin (formication) can be seen in delusional parasitosis. Tactile hallucinations are often seen in cocaine and amphetamine intoxication and in delirium tremens secondary to alcohol withdrawal.

■ ANXIETY

Anxiety has emotional, cognitive, motoric, and autonomic manifestations. *Emotional and cognitive disturbances* include excessive and unjustified apprehension, feelings of foreboding, and thoughts of impending doom. Patients are irritable, tense, have difficulty concentrating, and often have insomnia. *Motor abnor-malities* include tremor (typically seen as a high-frequency, low-amplitude tremor of the hands), an exaggerated startle response, and restlessness with frequent shifting of posture, pacing, and fidgeting. Facial expression conveys the patient's excessive concern. *Autonomic disturbances* of anxiety include sweating, palpitations, gastrointestinal distress (nausea, diarrhea), shortness of breath, dry mouth, chest pain, light-headedness, and frequent urination.

Several types of anxiety disorders are recognized, including panic disorder (discrete periods of intense fear or discomfort that is unexpected and unpredictable), agoraphobia (excessive fear of public spaces), social phobia (exaggerated fear of situations that expose one to scrutiny by others), specific phobia (abnormal fear of objects or situations, e.g., insects, snakes, blood, heights, or elevators), and generalized anxiety disorder (anxiety about routine life circumstances occurring on most days of a 6-month period). PTSD is classified in DSM-5 in a new category, "Trauma- and Stressor-Related Disorders," and occurs in individuals who have experienced severe psychological stress. PTSD is characterized by reliving the traumatic event, avoiding stimuli associated with the trauma or a generalized reduction in emotional responsiveness, and heightened arousal. This includes difficulty sleeping, irritability, hypervigilance, exaggerated startle response, and autonomic symptoms when exposed to events that resemble the traumatic event.

The neuroanatomical structures and neurophysiological mechanisms involved in anxiety have not yet been completely determined. Focal lesions associated with anxiety usually involve the limbic system, and more right-sided than left-sided lesions have been reported. Neurological conditions associated with anxiety include stroke, epilepsy (particularly temporal lobe epilepsy), Parkinson's disease, migraine, multiple sclerosis, encephalitis, and posttraumatic and post-concussive syndromes. Parkinsonian patients with the "on-off" syndrome frequently experience increased anxiety during off periods in concert with decreased mobility. Anxiety has been reported most often with poststroke depression in patients who have lesions of the left prefrontal cortex and in those with right temporal lobe lesions. Anxiety often accompanies hypoxia, hypoglycemia, hyperthyroidism, and mitral valve prolapse. It can be induced by amphetamines, cocaine, sympathomimetic agents, caffeine, lidocaine, procaine, and alcohol and drug withdrawal.

Anxiety disorder treatment includes behavioral therapy, mindfulness-based interventions, and pharmacotherapy with SSRIs, SNRIs, benzodiazepines, β-adrenergic receptor–blocking agents (e.g., propranolol), buspirone, gabapentin, and TCAs. Exposure therapy can be used for specific phobias.

■ OCD AND OTHER REPETITIVE BEHAVIORS

OCD is characterized by recurrent, intrusive ego-dystonic impulses, thoughts, or images (*obsessions*) and ritualistic behaviors (hand washing, checking, needing symmetry, doing tasks in a required order), mental acts (counting, repeating words), and obligatory ego-dystonic motor behaviors (touching, echoing actions of others) (*compulsions*). The person recognizes that the thoughts and actions are excessive and can engage in reality testing (i.e., not delusional). *Mood and behavior changes* tend to arise from exaggerated harm avoidance, often secondary to feelings of disgust or guilt. There can be a torturous sense of incompleteness and imperfection, and people with OCD are compelled to generate "just right" feelings through their compulsions. *Cognitive changes* can be appreciated, including delayed response inhibition, speed of information processing, and impaired attentional set shifting. OCD also has substantial comorbidity, with high association with anxiety disorders, mood disorders, eating disorders, and substance use disorders. Tics and Gilles de la Tourette syndrome often occur in both people with OCD and in their immediate family members.

PET studies of individuals with idiopathic OCD have demonstrated increased metabolic activity in the orbitofrontal cortex and caudate nuclei. Patients with OCD have more neurological soft signs than age-matched control subjects, subtle neuropsychological deficits, and nonspecific electroencephalographic abnormalities (e.g., decreased beta and increased theta oscillations).

OCD resulting from neurological causes typically includes more compulsions than obsessions. OCD can occur in disorders of the caudate nuclei, globus pallidus, or frontal lobes (Table 3–8). Frontotemporal dementias are often accompanied by atrophy of the caudate nuclei, and the compulsive behavior seen early in these disorders may reflect these subcortical abnormalities. Compulsive behaviors are sometimes difficult to separate from the impulsive behaviors, such as gambling, shop-

TABLE 3–8.	Neurological disorders associated with OCD or compulsions

Site of dysfunction	Etiology
Caudate nucleus	Anoxic-ischemic caudate lesions
	Frontotemporal dementia
	Gilles de la Tourette's syndrome
	Huntington's disease
	Idiopathic spasmodic torticollis
	Neuroacanthocytosis
	Parkinson's disease
	Pediatric acute-onset neuropsychiatric syndrome
	Sydenham's chorea
Globus pallidus	Anoxic-ischemic lesions
	Carbon monoxide toxicity
	Manganese intoxication
Midbrain	Encephalitis lethargica (postencephalitic parkinsonism)
	Myoclonus-dystonia
	Progressive supranuclear palsy

ping, eating, or sexual behaviors, that can be seen in Parkinson's disease. Patients with OCD (idiopathic and neurological) exhibit dysfunction of the orbitofrontal-subcortical circuit, which includes the orbitofrontal cortex, caudate nucleus, globus pallidus, and thalamus. Decreased pallidal inhibition of the thalamus with resultant thalamocortical excitation may be a causal association. Compulsive behavior may also be caused by psychostimulants and dopamine agonists. Other repetitive behaviors, some of which may share subcortical striatal mechanisms with the repetitive behaviors of OCD, occur in patients with brain dysfunction, as listed in Table 3–9.

OCD is treated with behavioral therapy and pharmacologically with serotonergic agents or TCAs (clomipramine). Neurosurgery is useful for individuals with treatment-resistant illness; anterior capsulotomy with lesions placed in the anterior limb of the internal capsule has produced the highest rate of improvement. Deep brain stimulation targeting the ventral capsule and the ventral striatum has also been used for treatment-

TABLE 3–9. Repetitive behaviors observed in patients with brain dysfunction

Repetitive behavior	Description	Etiologies
Carphologia	Handling, picking	Advanced dementia, delirium
Coprolalia	Cursing	GTS, neuroacanthocytosis, basal ganglia disorders
Copropraxia	Obscene gesturing	GTS, basal ganglia disorders
Echolalia	Repetition of what is heard	GTS, DD, TBI, advanced dementia
Echopraxia	Imitating the actions of others	GTS, hyperekplexias
Excoriation	Compulsive skin picking	OCD, cocaine, dopaminergic agents
Exhibitionism	Removing clothing	GTS, idiopathic paraphilia, Huntington's disease, postencephalitic parkinsonism, delirium
Hypermetamorphosis	Exploration of environmental stimuli	Klüver-Bucy syndrome with bilateral temporal lobe lesions
Lip biting	Self-inflicted perioral bites	Lesch-Nyhan syndrome, neuroacanthocytosis
Logoclonia	Repetition of the final syllable of words	Logopenic variant primary progressive aphasia, advanced AD
Mannerisms	Repetitive goal-directed movements	Psychosis (idiopathic or with neurological disease), ASD
Oculogyric crises	Forced eye deviation	Postencephalitic parkinsonism, neuroleptic-induced parkinsonism
Palilalia	Repetition of one's own words	GTS, DD, advanced dementia, basal ganglia disorders

TABLE 3–9. Repetitive behaviors observed in patients with brain dysfunction (*continued*)

Repetitive behavior	Description	Etiologies
Perseveration	Repetition of the last or a recently performed motor act	Frontal lobe disorders; dementia, delirium
Repetitive questioning	Asking same question repeatedly	Dementia with memory loss
Rumination	Repeated regurgitation	ASD, DD
Self-injurious behavior	Cutting oneself, drug overdose, or other wounding	Epilepsy, GTS, personality disorders, learning disability, DD
Stereotypy	Repetitive non-goal-directed movements	Psychosis (idiopathic or with neurological disease), Rett's syndrome, ASD, nonverbal DD
Trichotillomania	Pulling out one's hair	GTS, idiopathic

AD=Alzheimer's disease; ASD=autism spectrum disorder; DD=developmental delay; GTS=Gilles de la Tourette's syndrome; TBI=traumatic brain injury.

resistant cases. Transcranial magnetic stimulation and exposure and response prevention therapies may also be tried.

■ PERSONALITY CHANGE

Brain dysfunction may be associated with a variety of personality changes. There is often an exaggeration of previous personality traits plus new behavioral patterns associated with regional brain dysfunction. Irritability, apathy, and exaggerated emotionality are behavioral alterations common to many neurological disorders.

Table 3–10 lists the personality changes that are often seen in the context of neurological disease. Most types of personality change are refractory to pharmacological treatment; aggressive or agitated behavior may respond to neuroleptic agents, trazodone, carbamazepine, valproate, benzodiazepines, antidepressants, or behavioral treatment. Apathy is sometimes treated with psychostimulants or amantadine; apathy in Alzheimer's disease may improve some with cholinesterase inhibitors (see Chapter 22).

■ DISSOCIATIVE DISORDERS

Dissociative disorders are characterized by disruption in the normal integration of consciousness, memory, identity, emotion, body representation, or behavior and tend to occur in the setting of a history of trauma, PTSD, or panic. *Dissociative (psychogenic) amnesia* for autobiographical details may present as periodic lapses or generalized amnesia and may include travel or wandering (*fugue*). Memory lapses are associated with disruption in one's identity in *dissociative identity disorder* and may be associated with periodic functional neurological symptoms. *Depersonalization* is associated with feelings of unreality or detachment from one's self or body, and *derealization* includes feelings of unreality and detachment from one's surroundings.

Dissociative amnesia must be distinguished from *transient global amnesia*. In the former condition, learning is intact, although patients are unable to recall previously known information, with remote recall of personal details disproportionately affected. In the latter condition, patients have anterograde amnesia and cannot learn new information, with recent memory more affected than remote recall. MRI with diffusion-weighted imaging performed during active symptoms may show restricted diffusion in the hippocampus. Psychogenic fugue must be distinguished from "twilight states" and poriomania (aimless wandering) occurring in the setting of recurrent complex partial

TABLE 3-10. Personality alterations in neurological disorders

Personality symptom	Neurological causes
Alexithymia	Right-hemisphere lesions
Apathy	FTDs, AD, medial frontal lesions, PD, HD, other basal ganglia disorders, thalamic lesions, vascular dementia, HIV encephalopathy, TBI, pituitary tumors
Disinhibition	Orbitofrontal lesions (neurodegeneration including behavioral variant FTD, tumors, TBI), caudate disorders (including HD), MS, frontal epilepsy, ACA stroke, Pick's disease
Irritability	Orbitofrontal lesions, caudate disorders (particularly HD), TBI, ASD
Suspiciousness	Epilepsy, HD, pure word deafness, TBI, Wernicke's aphasia

Personality syndrome	Syndrome characteristics
Dorsolateral prefrontal syndrome	Apathetic, abulia (lack of will or initiative), unmotivated; psychomotor slowing; deficits in working memory, rule-learning, planning, multitasking, and maintenance of attention; concrete; stimulus bound; poor problem solving; perseverative
Kleine-Levin syndrome	Abrupt onset hypersomnolence, hyperphagia, spacey appearance, confusion, child-like affect, anergia, apathy, hypersexuality, noise and light sensitivity in episodes lasting days to months, typically late adolescence through young adulthood; normal between episodes
Klüver-Bucy syndrome	Placidity, hyperorality with alteration in diet, altered sexual behavior, hypermetamorphosis (compulsive attention/reaction to visual stimuli in environment), "psychic blindness" (visual agnosia, generally prosopagnosia), decreased fear/anxiety

TABLE 3–10. Personality alterations in neurological disorders *(continued)*

Personality syndromes *(continued)*	Syndrome characteristics *(continued)*
Medial frontal syndrome	Paucity of verbal output and spontaneous movement; akinetic mutism may develop; apathy, abulia, "emotional emptiness;" false sense of well-being, incontinence, gait disturbance
Orbitofrontal syndrome	Lack of appreciation of social nuance; social disinhibition; impaired judgment, tact, foresight; distractible; shallow; affective lability; facetiousness (*Witzelsucht*); child-like euphoria (*moria*); difficulty maintaining set
Right hemisphere syndrome	Anosognosia (denial of deficit), delusional misidentification syndromes; emotional aprosodia; left hemi-inattention/neglect; impaired regulation of affect; difficulty interpreting pun, sarcasm, double-entendre; impaired pragmatic communication (eye contact, turn taking); impaired comprehension of metaphor; impaired attention to detail, sustained attention
Temporal lobe epilepsy interictal behavior syndrome (Gastaut-Geschwind syndrome)	Hyposexuality, viscosity (circumstantiality, interpersonal "stickiness"), hyperreligiosity, hypermoralism, hypergraphia, exaggerated philosophical concern, humorlessness, obsessional, dependence, mood lability

ACA=anterior cerebral artery; AD=Alzheimer's disease; ASD=autism spectrum disorder; DD=developmental delay; FTD=frontotemporal dementia; HD=Huntington's disease; MS=multiple sclerosis; PD=Parkinson's disease; TBI=traumatic brain injury.

seizures. Patients with dissociative amnesia exhibit integrated behavior during the episode, whereas patients with transient global amnesia are usually in confusional states and may have other seizure-related phenomena (automatisms, lip smacking, incontinence, generalized seizures).

Depersonalization and *derealization*, which can occur in primary psychotic disorders, occur in various neurological disorders, including partial complex seizures, migraine with aura, postconcussive states, encephalitis, and acute confusional states accompanying toxic-metabolic disorders.

■ ALTERED SEXUAL BEHAVIOR AND PARAPHILIC DISORDERS

Various changes in sexual behavior can be seen in neuropsychiatric conditions. Diminished libido with decreased interest in sexual behavior is the most common alteration. Hyposexuality occurs in epilepsy, stroke (particularly right hemispheric), Parkinson's disease and parkinsonian syndromes, Alzheimer's disease, and multiple sclerosis in addition to depression, which itself may be due to neurological dysfunction (see Table 3–1). Reduced sexual behavior follows injury or surgery to the posterior hypothalamus. Many medications reduce libido or interfere with erectile, ejaculatory, or orgasmic function.

Increased libido with a heightened interest in sexual activity has been reported in conjunction with secondary mania (as discussed earlier); right thalamic stroke involving the dorsal medial nucleus; orbitofrontal dysfunction; septal injury (following placement of ventriculoperitoneal shunts); right temporal stroke; lesions of the striatum, ventral striatum, and pallidum; hypothalamic dysfunction, as in *Klein-Levin syndrome*; and in *Klüver-Bucy syndrome*. The latter condition, which may develop early in behavioral variant frontotemporal dementia and later in the course of Alzheimer's disease, consists of hypersexuality, emotional placidity, hypermetamorphosis (i.e, compulsive exploration of one's environment), hyperorality (i.e., tendency to put items into one's mouth), and dietary changes. Disorders with bilateral medial temporal lobe involvement also produce Klüver-Bucy syndrome (Table 3–11). Several classes of drugs (e.g., stimulants, testosterone-containing agents, sildenafil, and dopaminergic agents) may increase libido. Hypersexuality in males may respond to estrogens or to testosterone antagonists; Klüver-Bucy syndrome has been reported to improve with carbamazepine.

Paraphilic disorders are characterized by intense sexual urges or sexually arousing fantasies that involve non-human objects, the suffering or humiliation of oneself or one's partner, or children or non-consenting adults. Some examples of paraphilias include exhibitionism (exposing one's genitals), fetishism (non-living objects), frotteurism (touching/rubbing against a non-consenting person), pedophilia (prepubescent children), sexual masochism (being humiliated, beaten, or bound), sexual

TABLE 3–11. Causes of Klüver-Bucy syndrome
Adrenoleukodystrophy
Alzheimer's disease
Amygdalotomy (bilateral)
Bilateral temporal lobe damage due to stroke
Bilateral temporal lobectomy (for seizures) or unilateral temporal lobectomy combined with pathology of the opposite temporal lobe
Delayed postanoxic leukoencephalopathy
Frontotemporal dementias
Herpes encephalitis
Hypoglycemia
Paraneoplastic limbic encephalitis
Posttraumatic encephalopathy
Status epilepticus with bitemporal foci
Toxoplasmosis
Trauma

sadism (the psychological or physical suffering of a victim), and voyeurism (observing an unsuspecting person who is naked, disrobing, or engaging in sexual activity). Some rarer types involving uncommon stimuli to induce sexual arousal have also been described. Paraphilic behavior has been reported in conjunction with temporal lobe epilepsy, postencephalitic parkinsonism, Huntington's disease, multiple sclerosis, and frontal lobe disorders.

■ AGGRESSIVE BEHAVIOR

Aggressive behavior occurs in many psychiatric and neurological disorders and should be treated only after considering its characteristics and cause. New-onset aggressive behavior toward oneself, others, or physical objects merits evaluation. In nonverbal persons, new-onset aggression may be a sign of pain; psychiatric, medical, or neurological problems; or a medication side effect. Aggression toward others or objects may be due to brain stem, diencephalic, limbic, or neocortical pathology. For example, pseudobulbar palsy can include brief explosive outbursts. Third ventricle tumors that compress the hypothalamus can result in territorial aggression or tactile defensiveness that may be combined with disruption of eating, drinking, sleep, or sexual behaviors. Temporolimbic seizures may be associated with interic-

tal or postictal aggression. Ictal aggression, on the rare occasions
it occurs, is unplanned and generally untargeted and may consist
of spitting at, kicking, or hitting anyone nearby. Postictal aggression varies from irritability to more serious behaviors. Orbitofrontal dysfunction may be associated with explosive outbursts in
response to trivial stimuli and may be associated with disinhibited behavior. Bilateral dorsolateral prefrontal dysfunction may
result in occasional outbursts in the setting of apathy. Broca's
aphasia may be associated with catastrophic outbursts as well.
Right hemisphere syndromes can result in aggression due to the
failure to correctly interpret nonverbal communication or nu-
anced communication, such as sarcasm or double entendre.

A few genetic syndromes have been associated with a predisposition to aggressive behavior. Early-onset male alcoholism
has been associated with glucose intolerance, low cerebrospinal
fluid levels of serotonin metabolites, and a propensity to violent
behavior toward self or others. A monoamine oxidase-A deficiency syndrome has been described in which male offspring
with mild intellectual disability develop shy, withdrawn behavior; aberrant sexual behavior; interrupted sleep with night ter-
rors; stereotyped hand movements; elevated serotonin levels;
and 3-day clusters of aggressive outbursts that are magnified
in intensity if there is a history of childhood maltreatment. Self-
injurious behavior occurs in personality disorders, in some adolescents, and in neurodevelopmental disabilities (Table 3–12)
and can occur in the context of increased stimulation or as a self-
stimulatory behavior.

TABLE 3–12. **Neurodevelopmental disorders associated with self-injurious behavior**

Angelman syndrome	Lowe syndrome
Autism spectrum disorder	Prader-Willi syndrome
Cornelia de Lange syndrome	Rett syndrome
Cri du Chat syndrome	Smith-Magenis syndrome
Down syndrome	Tuberous sclerosis
Fragile X syndrome	Williams-Beuren syndrome
Lesch-Nyhan syndrome	

∎ REFERENCES

American Psychiatric Association: Diagnostic and Statistical Manual of Mental Disorders, 5th Edition. Arlington, VA, American Psychiatric Association, 2013

Arciniegas DB, Yudofsky SC, Hales RE: The American Psychiatric Association Publishing Textbook of Neuropsychiatry and Clinical Neurosciences, 6th Edition. Washington, DC, American Psychiatric Association Publishing, 2018

Bandelow B, Baldwin D, Abelli M, et al: Biological markers for anxiety disorders, OCD and PTSD: a consensus statement. Part I: neuroimaging and genetics. World J Biol Psychiatry 17(5):321–365, 2016 27403679

Barnes DE, Yaffe K, Byers AL, et al: Midlife vs late-life depressive symptoms and risk of dementia: differential effects for Alzheimer disease and vascular dementia. Arch Gen Psychiatry 69(5):493–498, 2012 22566581

Baxter LR Jr, Schwartz JM, Bergman KS, et al: Caudate glucose metabolic rate changes with both drug and behavior therapy for obsessive-compulsive disorder. Arch Gen Psychiatry 49(9):681–689, 1992 1514872

Bear DM, Fedio P: Quantitative analysis of interictal behavior in temporal lobe epilepsy. Arch Neurol 34(8):454–467, 1977 889477

Benjamin S: Treatment of aggressive behavior in brain damage. Focus Am Psychiatr Publ 14(4):473–476, 2016 31975827

Benjamin S, Lauterbach MD: The Brain Card, 3rd Edition. Boston, MA, Brain Educators LLC, 2016

Benjamin S, Lauterbach MD: The neurological examination adapted for neuropsychiatry. CNS Spectr 23(3):219–227, 2018 29789033

Benjamin S, Lauterbach MD: The neurological examination for neuropsychiatric assessment, in Textbook of Medical Psychiatry. Edited by Summergrad P, Silbersweig DA, Muskin PR, Querques J. Washington, DC, American Psychiatric Association Publishing, 2020, pp 15–30

Bertram K, Williams DR: Visual hallucinations in the differential diagnosis of parkinsonism. J Neurol Neurosurg Psychiatry 83(4):448–452, 2012 22228724

Chavez-Castillo M, Nunez V, Nava M: Depression as a neuroendocrine disorder: emerging neuropsychopharmacological approaches beyond monoamines. Adv Pharmacol Sci 2019:7943481, 2019

Cummings JL: Frontal-subcortical circuits and human behavior. Arch Neurol 50(8):873–880, 1993 8352676

Cummings JL, Mega M, Gray K, et al: The Neuropsychiatric Inventory: comprehensive assessment of psychopathology in dementia. Neurology 44(12):2308–2314, 1994 7991117

Feinstein A, Magalhaes S, Richard JF, et al: The link between multiple sclerosis and depression. Nat Rev Neurol 10(9):507–517, 2014 25112509

Gurin L, Blum S: Delusions and the right hemisphere: a review of the case for the right hemisphere as a mediator of reality-based belief. J Neuropsychiatry Clin Neurosci 29(3):225–235, 2017 28347214

Hauptman A, Benjamin S: Neurodevelopmental disorders, in Textbook of Medical Psychiatry. Edited by Summergrad P, Silbersweig DA, Muskin PR, Querques J. Washington, DC, American Psychiatric Association Publishing, 2020, pp 481–498

Hurwitz TA, Lee WT: Casebook of Neuropsychiatry. Washington, DC, American Psychiatric Publishing, 2013

Jellinger KA: Cerebral correlates of psychotic syndromes in neurodegenerative diseases. J Cell Mol Med 16(5):995–1012, 2012 21418522

Lee CH, Giuliani F: The role of inflammation in depression and fatigue. Front Immunol 10:1696, 2019 31379879

Lilly R, Cummings JL, Benson DF, Frankel M: The human Klüver-Bucy syndrome. Neurology 33(9):1141–1145, 1983 6684248

Marsh L: Depression and Parkinson's disease: current knowledge. Curr Neurol Neurosci Rep 13(12):409, 2013 24190780

Mendez MF: Mania in neurologic disorders. Curr Psychiatry Rep 2(5):440–445, 2000 11122994

Miller BL, Cummings JL, McIntyre H, et al: Hypersexuality or altered sexual preference following brain injury. J Neurol Neurosurg Psychiatry 49(8):867–873, 1986 3746322

Robinson RG, Jorge RE: Post stroke depression: a review. Am J Psychiatry 173(3):221–231, 2016 26684921

Satzer D, Bond DJ: Mania secondary to focal brain lesions: implications for understanding the functional neuroanatomy of bipolar disorder. Bipolar Disord 18(3):205–220, 2016 27112231

Signer S, Cummings JL, Benson DF: Delusions and mood disorders in patients with chronic aphasia. J Neuropsychiatry Clin Neurosci 1(1):40–45, 1989 2535428

Silbersweig D, Safar LT, Daffner KR: Neuropsychiatry and Behavioral Neurology: Principles and Practice. New York, McGraw Hill, 2021

Sommer IE, Koops S, Blom JD: Comparison of auditory hallucinations across different disorders and syndromes. Neuropsychiatry (London) 2:57–68, 2012

Teeple RC, Caplan JP, Stern TA: Visual hallucinations: differential diagnosis and treatment. Prim Care Companion J Clin Psychiatry 11(1):26–32, 2009 19333408

Trimble MR, Mendez MF, Cummings JL: Neuropsychiatric symptoms from the temporolimbic lobes. J Neuropsychiatry Clin Neurosci 9(3):429–438, 1997 9276844

Weintraub D, Claassen DO: Impulse control and related disorders in Parkinson's disease. Int Rev Neurobiol 133:679–717, 2017 28802938

Wright A, Rickards H, Cavanna AE: Impulse-control disorders in Gilles de la Tourette syndrome. J Neuropsychiatry Clin Neurosci 24(1):16–27, 2012 22450610

4

FUNCTIONAL NEUROLOGICAL SYMPTOMS DISORDER

Sepideh N. Bajestan, M.D., Ph.D.
Gaston Baslet, M.D.

Functional neurological symptoms disorder (FNSD), also called conversion disorder, is diagnosed when there is an alteration of motor or sensory function that is inconsistent with altered physiological processes in known neurological or medical conditions. Per DSM-5 criteria, the symptoms of FNSD cannot be better explained by another medical or psychiatric disorder and cause significant distress or impairment in social, occupational, or other important areas of functioning. Psychological stressors are frequently associated with the onset of FNSD symptoms; however, their presence or identification is not required to establish a diagnosis of FNSD. This represents a change from the previous edition of DSM.

There are a number of phenotypic presentations of FNSD: weakness or paralysis, abnormal movements, gait difficulties, seizure-like episodes (called *psychogenic nonepileptic seizures* or PNES), speech symptoms, and swallowing symptoms. Functional neurological disorder is included in the "Somatic Symptom and Related Disorders" chapter in DSM-5. *Somatic symptom disorder* (SSD) is a separate diagnosis from FNSD, and both are included in the same DSM-5 chapter. SSD is diagnosed when a physical symptom is the primary complaint, and there is accompanying psychobehavioral criteria (i.e., excessive thinking, behaviors, and emotional responses) related to the primary somatic symptom. To meet DSM-5 diagnostic criteria for SSD, patients must have one or more somatic symptoms for a duration of ≥6 months, and these symptoms must be distressing and result in significant impairment. A medically diagnosed condition may (or may not) explain the somatic symptoms. Patients with

SSD or FNSD do not fabricate their symptoms as is the case in factitious disorder.

Medically unexplained symptoms (MUS) is a term that implies physical complaints without a clear physiological explanation and is used to cover many disorders that lack a known pathophysiological process, including many cases of SSD and FNSD. MUS is not a DSM-5 diagnosis.

■ EPIDEMIOLOGY

MUS compose up to one-third of new referrals to an ambulatory neurology clinic, and many of these patients in fact have FNSD. Large epidemiological studies are lacking, and existing studies provide gross underestimates given many factors that limit documentation of the FNSD diagnosis. In this context, a review of studies provides an overall incidence rate of 4–12 per 100,000 per year. In a study of 3,781 ambulatory referrals to a neurology clinic in the United Kingdom, 16% were diagnosed during the initial neurology visit with FNSD, the second most common diagnosis after headache. The incidence rate of PNES in the U.S. population has been estimated to be between 1.4 and 4.9 per 100,000. PNES accounted for 7.4% of new neurology visits to a large ambulatory practice, according to one study. The prevalence rates of FNSD and PNES in the United States are approximately 50 per 100,000 and 2–33 per 100,000, respectively. Of patients presenting to epilepsy monitoring units (EMUs) with drug-resistant seizures, approximately 20%–40% of adults and 10%–23% of children are ultimately diagnosed with PNES.

■ RISK FACTORS

FNSD is more frequently diagnosed in females at a ratio of two or three females per one male. Differences in prevalence by sex are less pronounced in prepubertal and late-onset subgroups. Although FNSD can occur at any age, onset most commonly occurs between 35 and 50 years of age, and PNES tends to present earlier (mid-20s) than other subtypes of FNSD.

FNSD is associated with substantial healthcare utilization, even more than patients with "organic" disorders. Rates of disability are similar or higher than in other neurological disorders.

A prior neurological and medical history is a risk factor for FNSD. Mild traumatic brain injury, epilepsy, intellectual/learning disabilities, prior brain surgery, chronic pain syndromes (including headache), and other MUS are well-established neurological comorbidities in FNSD. In the case of PNES, more than 40% of patients have comorbid neurological diagnoses, and 10%–20% have comorbid epilepsy.

Psychiatric comorbidities commonly encountered in FNSD include depression, PTSD, personality disorders, anxiety disorders, and dissociative disorders. Stressful life events and maltreatment (e.g., physical abuse, sexual abuse, emotional neglect) are present in FNSD at a frequency that is significantly higher than in healthy, neurological, and psychiatric control groups. More specifically, at least one-third of FNSD patients report past traumatic experiences. Physical and sexual abuse are more frequently reported by females. PNES is associated with a higher rate of sexual abuse compared with other subtypes of FNSD. School failure, bullying, and family history of neurological disease are relevant risk factors in pediatric FNSD populations.

■ PSYCHOLOGICAL AND NEUROBIOLOGICAL MECHANISMS

Psychological theories offer hypothetical mechanisms for the development of FNSD. Sigmund Freud proposed that intolerable affect (usually from an intrapsychic conflict, mostly unconscious to the patient) is converted into neurological symptoms (therefore the name "conversion disorder"). This conversion leads to reduction of affective distress. Freud also proposed that the ensuing physical symptoms further reduce stress by altering the person's circumstances (e.g., weakness makes the person unable to return to work, which is where the source of the conflict originated). Pierre Janet postulated that dissociative mechanisms such as compartmentalization and detachment are originally adaptive in the face of traumatic experiences but become dysfunctional over time and lead to FNSD symptoms. According to the dissociative hypothesis, FNSD is an "autosuggestive disorder" with symptoms akin to those seen in hypnotic states.

Modern cognitive hierarchical models explain FNSD as the result of a change in the allocation of attentional resources and the activation of dysfunctional beliefs about sensory or motor function, with reinforcing feedback into dysfunctional mental representations. The symptoms themselves lead to avoidance and other behavioral changes that further reinforce and perpetuate symptoms and lead to disability. These dysfunctional mental representations are developed via a number of mechanisms, including autosuggestion, prior experiences, and learned models. Adaptations of this cognitive hierarchical hypothesis use a Bayesian computational model in which the feedback and feedforward processes of a predictive coding system are disturbed. As a result, a prediction error is not corrected, and the incorrect prediction ("prior") is reinforced, leading to the functional symptom.

Neurobiologically, primary sensory and motor pathways are not altered in FNSD, according to electromyographic studies. Instead, cortical inhibitory processes are presumed to explain motor and sensory dysfunction in FNSD. In PNES, lower parasympathetic activity at baseline signals stress vulnerability and a reduced capacity for restoration during periods of stress.

Individuals with FNSD show differences in neuroanatomy compared with healthy control subjects in volumetric MRI studies. For example, increased thickness in premotor cortex and decreased volumes in subcortical nuclei have been reported in functional motor disorders. However, these minimal changes are not detectable in regular structural MRI and are not used for clinical care.

Differences between patients with FNSD and healthy subjects in brain activity and connectivity have been demonstrated in functional neuroimaging studies. Some examples of these abnormalities include 1) increased functional connectivity between emotion processing and motor planning regions (specifically amygdala and supplementary motor area) during emotion-laden tasks and between self-monitoring regions (ventromedial prefrontal cortex) and motor cortex; 2) increased activity in the amygdala and insula at different stages of motor planning in motor FNSD; and 3) lower temporoparietal junction activity in functional tremor and lower supramarginal gyrus activity in functional paralysis, which implicate alterations at the level of agency and sensorimotor integration in FNSD.

In summary, alterations at levels of sensory, cognitive, emotional, and motor complex processing are implicated in FNSD.

■ CLINICAL PRESENTATION, ASSESSMENT, AND DIFFERENTIAL DIAGNOSES

FNSD includes a number of phenotypes, such as functional weakness, paralysis, seizures (or PNES), vertigo, and tremors. The diagnosis is made by documenting symptoms that are incompatible with a known medical or neurological disorder and then ruling out the most common neurological disorders that produce those symptoms. A patient may have more than one functional symptom. It is also possible to have functional symptoms combined with a known neurological disorder; for example, 10%–20% of patients with PNES also have epilepsy.

Normal test results rule out neurological disorders; however, tests are not always feasible or available. In PNES, capturing a typical seizure episode on video electroencephalogram (V-EEG) without abnormal electroencephalographic correlates is the gold standard for diagnosing PNES. However, in many cases V-EEG is not available. Given this limitation, the history, semiology of symptoms, neurological examination, and presence of specific medical and psychiatric comorbidities increase the diagnostic certainty of FNSD. For example, the semiology of seizures can increase the clinical suspicion for PNES. Symptoms such as side-to-side head movements, pelvic thrusting, or eye closure are highly specific for PNES (Table 4–1).

Some medical conditions, such as obesity, asthma, chronic fatigue, presence of several allergies, learning disabilities, history of traumatic brain injury, and chronic pain, are reported to be more common in patients with FNSD. Having one disorder of interest (i.e., associated comorbidity) confers a positive predictive value of 75.5% for a diagnosis of PNES; increasing the number of disorders increases specificity.

The presence of psychiatric comorbidities increases suspicion for FNSD. For example, exposure to traumatic experiences, PTSD, and Cluster A or B personality disorders are the most distinguishing features for PNES. Some psychological traits such as alexithymia, emotion dysregulation, avoidance, somatization, and dissociation are also more reported in PNES.

Specific neurological examinations can show the incompatibility with a known neurological disorder and confirm the diagnosis (Table 4–2).

For each type of FNSD, specific types of tests could be done, such as nerve conduction studies for paralysis or electroencephalography in case of PNES. In each type of FNSD, some strategies can be adapted to yield better diagnostic clarity. For example, ethically acceptable induction strategies (e.g., photo stimulation, hyperventilation, hypnosis) increase the chances of capturing seizures with typical semiology on EEG, and a spot or 24-hours EEG could be sufficient. Hypnosis can serve the diagnostic purpose and, if taught as self-hypnosis, can be utilized as a treatment tool by patients.

TABLE 4–1. Semiological signs suggestive of psychogenic nonepileptic seizures (PNES)

When observing a seizure one should	PNES sign	Studies, N	Sensitivity, %	Specificity, %
Measure the time	>2 minutes	8	65	93
Observe the ictal course	Waxing and waning	3	36–90	96–100
Synchrony of the limbs	Asynchronous	5	43–96	82–100
Pelvic movements	Pelvic thrusting	8	8–60	88–100
Body posture	Arc de cercle	2	6–33	98–100
Head movement	Side-to-side movements	4	25–70	92–100
Eyes	Eyes closed	4		98–100
	Eyelid fluttering	5	0–19	88–100
Vocalizations	Ictal crying/weeping	7	7–32	98–100
Try to open the eyes	Forced closure	1		100
Give an item to be remembered	Recall OK	3	50–88	94–100
Test for responsiveness	Eye response or others can alleviate seizure or preserved awareness	4	0–83	77–100

TABLE 4–1. Semiological signs suggestive of psychogenic nonepileptic seizures (PNES) (*continued*)

When observing a seizure one should	PNES sign	Studies, *N*	Sensitivity, %	Specificity, %
After the seizure:				
Observe return of cognitive functions	Rapid recovery, no confusion	4	15–73	38–85
Observe breathing	No stertorous	2		
	Shallow	1	3	98
	Long duration (>94 seconds)	1		
Test plantar reflex	No Babinski			
Check for urine loss	No urinary incontinence	4		
Check mouth/oral cavity	No oral ulceration	1		

Source. Baslet G, Bajestan SN, Aybek S, et al: "Evidence-Based Practice for the Clinical Assessment of Psychogenic Nonepileptic Seizures: A Report From the American Neuropsychiatric Association Committee on Research." *Journal of Neuropsychiatry and Clinical Neurosciences* 33(1):27–42, 2021. Copyright © 2021, American Psychiatric Association Publishing, Inc. Used with permission.

TABLE 4–2. Neurological examination findings that help confirm the diagnosis of functional neurological symptoms disorder

Sign	Definition and examples
Motor	
Variable strength (give-away weakness)	As examiner applies different levels of force, patient varies resistance. **Example:** Limb collapses from a normal position with a light touch, or normal strength is developed and then suddenly collapses (or gives way).
Hoover sign	Hip extension weakness returns to normal with contralateral hip flexion against resistance. **Example:** Examiner compares felt pressure in his/her hand under weak leg's heel when weak leg pushes downward versus when normal leg pushes upward. Positive sign: less strength when weak leg pushing downward.
Tremor	
Entrainment	Tremor frequency switches to match the frequency of voluntary rhythmical movement performed by unaffected limb. **Example:** Patient with unilateral tremor is asked to copy a rhythmic movement with unaffected limb. Tremor in the affected hand either "entrains" to rhythm of unaffected hand or stops completely or patient is unable to copy the simple rhythmic movement.
Distraction	Tremor changes when examiner has patient engage in cognitively distracting tasks (e.g., counting backward).
Variability	Characteristics of tremor (e.g., amplitude) vary during examination.
Sensory	
Nonanatomical sensory loss	**Example:** Sensation normalizes at hip or shoulder; unilateral glove or sock distribution.
Midline splitting	Exact splitting of sensation in midline; sensory nerves do not end exactly at midline.

TABLE 4–2.	Neurological examination findings that help confirm the diagnosis of functional neurological symptoms disorder *(continued)*
Sign	**Definition and examples**
Sensory *(continued)*	
Splitting of vibration	Difference in sensation of a tuning fork placed over left compared with right side of sternum or frontal bone (frontalis is a single bone, so vibration sense should be the same bilaterally).
Gait	
Dragging leg	Leg dragged at the hip behind the body.
Excessively slow gait	Slowness observed in all aspects of gait.
Psychogenic Romberg	Consistently falls toward or away from examiner when performing Romberg test.

The International League Against Epilepsy (ILAE) proposed different levels of diagnostic certainty for PNES that take into account the history, phenomenology, and electrophysiological findings. Given the obstacles to PNES diagnosis, the ILAE's Nonepileptic Seizure Task Force published a staged approach to PNES diagnosis. Three components—history and seizure semiology consistent with PNES and ictal EEG recordings without epileptiform activity—together inform the diagnosis levels, which include possible, probable, clinically established, and documented PNES. Adding psychological traits, psychiatric and medical comorbidities, and provoking methods as mentioned earlier can further increase the diagnostic certainty.

While ruling out other neurological or medical conditions, clinicians should be mindful of the differential diagnosis for FNSD to avoid misdiagnosis. Figure 4–1 shows several possible differential diagnoses for PNES.

The biopsychosocial formulation is commonly used for conceptualizing psychiatric disorders. Adding the predisposing, precipitating, and perpetuating (PPP) factors reflects the development and persistence of symptoms. The biopsychosocial/PPP model details the factors involved in the development of a reflexive way of maladaptive coping occurring in the context of past traumatic experiences, current life challenges, and physical health issues. This model can then inform treatment.

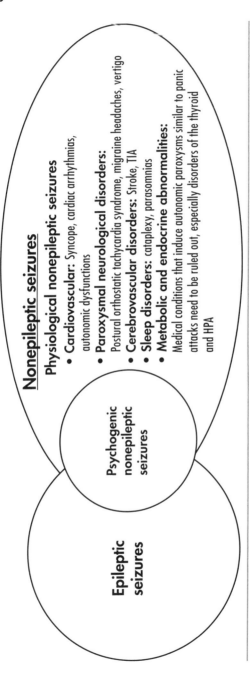

Nonepileptic seizures

<u>Physiological nonepileptic seizures</u>

- **Cardiovascular:** Syncope, cardiac arrhythmias, autonomic dysfunctions
- **Paroxysmal neurological disorders:** Postural orthostatic tachycardia syndrome, migraine headaches, vertigo
- **Cerebrovascular disorders:** Stroke, TIA
- **Sleep disorders:** cataplexy, parasomnias
- **Metabolic and endocrine abnormalities:** Medical conditions that induce autonomic paroxysms similar to panic attacks need to be ruled out, especially disorders of the thyroid and HPA

Psychogenic nonepileptic seizures

Epileptic seizures

FIGURE 4–1. **Differential diagnosis of psychogenic nonepileptic seizures (PNES).**

HPA=hypothalamic-pituitary-adrenal; TIA=transient ischemic attack.

Source. Bajestan SN, LaFrance WC Jr: "Clinical Approaches to Psychogenic Nonepileptic Seizures." *Focus* 14(4):422–431, 2016. Copyright © 2016 American Psychiatric Association Publishing, Inc. Used with permission.

TABLE 4–3. Example of biopsychosocial neuropsychiatric case formulation with predisposing, precipitating, and perpetuating (PPP) factors

	Bio	Psycho	Social
Predisposing factors	Family history of psychiatric disorders, developmental delay, increased resting levels of bodily arousal	Childhood adversity, alexithymia, dissociative tendencies, dysfunctional attachment	Dysfunctional and chaotic upbringing
Precipitating factors	Traumatic brain injury, traumatic or prolonged medical procedures	Recent sexual or psychological trauma	Interpersonal conflicts, unemployment
Perpetuating factors	Chronic medical problems, medication side effects, undertreated pain	Untreated comorbid psychiatric disorders, avoidant behavior, sick identity	Ongoing litigations, ongoing interpersonal conflicts, primary gain in frequent hospital admissions

Source. Baslet G, Bajestan SN, Aybek S, et al: "Evidence-Based Practice for the Clinical Assessment of Psychogenic Nonepileptic Seizures: A Report From the American Neuropsychiatric Association Committee on Research." *Journal of Neuropsychiatry and Clinical Neurosciences* 33(1):27–42, 2021. Copyright © 2021, American Psychiatric Association Publishing, Inc. Used with permission.

An example of a biopsychosocial/PPP formulation is provided in Table 4–3.

■ TREATMENT

Informing patients about their FNSD diagnosis can lead to improvement in symptoms and medical utilization for some. The communication strategy usually consists of 1) reassuring patients that the symptoms are genuine and not considered fake; 2) providing a name for the disorder and explaining how the diagnosis was confirmed; 3) highlighting PPP factors and a mechanism for the disease (even if hypothetical); and 4) stating that effective treatments are available. Many patients have a difficult time adhering to treatment recommendations, as shown by a longitudinal study of adherence rates in PNES. Multidisciplinary collaboration among neurologists, psychiatrists, psychotherapists, physical therapists, primary care physicians, and community supports is essential throughout treatment. Educating patients, families, and involved clinicians about FNSD is an essential part of treatment.

Functional motor disorders that present with gait abnormalities, weakness, or abnormal movements are recommended to be referred for physical therapy. Physical therapy for motor and gait manifestations of FNSD has been evaluated in both inpatient and outpatient settings; the basic principles for therapy are education, movement retraining, and an emphasis on self-management. Evidence-based psychotherapy should be considered first-line treatment in PNES and other nonmotor FNSD phenotypes. It should also be considered in motor FNSD in addition to physical therapy.

Cognitive-behavioral therapy (CBT) has proven effective in the treatment of PNES and other FNSD in randomized controlled trials. CBT programs for FNSD include the following: 1) education about the disorder, 2) training on stress management techniques, 3) incorporation of new behaviors that address avoidance patterns, and 4) identification and change of unhelpful thoughts that reinforce symptoms. CBT treatment workbooks can be recommended to patients and mental health providers.

Other psychotherapy modalities have been studied in different FNSD populations with positive results, including manualized hypnosis for motor FNSD, mindfulness-based therapy for PNES, prolonged exposure for PNES and comorbid PTSD, inpatient programs, and psychodynamic psychotherapies.

Psychopharmacological intervention should be limited to treatment of comorbid psychiatric conditions. There are few uncontrolled studies of antidepressants in FNSD and PNES with positive results. The only randomized, double-blind, placebo-controlled trial in PNES did not find sertraline to be superior to placebo, although the study may have been underpowered.

Case reports and case series have supported the use of noninvasive stimulation therapies (electroconvulsive therapy or repetitive transcranial magnetic stimulation [rTMS]) in functional weakness and PNES. Use of rTMS over the contralateral motor cortex in functional weakness is supported by an uncontrolled retrospective study and a single-blinded, placebo-controlled crossover study. Noninvasive stimulation therapies lack sufficient evidence for the treatment of FNSD at this time.

■ OUTCOMES

Most outcome studies in FNSD show a variable degree of symptomatic improvement years after the diagnosis. In psychogenic motor disorders, studies indicate that most patients remain the same or have become worse an average of 7.4 years after diagnosis. In PNES, outcome studies at a minimum of 1 year after diagnosis (many with a mean of 5 years after diagnosis) reveal that most patients continue to experience episodes. Most long-term outcome studies in FNSD have not considered the use of evidence-based treatments. Studies that more closely monitored participation in treatment show more favorable outcomes for those attending treatment.

Functional recovery is poor. Many patients remain disabled after an FNSD diagnosis, whether the symptoms improve or remit. Disability is therefore thought to be driven by factors that are independent of symptom occurrence.

Prognostic factors have been identified in various studies. Some of the negative prognostic factors more consistently replicated include longer duration of symptoms, psychiatric comorbidities, and pending litigation, whereas positive prognosis tends to be associated with employment, patient confidence in the clinician, and younger age at onset or diagnosis.

■ REFERENCES

Akagi H, House A: The clinical epidemiology of hysteria: vanishingly rare, or just vanishing? Psychol Med 32(2):191–194, 2002 11866315

American Psychiatric Association: Diagnostic and Statistical Manual of Mental Disorders, 5th Edition. Arlington, VA, American Psychiatric Association, 2013

Asadi-Pooya AA, Emami M: Demographic and clinical manifestations of psychogenic non-epileptic seizures: the impact of co-existing epilepsy in patients or their family members. Epilepsy Behav 27(1):1–3, 2013 23352998

Aybek S, Nicholson TRJ, Draganski B, et al: Grey matter changes in motor conversion disorder. J Neurol Neurosurg Psychiatry 85(2):236–238, 2014 23236016

Bajestan SN, LaFrance WC Jr: Clinical approaches to psychogenic nonepileptic seizures. Focus Am Psychiatr Publ 14(4):422–431, 2016 31975822

Baslet G, Ehlert A, Oser M, Dworetzky BA: Mindfulness-based ther apy for psychogenic nonepileptic seizures. Epilepsy Behav 103(pt A):106534, 2020 31680023

Baslet G, Bajestan SN, Aybek S, et al: Evidence-based practice for the clinical assessment of psychogenic nonepileptic seizures: a report from the American Neuropsychiatric Association Committee on Research. J Neuropsychiatry Clin Neurosci 33(1):27–42, 2021 32778006

Benbadis SR, Allen Hauser W: An estimate of the prevalence of psychogenic non-epileptic seizures. Seizure 9(4):280–281, 2000 10880289

Benbadis SR, Agrawal V, Tatum WO 4th: How many patients with psychogenic nonepileptic seizures also have epilepsy? Neurology 57(5):915–917, 2001 11552032

Broersma M, Koops EA, Vroomen PC, et al: Can repetitive transcranial magnetic stimulation increase muscle strength in functional neurological paresis? A proof-of-principle study. Eur J Neurol 22(5):866–873, 2015 25708187

Carson A, Lehn A: Epidemiology. Handb Clin Neurol 139:47–60, 2016 27719864

Carson AJ, Ringbauer B, Stone J, et al: Do medically unexplained symptoms matter? A prospective cohort study of 300 new referrals to neurology outpatient clinics. J Neurol Neurosurg Psychiatry 68(2):207–210, 2000 10644789

Chastan N, Parain D: Psychogenic paralysis and recovery after motor cortex transcranial magnetic stimulation. Mov Disord 25(10):1501–1504, 2010 20568093

Czarnecki K, Thompson JM, Seime R, et al: Functional movement disorders: successful treatment with a physical therapy rehabilitation protocol. Parkinsonism Relat Disord 18(3):247–251, 2012 22113131

Deleuran M, Nørgaard K, Andersen NB, Sabers A: Psychogenic nonepileptic seizures treated with psychotherapy: long-term outcome on seizures and healthcare utilization. Epilepsy Behav 98(pt A):195–200, 2019 31377661

Dixit R, Popescu A, Bagic A, et al: Medical comorbidities in patients with psychogenic nonepileptic spells (PNES) referred for video-EEG monitoring. Epilepsy Behav 28(2):137–140, 2013 23747495

Driver-Dunckley E, Stonnington CM, Locke DEC, Noe K: Comparison of psychogenic movement disorders and psychogenic nonepileptic seizures: is phenotype clinically important? Psychosomatics 52(4):337–345, 2011 21777716

Duncan R: Long-term outcomes, in Psychogenic Nonepileptic Seizures: Toward the Integration of Care. Edited by Dworetzky BA, Baslet GC. New York, Oxford University Press, 2017, pp 279–289

Duncan R, Oto M, Martin E, Pelosi A: Late onset psychogenic nonepileptic attacks. Neurology 66(11):1644–1647, 2006 16769934

Duncan R, Anderson J, Cullen B, Meldrum S: Predictors of 6-month and 3-year outcomes after psychological intervention for psychogenic non epileptic seizures. Seizure 36:22–26, 2016 26874857

Durrant J, Rickards H, Cavanna AE: Prognosis and outcome predictors in psychogenic nonepileptic seizures. Epilepsy Res Treat 2011:274736, 2011 22937230

Edwards MJ: Neurobiologic theories of functional neurologic disorders. Handb Clin Neurol 139:131–137, 2017 27719834

Espay AJ, Ries S, Maloney T, et al: Clinical and neural responses to cognitive behavioral therapy for functional tremor. Neurology 93:e1787–e1798, 2019

Gelauff J, Stone J, Edwards M, Carson A: The prognosis of functional (psychogenic) motor symptoms: a systematic review. J Neurol Neurosurg Psychiatry 85(2):220–226, 2014 24029543

Goldstein LH, Mellers JDC, Landau S, et al: Cognitive behavioural therapy vs standardised medical care for adults with Dissociative non-Epileptic Seizures (CODES): a multicentre randomised controlled trial protocol. BMC Neurol 15:98, 2015 26111700

Hall-Patch L, Brown R, House A, et al: Acceptability and effectiveness of a strategy for the communication of the diagnosis of psychogenic nonepileptic seizures. Epilepsia 51(1):70–78, 2010 19453708

Jirsch JD, Ahmed SN, Maximova K, Gross DW: Recognition of psychogenic nonepileptic seizures diminishes acute care utilization. Epilepsy Behav 22(2):304–307, 2011 21813334

Jordbru AA, Smedstad LM, Klungsøyr O, Martinsen EW: Psychogenic gait disorder: a randomized controlled trial of physical rehabilitation with one-year follow-up. J Rehabil Med 46(2):181–187, 2014 24248149

Kompoliti K, Wilson B, Stebbins G, et al: Immediate vs. delayed treatment of psychogenic movement disorders with short term psychodynamic psychotherapy: randomized clinical trial. Parkinsonism Relat Disord 20(1):60–63, 2014 24120952

Kotagal P, Costa M, Wyllie E, Wolgamuth B: Paroxysmal nonepileptic events in children and adolescents. Pediatrics 110(4):e46, 2002 12359819

Kuyk J, Siffels MC, Bakvis P, Swinkels WAM: Psychological treatment of patients with psychogenic non-epileptic seizures: an outcome study. Seizure 17(7):595–603, 2008 18395473

LaFrance WCJ Jr, Keitner GI, Papandonatos GD, et al: Pilot pharmacologic randomized controlled trial for psychogenic nonepileptic seizures. Neurology 75(13):1166–1173, 2010 20739647

LaFrance WCJ Jr, Deluca M, Machan JT, Fava JL: Traumatic brain injury and psychogenic nonepileptic seizures yield worse outcomes. Epilepsia 54(4):718–725, 2013 23281644

LaFrance WCJ Jr, Baird GL, Barry JJ, et al: Multicenter pilot treatment trial for psychogenic nonepileptic seizures: a randomized clinical trial. JAMA Psychiatry 71(9):997–1005, 2014 24989152

Lesser RP: Psychogenic seizures. Neurology 46(6):1499–1507, 1996 8649537

Liepert J, Hassa T, Tüscher O, Schmidt R: Electrophysiological correlates of motor conversion disorder. Mov Disord 23(15):2171–2176, 2008 18785215

Ludwig L, Pasman JA, Nicholson T, et al: Stressful life events and mal-treatment in conversion (functional neurological) disorder: systematic review and meta-analysis of case-control studies. Lancet Psychiatry 5(4):307–320, 2018 29526521

Martin R, Burneo JG, Prasad A, et al: Frequency of epilepsy in patients with psychogenic seizures monitored by video-EEG. Neurology 61(12):1791–1792, 2003 14694050

Matin N, Young SS, Williams B, et al: Neuropsychiatric associations with gender, illness duration, work disability, and motor subtype in a U.S. functional neurological disorders clinic population. J Neuropsychiatry Clin Neurosci 29(4):375–382, 2017 28449634

Mayor R, Howlett S, Grünewald R, Reuber M: Long-term outcome of brief augmented psychodynamic interpersonal therapy for psychogenic nonepileptic seizures: seizure control and health care utilization. Epilepsia 51(7):1169–1176, 2010 20561022

McKenzie PS, Oto M, Graham CD, Duncan R: Medically unexplained symptoms in patients with PNES: do they explain poor employment outcome in patients with good seizure outcomes? Epilepsy Behav 59:9–12, 2016 27084977

Moene FC, Spinhoven P, Hoogduin KAL, van Dyck R: A randomized controlled clinical trial of a hypnosis-based treatment for patients with conversion disorder, motor type. Int J Clin Exp Hypn 51(1):29–50, 2003 12825917

Myers L, Vaidya-Mathur U, Lancman M: Prolonged exposure therapy for the treatment of patients diagnosed with psychogenic non-epileptic seizures (PNES) and post-traumatic stress disorder (PTSD). Epilepsy Behav 66:86–92, 2017 28038392

Nicholson TR, Aybek S, Kempton MJ, et al: A structural MRI study of motor conversion disorder: evidence of reduction in thalamic volume. J Neurol Neurosurg Psychiatry 85(2):227–229, 2014 24039028

Nicholson TR, Aybek S, Craig T, et al: Life events and escape in conversion disorder. Psychol Med 46(12):2617–2626, 2016 27377290

Nielsen G, Stone J, Edwards MJ: Physiotherapy for functional (psychogenic) motor symptoms: a systematic review. J Psychosom Res 75(2):93–102, 2013 23915764

Nielsen G, Ricciardi L, Demartini B, et al: Outcomes of a 5-day physiotherapy programme for functional (psychogenic) motor disorders. J Neurol 262(3):674–681, 2015 25557282

Oto M, Conway P, McGonigal A, et al: Gender differences in psychogenic non-epileptic seizures. Seizure 14(1):33–39, 2005 15642498

Park EG, Lee J, Lee BL, et al: Paroxysmal nonepileptic events in pediatric patients. Epilepsy Behav 48:83–87, 2015

Perez DL, Dworetzky BA, Dickerson BC, et al: An integrative neurocircuit perspective on psychogenic nonepileptic seizures and functional movement disorders: neural functional unawareness. Clin EEG Neurosci 46(1):4–15, 2015 25432161

Peterson KT, Kosior R, Meek BP, et al: Right temporoparietal junction transcranial magnetic stimulation in the treatment of psychogenic nonepileptic seizures: a case series. Psychosomatics 59(6):601–606, 2018 29628295

Pick S, Mellers JDC, Goldstein LH: Dissociation in patients with dissociative seizures: relationships with trauma and seizure symptoms. Psychol Med 47(7):1215–1229, 2017 28065191

Pintor L, Baillés E, Matrai S, et al: Efficiency of venlafaxine in patients with psychogenic nonepileptic seizures and anxiety and/or depressive disorders. J Neuropsychiatry Clin Neurosci 22(4):401–408, 2010 21037125

Razvi S, Mulhern S, Duncan R: Newly diagnosed psychogenic nonepileptic seizures: health care demand prior to and following diagnosis at a first seizure clinic. Epilepsy Behav 23(1):7–9, 2012 22093246

Reinsberger C, Sarkis R, Papadelis C, et al: Autonomic changes in psychogenic nonepileptic seizures: toward a potential diagnostic biomarker? Clin EEG Neurosci 46(1):16–25, 2015 25780264

Reiter JM, Andrews D, Reiter C, LaFrance WC: Taking Control of Your Seizures Workbook. New York, Oxford University Press, 2015

Reuber M, Brown RJ: Understanding psychogenic nonepileptic seizures: phenomenology, semiology and the integrative cognitive model. Seizure 44:199–205, 2017 27988107

Reuber M, Fernández G, Helmstaedter C, et al: Evidence of brain abnormality in patients with psychogenic nonepileptic seizures. Epilepsy Behav 3(3):249–254, 2002 12662605

Reuber M, Pukrop R, Bauer J, et al: Multidimensional assessment of personality in patients with psychogenic non-epileptic seizures. J Neurol Neurosurg Psychiatry 75(5):743–748, 2004 15090571

Roelofs K, Pasman J: Stress, childhood trauma, and cognitive functions in functional neurologic disorders. Handb Clin Neurol 139:139–155, 2016 27719835

Sar V, Akyüz G, Kundakçi T, et al: Childhood trauma, dissociation, and psychiatric comorbidity in patients with conversion disorder. Am J Psychiatry 161(12):2271–2276, 2004 15569899

Schönfeldt-Lecuona C, Lefaucheur J-P, Lepping P, et al: Non-invasive brain stimulation in conversion (functional) weakness and paralysis: a systematic review and future perspectives. Front Neurosci 10:140, 2016 27065796

Sigurdardottir KR, Olafsson E: Incidence of psychogenic seizures in adults: a population-based study in Iceland. Epilepsia 39(7):749–752, 1998 9670904

Stone J, Carson A: An integrated approach to other functional neurological symptoms and related disorders, in Psychogenic Nonepileptic Seizures: Toward the Integration of Care. Edited by Dworetzky BA, Baslet G. New York, Oxford University Press, 2017, pp 290–307

Stone J, Carson A, Duncan R, et al: Symptoms 'unexplained by organic disease' in 1144 new neurology out-patients: how often does the diagnosis change at follow-up? Brain 132(pt 10):2878–2888, 2009 19737842

Stone J, Carson A, Duncan R, et al: Who is referred to neurology clinics? The diagnoses made in 3781 new patients. Clin Neurol Neurosurg 112(9):747–751, 2010 20646830

Stone J, Warlow C, Sharpe M: Functional weakness: clues to mechanism from the nature of onset. J Neurol Neurosurg Psychiatry 83(1):67–69, 2012 21836030

Szaflarski JP, Szaflarski M, Hughes C, et al: Psychopathology and quality of life: psychogenic non-epileptic seizures versus epilepsy. Med Sci Monit 9(4):CR113–CR118, 2003 12709668

Thomas AA, Preston J, Scott RC, Bujarski KA: Diagnosis of probable psychogenic nonepileptic seizures in the outpatient clinic: does gender matter? Epilepsy Behav 29(2):295–297, 2013 24021495

Tolchin B, Dworetzky BA, Baslet G: Long-term adherence with psychiatric treatment among patients with psychogenic nonepileptic seizures. Epilepsia 59(1):e18–e22, 2018 29218816

Tolchin B, Dworetzky BA, Martino S, et al: Adherence with psychotherapy and treatment outcomes for psychogenic nonepileptic seizures. Neurology 92(7):e675–e679, 2019 30610097

Voon V, Lang AE: Antidepressant treatment outcomes of psychogenic movement disorder. J Clin Psychiatry 66(12):1529–1534, 2005 16401153

Voon V, Cavanna AE, Coburn K, et al: Functional neuroanatomy and neurophysiology of functional neurological disorders (conversion disorder). J Neuropsychiatry Clin Neurosci 28(3):168–190, 2016 26900733

Williams C, Kent C, Smith S, et al: Overcoming Functional Neurological Symptoms: A Five Areas Approach. London, Routledge, 2011

Wong VSS, Salinsky MC: Neurological and medical factors, in Psychogenic Nonepileptic Seizures: Toward the Integration of Care. Edited by Dworetzky BA, Baslet G. New York, Oxford University Press, 2017, pp 67–85

5

FRONTAL LOBE SYNDROMES

Simon Ducharme, M.D.
Lisa Koski, Ph.D.

The frontal lobes are the largest lobes of the brain, composing almost one-third of the total cortical surface area. They are among the latest evolutionary additions to the brain and are larger in humans than in any other species. They complete myelination late in the maturation cycle and become functional in the final phases of ontogenetic development. The frontal lobes receive information about the external environment from the posterior sensory association cortices and information about the individual's emotional state and internal milieu from the limbic system and hypothalamus. They are anatomically poised to integrate environmental and emotional information and to formulate and execute an action plan. They initiate volitional activity and control the motor system, thus mediating the action of the individual on the environment. The frontal lobes bestow many of the uniquely human characteristics of behavior, and diseases of the frontal lobes are among the most dramatic in neuropsychiatry. Frontal lobe anatomy is described in Chapter 2, "Behavioral Neurobiology."

■ FRONTAL LOBE SYNDROMES

The frontal lobes are divided into the motor cortex adjacent to the Rolandic fissure, the premotor cortex (PMC) anterior to the motor cortex, and the prefrontal cortex (PFC) comprising the region anterior to the premotor areas. Contralateral weakness, brisk reflexes, and Babinski signs occur with lesions of the motor strip; Broca's aphasia and executive aprosodia (see Chapter 6, "Aphasia and Related Syndromes") follow lesions of the left and right inferior frontal gyrus, respectively; and alterations in cognition, demeanor, and mood are most associated with prefrontal dysfunction.

The PFC is a central brain structure in the mediation of complex human behavior. It is subdivided anatomically into the dorsolateral, ventrolateral, orbitofrontal, and medial frontal heteromodal association areas; the latter includes the ventromedial PFC and paralimbic anterior cingulate cortex. Each of these regions is involved in a complex set of cognitive and behavioral functions. Regarding cognitive functions, studies based on lesion mapping have identified three functional clusters that partially overlap with anatomical definitions: lateral PFC (i.e., selective attention, working memory, inhibitory control), ventromedial PFC (i.e., decision making, reward-based learning, value-based decisions, self-awareness), and dorsomedial PFC (i.e., conflict monitoring, optimal response threshold). These functions can be assessed with neuropsychological testing (Table 5–1).

Historically, *frontal lobe syndromes* is a term used to describe the three major behavioral syndromes associated with prefrontal dysfunction. These have been described in relationship to three critical prefrontal regions: the dorsolateral prefrontal area, anterolateral orbitofrontal area, and ventromedial/anterior cingulate area (including the dorsomedial PFC). These three regions are the origins of distinct frontal-subcortical circuits that mediate circuit-specific behaviors (see Chapter 2). Typical predominant symptoms of these regions and of their associated subcortical circuits are executive dysfunction (dorsolateral prefrontal syndrome), disinhibition (orbitofrontal syndrome), and apathy (medial frontal/anterior cingulate syndrome).

Although these distinct syndromes have some heuristic clinical value, most lesions or diseases affecting the frontal lobes involve multiple frontal lobe regions, and combinations of the three syndromes are the rule in clinical practice. Clinically, patients rarely fail all tests of functions ascribed to a particular region; the overall pattern of successes and failures is what leads to recognition of a frontal lobe syndrome, rather than performance on any individual test. In addition, the prefrontal regions are part of larger intrinsic connectivity networks that have clinical relevance. For example, the dorsolateral PFC is part of the larger executive control network including several parietal areas (this network is also referred to as "frontoparietal"). Consequently, tests typically considered as evaluating frontal lobe functions may be disrupted by lesions outside the frontal lobes and frontal-subcortical circuits. In some situations, it is only when failure occurs in the absence of dysfunction in other areas that the performance deficits can be correlated with frontal lobe

TABLE 5–1. Frontal lobe syndromes and their assessment

Frontal region	Characteristic abnormality	Assessment	Examples of specific tests
Dorsolateral prefrontal cortex	Reduced verbal fluency	Word generation tasks	Letter fluency, category fluency*
	Reduced nonverbal fluency	Design generation tasks	Five-point test; design fluency test*
	Poor mental flexibility	Set-shifting	WCST, BADS Rule-Shift Cards Test; Trail Making Test*
	Impaired concept formation	Tests of abstract reasoning, cognitive estimates	Similarities, Proverbs, BADS Temporal Judgment Test; Clock Drawing Test*
	Poor judgment	Understanding of societal conventions; clinical evaluation of insight and plans*	WAIS-IV Comprehension
	Poor response inhibition	Cognitive interference tasks; commission errors on Go/No go tasks	Stroop Color-Word Interference Test; Connors CPT commissions
	Reduced spontaneous recall of word list, designs, stories	Delayed-recall vs. recognition test*	Brief Visual Memory Test, CVLT, Wechsler Memory Scale Logical Memory
	Poor memory organization	Clustering of similar items	CVLT semantic clustering score
	Poor planning	Copy of complex figure; concrete problem-solving tasks	Rey-Osterreith or Taylor Complex Figures; Tower of London, Mazes; BADS Zoo Map

TABLE 5–1. Frontal lobe syndromes and their assessment *(continued)*

Frontal region	Characteristic abnormality	Assessment	Examples of specific tests
Dorsolateral prefrontal cortex *(continued)*	Reduced divided attention	Multitasking tests	Brown-Petersen Consonant Trigrams test; BADS Modified Six-Elements Test
	Reduced sustained attention	Decline in accuracy, speed, or reliability with increasing time on task	Connors CPT Block Change scores; WCST Failure to Maintain Set
	Perseveration on sequential motor tasks	Alternating programs, reciprocal programs, multiple loops, serial hand sequences*	"MNO" test*
Orbitofrontal	Disinhibition	Clinical evaluation of impulsive or tactless behavior; tests of risk-taking	Social Norms Questionnaire, Cambridge Gambling Task, Iowa Gambling Task
	Unable to change behavior	Assess response to a change in reward contingency	CANTAB intra/extradimensional set-shifting
	Social cognitive deficits	Facial emotion recognition*	Ekman 60 faces, Mind in the Eyes, Faux Pas Test, Mini-SEA, Social Norms Questionnaire
	Anosmia	Tests of olfaction*	

TABLE 5–1. Frontal lobe syndromes and their assessment (*continued*)

Frontal region	Characteristic abnormality	Assessment	Examples of specific tests
Medial prefrontal	Apathy	Clinical evaluation of reduced motivation, interest, and activity*	Apathy Evaluation Scale, Philadelphia Apathy Computerized Test
	Decreased generation	Word or design generation tasks	Letter fluency*, design fluency test*
	Social cognitive deficits	Facial emotion recognition*; social-moral reasoning; sensitivity to future consequences of action	Ekman 60 faces, Mind in the Eyes Faux Pas Test, Mini-SEA, Social Norms Questionnaire

BADS=Behavioral assessment of the dysexecutive syndrome; CANTAB=Cambridge Neuropsychological Test Automated Battery; CPT=Continuous performance task; CVLT=California Verbal Learning Test; SEA=Social and Emotional Assessment; WAIS=Wechsler Adult Intelligence Scale; WCST=Wisconsin Card Sorting Test.
*These tests are particularly useful for bedside testing.

or frontal systems dysfunction (e.g., reduced verbal fluency can be attributed to prefrontal dysfunction only in patients with otherwise intact language function).

■ DORSOLATERAL PREFRONTAL SYNDROME

Executive function includes planning, initiating, sequencing (maintaining, alternating, stopping), and monitoring behavior. Dorsolateral prefrontal disorders are marked by predominant working memory and executive function deficits as opposed to emotional or behavioral symptoms. Executive dysfunction of this syndrome is characterized by poor strategies, including impaired planning when copying constructions and when organizing material to be remembered or impaired set shifting in response to changing task contingencies, abnormalities of motor programming, compromised attention, and environmental dependency (see Table 5–1).

Compromised learning strategies and poor spontaneous recall are the primary memory disturbances typical of patients with prefrontal and frontosubcortical dysfunction (including but not restricted to the dorsolateral area). Poor learning is most evident on tests of new learning in which the patient is asked to learn a list of words. Patients with dorsolateral prefrontal dysfunction do not organize information efficiently and thus have difficulty with spontaneous recall after a delay. However, they usually learn a substantial amount of the information, and this can be seen by giving them the opportunity to choose the previously learned words from a multiple-choice list. This is referred to as a *retrieval deficit*, as evidenced by poor recall and preserved recognition memory. Amnestic syndromes characterized by poor recall and poor recognition occur with frontal lobe dysfunction only when deeply placed lesions affect the fornix as it courses through the frontal lobe on its trajectory from the hippocampus to the hypothalamus or when the lesion involves the basal forebrain, producing an interruption of cholinergic innervation of the hippocampus (see Chapter 2, Figure 2–1).

Impaired search of semantic memory and manipulation of knowledge are evident on tasks of verbal fluency in which the patient is asked to name as many members of a specific category (e.g., animals or words beginning with a specific letter of the alphabet) as possible in 1 minute. Patients with left-sided dorsolateral prefrontal dysfunction have disproportionate difficulty with this task. A normal performance is 18 animals per minute; fewer than 12 animals recalled in 1 minute is abnormal. An approximately equivalent nonverbal fluency task sensitive to right-sided dorsolateral prefrontal dysfunction requires the patient draw as many figures composed of four lines of equal length as possible in 1 minute. Each line must intersect at least one other line, and the figures must not be repeated. A normal performance is 10 figures per minute; fewer than 8 is abnormal. Figure 5–1 provides examples of normal and abnormal performances on the nonverbal fluency test. The test is particularly difficult for patients with right dorsolateral prefrontal dysfunction and can be a useful executive function test in patients with language deficits, such as in primary progressive aphasia.

In a formal testing environment, poor planning abilities are demonstrated using "tower" tests involving beads placed on pegs, in which the patient must move the beads from their starting positions to a target position using the smallest number of moves possible. Typical difficulties may include failure to anticipate the consequences of a move, making illegal moves, and losing track of a plan during its execution. A simpler bedside evaluation might use copying tasks to assess strategic planning by asking patients to copy a complex figure and observing their approach. They typically have a segmented approach, reproducing individual elements and failing to organize the drawing around the principal figure elements.

Poor set shifting is demonstrated by tasks such as Trails B and the Wisconsin Card Sorting Test, which require the patient to flexibly shift from one cognitive set to another. Several types of abnormalities may be observed on these tests: patients may be excessively slow, they may lose the set prematurely, or they may perseverate, repeating previous responses.

Motor programming tasks assess patients' ability to execute sequential motor acts. Examples of alternating programs (alternating between square and pointed figures) and multiple loops are shown in Figures 5–2 and 5–3. Reciprocal programs require patients to alternate performances with the examiner. For example, patients are asked to tap twice each time the examiner taps once and to tap once each time the examiner taps twice. In the go–no go test, which is a further elaboration of this task, patients are asked to tap once each time the examiner taps once and to withhold any response when the examiner taps twice. This test requires that patients inhibit a learned response.

Another example of a motor programming test is the performance of serial hand sequences with verbal guidance (e.g.,

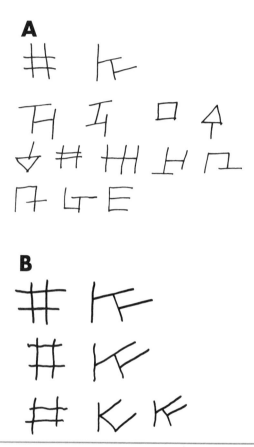

FIGURE 5–1. **Examples of a normal performance (*A*) and an abnormal performance (*B*) on the design fluency test.**

The patient who fails the task is unable to generate a normal number of designs and produces stereotyped figures. In each case, two sample figures (comprising four lines of equal length with each line touching at least one other line) are the first two figures and were provided by the examiner; the remaining figures were produced by the patient. The patient had a degenerative frontotemporal dementia.

having patients say "fist, slap, cut" aloud while executing the corresponding hand postures). Patients with dorsolateral prefrontal dysfunction have difficulty with verbal mediation of motor behavior and manifest verbal-manual dissociation, saying one sequence while executing another. Tests of motor program-

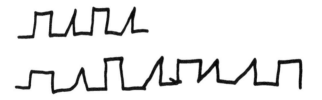

FIGURE 5–2. Example of abnormal performance on alternating programs.

The examiner's model is shown on the *top line*; the patient's attempt to reproduce the model is shown on the *bottom line*. Perseveration is evident in the patient's attempt to copy and extend the examiner's model. The patient had a frontal lobe degenerative disorder.

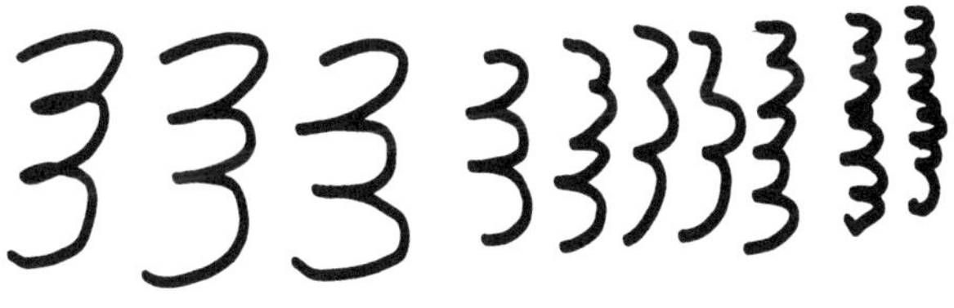

FIGURE 5–3. Examples of abnormal performance on the multiple loop test.

The examiner's models are the first three figures on the *left*; the patient's abnormal copies are on the *right*. Perseveration is evident as the patient tries to reproduce the examiner's model figures. This patient had a clinical syndrome consistent with a frontotemporal dementia.

ming evaluate patients' ability to perform a sequence of actions; impersistence, with failure to continue the required acts; perseveration, with repetition of a previous response; or failure to verbally guide motor behavior may be observed.

Compromised attention is also characteristic of individuals with dorsolateral prefrontal dysfunction. They may fail elementary tests of attention, such as digit span or continuous performance tasks. The former requires patients to repeat a series of digits that are read aloud by the examiner (normally, patients can repeat a series of at least five digits). The latter tests their ability to sustain attention over time; patients are asked to signal each time the letter A occurs in a series of letters that are read aloud by the examiner. The test continues for at least 1 minute. Lapses of attention result in errors of omission. Some patients perform these elementary tests satisfactorily but fail more complex attentional tests, such as mental control (repeating the months of the year in reverse order), response inhibition (as required by the Stroop Color-Word Interference Test, in which patients must name aloud the color of the ink in which a word is printed rather than read the word itself), and divided attention (e.g., consonant trigrams, which require patients to memorize three letters, count backward serially, and then repeat the three letters).

Environmental dependency is evident with severe frontal lobe dysfunction and may reflect attentional and motivational abnormalities. Patients' attention is inappropriately dominated by environmental stimuli. For example, when patients with dorsolateral prefrontal dysfunction are asked to set the hands of a clock to read 11:10, they may put one hand on the 11 and one on the 10. The 10 is an environmental stimulus that attracts their attention and creates an erroneous behavior. Imitative behavior emerges when patients imitate the actions of others. Utilization behavior refers to patients' forced use of environmental objects, even in inappropriate circumstances (e.g., taking the examiner's glasses and putting them on).

Although cognitive deficits are predominant in this syndrome, depressive symptoms and anxiety are also common in patients with dorsolateral prefrontal lesion. For example, acute poststroke depression tends to be more frequent in those with more anterior and left-sided lesions.

If the lesion or disease that is affecting the dorsolateral convexity extends sufficiently posterior to affect the inferior frontal gyrus area of the left dominant hemisphere, then expressive aphasia (Broca's aphasia) is present (see Chapter 6). A similarly placed lesion in the right hemisphere produces aprosodia, as evidenced by diminished inflection of spontaneous speech. A lesion affecting the motor strip produces contralateral hemiparesis with increased muscle stretch reflexes and an extensor response of the great toe with stimulation of the plantar surface of the foot (Babinski sign). Weakness is most marked in the extensor muscles of the arm (e.g., deltoid, triceps, brachioradialis; resulting in a tendency to keep the arm flexed) and in the flexor muscles of the leg (iliopsoas, hamstrings, peroneals; producing an extensor posture of the leg). When the frontal eye field is affected unilaterally, patients have ipsilateral gaze deviation or gaze preference, directed toward the side of the lesion. Prefrontal lesions can also produce contralateral neglect, usually manifested by a lack of action directed into the neglected space.

■ LATERAL ORBITOFRONTAL SYNDROME

The predominant behavioral change associated with orbitofrontal syndrome is social disinhibition; this lack of interpersonal restraint is manifested in many ways. Patients may ignore social conventions and display undue familiarity, talking to strangers and touching or fondling others without permission. Their behaviors can include being tactless in conversation and making uncivil or lewd remarks. Thesy tend to be impulsive, responding immediately and unpredictably to changing environmental circumstances. Patients may lack empathy and be unsympathetic to the needs of others. They sometimes lack conscientiousness and fail to complete assigned tasks. Given their decreased level of concern about the consequences of their behavior, they may engage in activities that endanger themselves or others. Risk assessment tends to be poor.

Mood alterations also accompany the orbitofrontal syndrome. Lability and irritability are the most common changes. Patients rapidly shift from happiness (sometimes a vacuous euphoria) to anger or sadness. Mood changes are rarely sustained, and anger can often be relieved by redirecting their attention to some new activity. Hypomania or mania may accompany orbitofrontal dysfunction, possibly more commonly in lesions that affect the right hemisphere.

Orbitofrontal syndromes are observed in frontotemporal dementia, in severe traumatic brain injuries, and after the rupture of anterior communication artery aneurysms. An elementary neurological examination of individuals with orbitofrontal syndrome reveals few abnormalities. Their olfaction may be impaired due to the proximity of the olfactory nerves, bulbs, and tracts to the inferior orbitofrontal surface. Cognitive changes on common cognitive tests can be absent in patients with lesions limited to the orbitofrontal cortex. Language, memory, and visuospatial skills are unaffected, although distractibility, irritability, and failure to cooperate may compromise test performance.

■ MEDIAL FRONTAL SYNDROME

Classic medial frontal syndrome is marked by apathy, which has emotional, cognitive, and motor dimensions. Emotionally, apathetic individuals are unmotivated to initiate new tasks; they have disinterest in establishing or accomplishing goals and little excites or stimulates them. Mood changes may include an emotional emptiness or indifference. Cognitively, apathetic individuals fail to formulate or implement plans and activities and have a loss of generative thought. Slowing of cognition may be evident. Patients with a left unilateral lesion may further have transcortical motor aphasia (see Chapter 6) characterized by transient mutism recovering to a nonfluent verbal output, with preserved repetition and comprehension. Contralateral neglect may occur in the period immediately following the onset of an acute cingulate lesion. Motorically, individuals with apathy have reduced activity; they may sit for long periods without participating in conversation or activities. In the most extreme form of apathy, akinetic mutism, patients are awake but motionless and mute. They will eat if fed, and they may occasionally move or speak briefly. They are not paralyzed, and the syndrome must be distinguished from locked-in syndrome (paralysis of all limbs secondary to a pontine lesion) and catatonia.

Frontal lobe disorders producing the apathetic syndrome involve the medial frontal region (ventral and dorsal), particularly the anterior cingulate cortex. Apathy also occurs in individuals with lesions of the caudate nucleus, globus pallidus, and thalamus; these structures are part of the medial frontal–subcortical circuit (see Chapter 2, Figure 2–3). Apathy is prominent in frontotemporal dementia and can be seen in several other neuropsychiatric conditions, including Alzheimer's disease and progressive supranuclear palsy.

Relatively few abnormalities of the elementary neurological examination accompany medial frontal lobe lesions. Frontal release reflexes, such as grasp reflex, can be present. Neuropsychologically, patients with medial frontal lesions may exhibit abnormalities on the go–no go test, echoing the examiner's actions instead of following instructions (e.g., patients are asked to hold up two fingers when the examiner holds up one finger and to make no response when the examiner holds up two fingers, but they exhibit echopraxia, reproducing the examiner's movements). A deficit in the letter fluency task in the absence of language abnormalities (referred to as executive function "generation") is often observed in patients with dorsomedial lesions. Medial prefrontal dysfunction (particularly ventromedial lesions) also leads to social cognitive deficits, which can be captured on social cognition tests such as facial emotion recognition tasks or the detection of *faux pas* in social situation vignettes (see Table 5–1).

■ FRONTAL LOBE DYSFUNCTION ASSOCIATED WITH WHITE MATTER INJURY

In addition to the three classical cortical prefrontal syndromes just described, similar behavioral and cognitive alterations can also occur with disorders of the frontal white matter connecting these different brain regions. These alterations may be seen with demyelinating (e.g., multiple sclerosis), ischemic (e.g., vascular dementia), or compression (e.g., normal-pressure hydrocephalus) syndromes. Gait abnormalities commonly accompany disorders involving the frontal white matter. The most typical gait change is vascular (or lower body) parkinsonism and comprises reduced step height and limited stride length. A foot grasp reflex may be present, producing a magnetic-type sticking of the foot to the floor. Poor balance and retropulsion may be evident. Urinary and occasionally fecal incontinence may be present.

■ DISEASES OF THE FRONTAL LOBES

Table 5–2 lists the major disorders that affect the frontal lobes and describes the frontal regions most likely to be affected by each process. These disorders are individually discussed in more detail in other chapters of this textbook. Of note, subcortical diseases that can produce overlapping symptoms to cortical frontal lobe syndromes are not included in this list.

■ TREATMENTS

Frontal lobe syndromes can be caused by several different diseases, thus, there is no single intervention for all syndromes. Treatments can be disease modifying (e.g., immunomodulation for autoimmune encephalitis) or preventive (e.g., blood pressure control in vascular neurocognitive disorder) or are most commonly aimed at nonspecific symptom control (e.g., low-dose antipsychotic medications for the behavioral management of dementia).

In terms of rehabilitation, a technique called goal management training (GMT) has shown to improve executive function deficits, including in patients with frontal lobe lesions. GMT is a standardized meta-cognitive training program that includes approximately 20 hours of training, comprising psychoeducation, narrative examples, mindfulness practice, and assignments

TABLE 5–2. Disorders of the frontal lobes

Class of disorder and examples	Frontal region affected
Degenerative	
Alzheimer's disease	Prefrontal (frontal variant or late-stage changes of typical amnestic presentation)
Behavioral variant FTD	Prefrontal
FTD-ALS	Prefrontal
Lewy body dementia	Prefrontal
Nonfluent variant PPA	Left inferior frontal gyrus and prefrontal
Vascular	
Anterior cerebral artery aneurysm rupture	Orbitofrontal
Anterior cerebral artery occlusion	Medial frontal
Middle cerebral artery occlusion	Lateral convexity
Subcortical vascular dementia (Binswanger's disease)	Subcortical and hemispheric white matter
Traumatic	
Closed head injury	Orbitofrontal contusion, diffuse axonal injury to white matter fibers
Penetrating injury	Local and diffuse
Demyelinating	
Marchiafava-Bignami disease	Corpus callosum (anteriorly)
Metachromatic leukodystrophy	White matter (begins frontally)
Multiple sclerosis	White matter (especially periventricular)
Neoplastic	
Glioblastoma, oligodendro-glioma, metastasis	Local with diffuse edema
Meningioma	
Subfrontal	Orbitofrontal
Convexity	Lateral convexity
Falcine	Medial frontal

TABLE 5–2. Disorders of the frontal lobes *(continued)*

Class of disorder and examples	Frontal region affected
Infectious	
Creutzfeldt-Jakob disease	Focal onset with rapid spread
Herpes encephalitis	Orbitofrontal and temporal
Neurosyphilis	Prefrontal
Inflammatory	
Autoimmune ("limbic") encephalitis	Medial prefrontal and orbitofrontal
Systemic lupus erythematosus and other inflammatory disorders	Diffuse

ALS=amyotrophic lateral sclerosis; FTD=frontotemporal dementia; PPA=primary progressive aphasia.

completed both between and within sessions. Meta-cognitive programs educate patients on how to gain awareness of their deficits, self-monitor, and regain control over their ability to perform activities of daily living.

The knowledge of frontal lobe functions in cognition and behavior has also led to the development of new treatments for idiopathic psychiatric disorders. One of the best examples is repetitive transcranial magnetic stimulation (rTMS) targeting the dorsolateral PFC, which has proven to have a beneficial effect in treating major depression. The initial target was in part selected based on studies using functional imaging that suggested patients with idiopathic depression have reduced activity in the dorsolateral PFC compared with patients without depression. Recent advances in our understanding of distinct systems within the frontal lobes have further prompted novel rTMS approaches that target different frontal regions to treat specific clinical manifestations of depression and other psychiatric conditions. For example, the clinical effectiveness of rTMS for the treatment of compulsive behaviors in OCD or negative symptoms in schizophrenia is currently being investigated. Another example is the neurosurgical procedure of anterior cingulotomy, which has been shown to have benefit in patients with treatment-refractory OCD, depression, and chronic pain. Of note, in recent years there has been significant interest in using deep brain stimulation to produce similar benefits with potentially less complications in several psychiatric disorders.

■ REFERENCES

Chapados C, Petrides M: Impairment only on the fluency subtest of the Frontal Assessment Battery after prefrontal lesions. Brain 136(Pt 10):2966–2978, 2013 24030949

Cocchi L, Zalesky A, Nott Z, et al: Transcranial magnetic stimulation in obsessive-compulsive disorder: a focus on network mechanisms and state dependence. Neuroimage Clin 19:661–674, 2018 30023172

Cummings JL: Frontal-subcortical circuits and human behavior. Arch Neurol 50(8):873–880, 1993 8352676

Ducharme S, Price BH, Dickerson BC: Apathy: a neurocircuitry model based on frontotemporal dementia. J Neurol Neurosurg Psychiatry 89(4):389–396, 2018 29066518

Eslinger PJ, Damasio AR: Severe disturbance of higher cognition after bilateral frontal lobe ablation: patient EVR. Neurology 35(12):1731–1741, 1985 4069365

Eslinger PJ, Geder L: Behavioral and emotional changes after frontal lobe damage, in Behavior and Mood Disorders in Focal Brain Lesions. Edited by Bogousslavsky T, Cummings JL. Cambridge, UK, Cambridge University Press, 2000, pp 217–260

Fellows LK: The functions of the frontal lobes: evidence from patients with focal brain damage. Handb Clin Neurol 163:19–34, 2019 31590730

Grattan LM, Bloomer RH, Archambault FX, et al: Cognitive flexibility and empathy after frontal lobe lesion. Neuropsychiatry Neuropsychol Behav Neurol 7:251–259, 1994

Levine B, Schweizer TA, O'Connor C, et al: Rehabilitation of executive functioning in patients with frontal lobe brain damage with goal management training. Front Hum Neurosci 5:9, 2011 21369362

Lhermitte F: Human autonomy and the frontal lobes. Part II: patient behavior in complex and social situations: the "environmental dependency syndrome." Ann Neurol 19(4):335–343, 1986 3707085

Lhermitte F, Pillon B, Serdaru M: Human autonomy and the frontal lobes. Part I: imitation and utilization behavior: a neuropsychological study of 75 patients. Ann Neurol 19(4):326–334, 1986 3707084

Marin RS: Apathy: a neuropsychiatric syndrome. J Neuropsychiatry Clin Neurosci 3(3):243–254, 1991 1821241

Mega MS, Cummings JL: The cingulate and cingulate syndromes, in Contemporary Behavioral Neurology. Edited by Trimble MR, Cummings JL. Boston, MA, Butterworth-Heinemann, 1997, pp 189–214

Miller BL, Cummings JL (eds): The Human Frontal Lobes: Functions and Disorders. 3rd Edition. New York, Guilford, 2018

Olney NT, Spina S, Miller BL: Frontotemporal dementia. Neurol Clin 35(2):339–374, 2017 28410663

Price BH, Daffner KR, Stowe RM, Mesulam MM: The comportmental learning disabilities of early frontal lobe damage. Brain 113(pt 5):1383–1393, 1990 2245302

Robinson RG, Spalletta G: Poststroke depression: a review. Can J Psychiatry 55(6):341–349, 2010 20540828

Seeley WW, Zhou J, Kim EJ: Frontotemporal dementia: what can the behavioral variant teach us about human brain organization? Neuroscientist 18(4):373–385, 2012 21670424

Stamenova V, Levine B: Effectiveness of goal management training in improving executive functions: a meta-analysis. Neuropsychol Rehabil 29(10):1569–1599, 2019 29540124

Stuss DT, Alexander MP, Benson DF: Frontal lobe functions, in Contemporary Behavioral Neurology. Edited by Trimble MR, Cummings JL. Boston, MA, Butterworth-Heinemann, 1997, pp 169–187

Zald DH, Andreotti C: Neuropsychological assessment of the orbital and ventromedial prefrontal cortex. Neuropsychologia 48(12):3377–3391, 2010 20728457

6

APHASIA AND RELATED SYNDROMES

Jeffrey L. Cummings, M.D., Sc.D.
Michael R. Trimble, M.D., FRCP, FRCPsych

This chapter addresses disorders of verbal output, including aphasia, aprosodia, amusia, dysarthria, mutism, and reiterative speech disturbances such as stuttering, echolalia, and palilalia. Neurobehavioral disorders occurring with left-hemisphere dysfunction and frequently observed in patients with aphasia (i.e., apraxia, acalculia, Gerstmann syndrome) are also described. The clinical features, anatomical correlates, and appropriate assessments and interventions appropriate for aphasias and related conditions are presented. First, however, the concepts of handedness, hemispheric specialization, and cerebral dominance are discussed because an understanding of these concepts is fundamental to understanding aphasia and related syndromes.

■ HEMISPHERIC SPECIALIZATION, CEREBRAL DOMINANCE, AND HANDEDNESS

A uniquely well-developed aspect of human brain organization is *hemispheric specialization*. This refers to the asymmetrical cerebral mediation of neuropsychological and behavioral functions. *Cerebral dominance* refers to the corresponding principle that one hemisphere is usually superior to the other with regard to a specific task and is dominant for that function. Neural organization in the right hemisphere tends to be more diffuse and less discrete than in the left hemisphere. Neither hemisphere is dominant for all functions; in general, the left is dominant for language-related tasks and the right for visuospatial tasks. This can be an overly simplistic dichotomy, however. First, the left brain has the capacity to mediate some visuospatial functions, and the right brain has at least some rudimentary language skills.

TABLE 6–1.	Skills and abilities mediated asymmetrically by the two hemispheres of the brain
Left hemisphere	**Right hemisphere**
Propositional speech	Facial discrimination and recognition
Language comprehension	Depth perception
Naming	Expressive and receptive prosody and intonation
Reading	
Writing	Emotion recognition
Praxis (skilled movements)	Self-awareness
	Music
Linear calculations	Proprioception
Processing of details	Constructional abilities
Verbal learning and memory	Mental rotation and spatial orientation
	Appreciation of humor
	Holistic processing
	Spatially mediated calculations
	Nonverbal learning and memory

Also, some visuospatial information lends itself to verbal descriptions or labeling and thus would not necessarily be classified as "nonverbal" or right hemisphere dominant. Table 6–1 provides an overview of tasks with known asymmetric hemispheric demands.

Anatomical asymmetries between the hemispheres have been identified. The hemispheres of most individuals include the following asymmetries: Sylvian fissures (more horizontal on the left, more vertical on the right), larger occipital horn of the left lateral ventricle, longer left hemisphere, wider right frontal lobe, increased left cortical area in Broca's area on the left, larger left pulvinar, and asymmetric decussation (the fibers descending from the left brain cross first) in the cerebral medulla. The anatomical differences are relatively modest compared with the marked functional differences between the hemispheres.

Handedness is related to cerebral dominance and is the most readily available means of assessing cerebral dominance for language. Ninety-nine percent of right-handed individuals have left-cerebral dominance for language. Among left-handed persons, approximately 70% are also left-brain dominant for language, 15% have language skills mediated primarily by the right hemisphere, and 15% have a bilateral representation of language.

■ APHASIA

Aphasia refers to an impairment in linguistic communication produced by brain dysfunction. It must be distinguished from other disorders of verbal output, such as dysarthria, mutism, and the abnormal language production of patients with formal thought disorders. Nine principal aphasia syndromes are recognized (Table 6–2); each has unique characteristics and occurs with brain dysfunction in specific brain regions. The three main features that differentiate the aphasias are fluency of verbal output, the ability to comprehend spoken language, and the ability to repeat phrases stated by the examiner. The rules guiding localization provided here apply to right-handed adults. Left-handed individuals can have atypical patterns of hemispheric dominance and manifest less predictable clinical syndromes with brain lesions. Children often have nonfluent verbal output regardless of lesion location.

Fluency refers to the flow of spontaneous speech. Aphasias are either fluent or nonfluent. *Fluent aphasias* are characterized by normal or increased rate of speech, preserved speech melody, normal phrase length, preserved grammatical constructions (minor grammatical errors may occur), empty speech with impoverished information content, and the presence of paraphasic errors. Paraphasias may be phonemic (substitution of a single phoneme or syllable), verbal (substitution of one word for another), or neologistic (production of novel words that have no meaning). Wernicke's, anomic, conduction, thalamic, and transcortical sensory aphasias are all fluent. Fluent aphasias occur with post-Rolandic lesions sparing anterior hemispheric regions.

Nonfluent aphasias feature sparse, effortful verbal output with reduced amount of speech, short phrase length, abnormal prosody (rhythm and melody of speech), and agrammatism (loss of short grammatical "functor" words such as *to*, *in*, and *then*). Informational content of speech is relatively preserved, and there are few paraphasic errors; dysarthria may be present. Global, Broca's, transcortical motor, and mixed transcortical aphasias are nonfluent. Nonfluent aphasias are associated with lesions that involve the pre-Rolandic brain regions.

Comprehension of spoken language is assessed by asking patients to follow commands, decipher yes-and-no questions, and

TABLE 6–2. Characteristics of the aphasia syndromes

Syndrome	Fluency	Comprehension	Repetition	Localization in left hemisphere
Anomic	Fluent	Intact	Intact	Anterior temporal; angular gyrus
Conduction	Fluent	Intact	Impaired	Arcuate fasciculus
Broca's	Nonfluent	Intact	Impaired	Inferior frontal
Transcortical sensory	Fluent	Impaired	Intact	Angular gyrus
Wernicke's	Fluent	Impaired	Impaired	Posterior superior temporal
Thalamic*	Fluent	Impaired	Intact	Thalamus
Global	Nonfluent	Impaired	Impaired	Wernicke's and Broca's areas
Mixed transcortical	Nonfluent	Impaired	Intact	Lesions of transcortical motor and transcortical sensory aphasias
Transcortical motor	Nonfluent	Intact	Intact	Medial frontal or superior to Broca's area

*Thalamic aphasia is usually distinguished from transcortical sensory aphasia associated with cortical lesions by the onset with mutism, co-occurring dysarthria, and prominent hemiparesis.

respond to sentences with complex grammatical constructions. Commands frequently request a pointing response ("point to the ceiling," "point to the door and then to the ceiling," "point to your nose, your wrist, and your chin"). Yes-and-no questions assess their ability to understand language content and grammar ("Are the lights in this room on?" "Do you put your shoes on before your socks?" "Do you have your lunch before your breakfast?"). More complex questions can also be formulated, such as "Is my wife's brother a man or a woman?" and "If a lion and a tiger were in a fight and the lion was killed by the tiger, which animal was dead?" Comprehension is impaired (but not necessarily completely absent) in patients with lesions that involve Wernicke's area and the angular gyrus region and is preserved in patients with lesions that spare these areas.

Repetition is evaluated by asking patients to repeat words, phrases, and sentences. The examination begins by asking patients to repeat single words to ensure that they understand the task ("Say after me: 'boy,'" "Say 'basketball player'"). Then they are asked to repeat phrases ("no ifs, ands, or buts") and sentences ("She went home early," "The truck rolled over the stone bridge," "The quick brown fox jumped over the lazy dog"). Repetition is impaired in patients with lesions involving structures abutting the Sylvian fissure (Wernicke's, conduction, Broca's, global aphasias) and is spared in patients with lesions removed from the peri-Sylvian area (anomic, transcortical motor, transcortical sensory, mixed transcortical, and thalamic aphasias).

Naming is impaired in all aphasic syndromes, and anomic aphasia may reflect the end stage of other resolving aphasia syndromes. Three types of anomia occur: word production aphasia, semantic anomia, and word selection anomia. Paraphasic naming errors may be observed in fluent aphasic disorders. Errors in *writing* generally reflect the disturbances observed in spontaneous speech. *Reading comprehension* is impaired in most patients with reduced auditory comprehension; *reading aloud* is impaired in Wernicke's, Broca's, conduction, global, and mixed transcortical aphasias. Singing, automatic speech (reciting the alphabet or counting), and cursing are preserved in many aphasias, even those with severe verbal output disturbances.

Aphasias occur in a wide variety of neurological disorders affecting the left hemisphere, such as stroke, tumors, trauma, infections (e.g., herpes encephalitis, Creutzfeldt-Jakob disease, abscesses), and degenerative diseases such as Alzheimer's disease and primary progressive aphasia (including semantic, logopenic, and agrammatic variants).

In addition to the bedside tests just described, formal aphasia evaluations can be performed by speech and language therapists or neuropsychologists. MRI is the optimal technique for demonstrating focal brain lesions associated with aphasia. CT will reveal most aphasia-producing lesions. PET and single-photon emission computed tomography usually reveal areas of functional impairment that are larger than the structural lesions demonstrated by MRI and CT in patients with aphasia.

Patients with acute aphasias secondary to stroke or trauma may be helped by speech and language therapy and should be referred to a speech therapist for evaluation and construction of a treatment program.

■ ALEXIAS AND AGRAPHIAS

Alexia is an acquired inability to read, and *agraphia* is an acquired inability to write. These terms are not applicable to illiterate individuals who never developed significant reading and writing skills. Four alexias are recognized. *Alexia with agraphia* occurs with lesions of the left angular gyrus. Patients can neither read nor write and are not aided by spelling the words aloud. They perform as if truly illiterate. *Alexia without agraphia* is observed with lesions of the medial left occipital cortex and the splenium of the corpus callosum or lesions of the left lateral geniculate body and splenium of the corpus callosum. Patients can often understand written words by spelling them aloud. *Frontal alexia* occurs with lesions of the left frontal lobe, and most patients with frontal alexia have Broca's aphasia. The reading deficit of frontal alexia involves an inability to name individual letters and disturbed comprehension of written language that is contingent on grammatical constructions and accurate interpretation of functor words (e.g., "put the red circle *on top of* the blue square"). Finally, *hemialexia* occurs hemispheric lesions that produce profound unilateral neglect.

Agraphia occurs several circumstances, including linguistic, spatial, apractic, and motor disturbances. *Linguistic agraphias* occur in all aphasias, as a part of Gerstmann syndrome and the angular gyrus syndrome (discussed later), and in the syndrome of alexia with agraphia (described in previous paragraph). In aphasia, patients' written output mirrors their spontaneous verbalizations. Anterior lesions result in nonfluent agraphia with agrammatism, whereas posterior lesions are associated with fluent agraphias characterized by written paraphasias and relative preservation of syntax.

Spatial agraphias are common with lesions of the posterior right hemisphere. The left side of the page is neglected, there is a gradually enlarging margin on the left, letters are omitted or repeated, and the spacing of the words and letters is uneven.

Apractic agraphia is a disorder of orthography that is manifest despite normal sensorimotor function and intact letter and word knowledge. Patients can type normally, establishing the integrity of their linguistic and motor functions. Manual writing, including copying letters produced by others, is disrupted. Lesions of the left superior parietal regions, the thalamus, and the cerebellum have been associated with the syndrome.

Mechanical agraphias accompany motor disorders that affect the limbs and are described in patients with parkinsonism (micrographia), choreas, dystonic disorders (writer's cramp), and cerebellar syndromes. Action tremors disrupt writing, and some tremors are elicited virtually only by the act of writing (primary writing tremors).

■ APROSODIA

Prosody refers to the melodic, intonational, and inflectional aspects of speech. Much of the informational content of speech is conveyed through prosody rather than through its propositional (verbal) components. Prosody plays a role in dialect (i.e., regional variations in word pronunciation), linguistic communication (e.g., differentiating a statement from a question), conveyance of attitude (e.g., sarcasm), and portrayal of emotion (e.g., sadness, anger). Prosody has executive and receptive aspects. *Executive prosody* refers to patients' ability to produce prosodically accurate utterances; *receptive prosody* refers to their ability to comprehend the prosodic aspects of another's speech (e.g., deduce the person's emotional state). Linguistic prosody is affected by left-hemisphere lesions, whereas affective and emotional prosody is impaired by right-hemisphere and basal ganglia lesions. Gesture is usually reduced in patients with affective dysprosody, and pantomime is impaired in patients with linguistic dysprosody. Damage to the region of the right hemisphere equivalent to Broca's area produces an executive affective aprosodia; injury to the right-hemisphere equivalent of Wernicke's area produces a receptive affective aprosodia.

Executive prosody is assessed by asking patients to state a neutral sentence (e.g., "I'm going to the store") with inflections denoting anger, happiness, surprise, and sadness. Prosodic comprehension is evaluated by asking patients to identify which emotion is present as the examiner says the sentence with each of the four different inflections.

Patients with executive aprosodia have difficulty communicating their feelings, and their emotional distress may be underestimated. Children who sustain right-hemisphere injuries that deprive them of the ability to communicate their emotions or to comprehend the emotions of others may develop an asocial or schizoid demeanor.

■ AMUSIA

The amusias encompass syndromes characterized by loss of ability to sing (executive amusia) and to recognize or appreciate features of heard music (receptive or sensory amusia). Several brain regions are involved in the processing of musical stimuli. Lesions of the right temporal lobe impair appreciation of timbre, pitch, and intensity as well as tonal memory. Lesions of the right frontal lobe impair tonal processing. In contrast, left anterior hemispheric lesions tend to produce rhythm disturbances. Changes in musical abilities resemble those involving prosody: right temporal lesions produce primarily receptive musical and prosodic deficits, whereas right and left frontal injuries impair different aspects of executive musical and prosodic abilities. The right temporal lobe has a greater role in processing unfamiliar melodic sequences, and the left temporal lobe has a greater role in processing familiar sequences.

■ DYSARTHRIA

Dysarthria refers to impairment of the motor aspects of speech. Dysarthria results from loss of speed, coordination, or strength, producing abnormalities of speech articulation, phonation, or timing. Flaccid, spastic, ataxic, hypokinetic, hyperkinetic, and dystonic dysarthrias are recognized. *Flaccid dysarthrias* result from lower motor neuron, peripheral nerve, and muscular disorders and are characterized by a breathy, hypernasal sound quality with imprecise consonants. *Spastic dysarthrias* feature slow speech, strained-strangled voicing, and a monotone execution. Spastic dysarthrias occur with upper motor neuron disease and are associated with an exaggerated gag reflex, brisk muscle stretch reflexes, and pseudobulbar palsy. *Ataxic dysarthrias* include abnormal rhythm and timing of speech with abnormal sound stress patterns. They occur with diseases of the cerebellum and of the cerebellar tracts in the midbrain. *Hypokinetic dysarthrias* occur in parkinsonian syndromes and evidence reduced speech volume, reduced syllable stress, variable rate, and monotone output. Festination of speech (i.e., speaking with increasing rapidity) may occur. *Hyperkinetic* and *dystonic dysarthrias* are present in choreiform and dystonic disorders. They are notable for distorted sounds, inappropriate silences, respiratory irregularities, loudness variations, imprecise consonants, and slow rate. Dystonic dysarthrias have a strained-strangled speech quality. Dysphagia may accompany any of the dysarthrias and can be life threatening if aspiration occurs. Dysarthria may improve with speech therapy, and patients should be referred to a speech therapist for evaluation and treatment.

■ MUTISM

Mutism is the inability or unwillingness to speak, resulting in an absence or marked paucity of verbal output. The term usually refers to a complete or nearly complete absence of speech and nonverbal utterances. Mutism has a wide differential diagnosis, occurring in both neurological and psychiatric disorders (Table 6–3).

Assessment of patients with mutism must include a careful review of the neurological and psychiatric history if available and a thorough examination to detect evidence of focal neurological dysfunction, catatonia, previous psychiatric treatment (e.g., tardive dyskinesia), or trauma. Medication trials of benzodiazepine for catatonia and akinetic mutism and dextromethorphan/quinidine for pseudobulbar affect may be helpful. An Amytal interview or the use of hypnosis may help in some cases, particularly if a conversion reaction with mutism is suspected.

■ REITERATIVE SPEECH DISTURBANCES

Reiterative speech disturbances include stuttering, palilalia (a complex tic), echolalia, logoclonia, and perseveration. There are also more complex repetitive disorders in which patients repeat the same story again and again. Stuttering may be congenital or acquired.

TABLE 6–3. Differential diagnosis of mutism

Psychiatric conditions

Conversion disorder

Depression with catatonia

Dissociation

Hysterical

Malingering

Reaction to severe stress

Schizophrenia with catatonia

Developmental conditions

Absence of speech development (developmental delay, autism, deafness)

Congenital or early onset infection

Selective mutism (e.g., mute only while at school)

Neurological disorders

Acute phase of aphemia*

Acute phase of a nonfluent aphasia (see Table 6–2)

Akinetic mutism—two types, vigilant and somnolents

Demyelination disorder

Epilepsy—postictal state after a generalized or partial seizure

Frontal lobe syndromes with marked abulia

Herpes encephalitis and other infectious processes

Locked-in syndrome

Neoplasms

Neurodegenerative disorder

Posttraumatic encephalopathy

Pseudobulbar palsy

Vascular

Medical conditions

Drug or alcohol intoxication and withdrawal

Endocrine hypothyroidism, diabetes, Addison's, etc.

Metabolic encephalopathies (delirium)

Neuroleptic effect

Toxins

*Aphemia is a syndrome of acute mutism followed by recovery to a hypo-phonic, breathy verbal output without aphasia; it is produced by a small lesion of Broca's area (called the "foreign accent syndrome").

Stuttering involves repetition of the initial or an internal phoneme of a word. *Acquired stuttering* occurs with lesions of either hemisphere that involve the basal ganglia or frontal lobe white matter of the internal capsule. Stuttering may occur transiently during recovery from aphasia and also is observed in basal ganglia disorders including Parkinson's disease. Patients with acquired stuttering have less frustration and grimacing than congenital stutterers. Other speech characteristics in patients who stutter include increased pause time, syllable prolongations, fast speech rate, and aprosodia.

Palilalia refers to the repetition of spontaneous utterances. It is manifest by repetition of the final phrase or last few words of a phrase (e.g., "I had eggs for breakfast, for breakfast, for breakfast"). It occurs in advanced stages of cortical dementias and in basal ganglia disorders.

Echolalia is a syndrome featuring repetition of words and phrases that patients hear from others (e.g., when greeted with "Hello, Mr. Brown," the patient may echo "Hello, Mr. Brown"). It occurs in patients with advanced cortical dementias, basal ganglia disorders, Gilles de la Tourette's syndrome, mental retardation syndromes, and schizophrenia.

Logoclonia is the term for repetitions limited to the final phoneme or two of a word (e.g., "Methodist Episcopal-copal-copal" or "hopping hippopotamus-amus-amus"). Logoclonia is particularly prominent in general paresis resulting from syphilitic encephalitis but can occur in patients who exhibit palilalia or echolalia.

Verbal perseveration, which occurs most often in patients with fluent aphasia, is marked by the frequent reappearance of the same word in the patient's spontaneous speech.

Gramophone syndrome is a disorder characterized by the repetition of a greeting or story. Each time the story is told, it is repeated in the same way regardless of whether the listener has heard it before. The syndrome occurs in frontotemporal dementias, such as Pick's disease. The speech of patients with schizophrenia is often characterized by the tendency to return to the same themes, but these discussions lack the rigid stereotypy of the gramophone syndrome.

■ APRAXIA

Apraxia is a form of motor agnosia, a dysfunction of motor planning. Stroke and dementias are the usual causes. Three varieties are recognized: limb-kinetic apraxia, ideomotor apraxia, and ideational apraxia. Other subtypes exist, such as gaze, speech, conceptual, and conduction apraxias.

Limb-kinetic apraxia refers to a loss of dexterity and coordination of distal limb movements that cannot be accounted for by weakness or sensory loss. The impairment is evident in pantomime, imitation, and use of objects. It occurs contralateral to a hemispheric lesion.

Ideomotor apraxia refers to an inability to perform learned movement on command that cannot be attributed to abnormalities of strength, coordination, sensory loss, or impaired comprehension. The defect is most obvious when pantomiming the use of objects (e.g., comb, toothbrush, lipstick, hammer, saw); however, it remains even after the movement has been demonstrated by the examiner, when patients attempt to imitate the movement. It also may be evident when patients attempt to use the object itself. Errors include abnormal sequencing of movement with perseveration of components of the movements, poor positioning of the limbs with regard to the imagined object during pantomime, and impaired execution of the object-related movement.

There are three types of ideomotor apraxia (Table 6–4). *Parietal apraxia* occurs with lesions of the inferior parietal region and underlying fibers of the arcuate fasciculus. Both limbs are apraxic, and patients usually have conduction aphasia; typically, there is no associated hemiparesis. *Sympathetic apraxia* is a syndrome comprising apraxia of the left limbs in patients with a right hemiparesis and Broca's aphasia. It occurs with lesions of the left frontal lobe. *Callosal apraxia* is characterized by apraxia of the left limbs only. There is no aphasia or hemiparesis. The corresponding lesion is in the fibers of the anterior corpus callosum.

Most patients with limb apraxia will also evidence buccal-lingual apraxia, with difficulty executing oral and facial movements on command (e.g., "stick out your tongue," "blow out a match," "sniff a flower," "cough"). These apraxic syndromes are less predictable in left-handed than in right-handed people; left-handed individuals are right dominant for praxis regardless of which hemisphere is dominant for language. Apraxia in right-handed individuals is almost always associated with a left-hemisphere lesion, but only about half of patients with aphasia exhibit apraxia, which suggests that the right hemisphere compensates more readily for apraxia than for aphasia.

TABLE 6–4.	Characteristics of ideomotor apraxias		
	Parietal	Sympathetic	Callosal
Aphasia	Conduction	Broca's	None
Apraxic limbs	Right and left	Left	Left
Hemiparesis	None	Right	None
Lesion location	Inferior parietal, arcuate fasciculus	Left frontal lobe	Anterior callosal fibers

Ideational apraxia features loss of the ability to pantomime execution of an act that requires multiple steps to complete. For example, patients cannot demonstrate how they would fold a letter, place it in an envelope, seal it, place a stamp, and address the envelope. Pantomiming other complex acts is similarly compromised (e.g., filling and lighting a pipe, filling a pitcher and pouring a glass of liquid). This unusual disorder occurs in patients with diffuse brain injuries and dementia.

■ ACALCULIA

Three types of acalculia have been described. The first occurs with lesions of the posterior left hemisphere that produce fluent aphasia and paraphasic errors. When paraphasic intrusions affect numbers, patients substitute one number for another, making accurate computation impossible. The second occurs with lesions of the angular gyrus region and is a true anarithmetria with disruption of primary calculation concepts (i.e., addition, subtraction, division, multiplication). The third is seen in patients with lesions of the posterior right hemisphere and reflects compromised spatial abilities, disrupting proper alignment of numbers and subverting multiple-digit manipulations.

■ GERSTMANN AND ANGULAR GYRUS SYNDROMES

Gerstmann syndrome consists of agraphia, acalculia, right-left disorientation, and finger agnosia. Many patients have a mild constructional disturbance. Agraphia and acalculia are demonstrated easily with tests of writing and arithmetic. Right-left disorientation may be subtle and should be assessed by asking patients to touch their own right and left limbs, to touch their right or left side with the opposite limb, and to indicate which is the clinician's right and left side as the clinician faces them. The last test requires patients to make a mental reversal of right and left. Finger agnosia, if severe, can be shown by asking patients to name their own fingers or to indicate fingers named by the examiner. If the disturbance is more subtle, it can be demonstrated by asking patients to show on one hand the finger that is equivalent to that touched by the examiner on the other hand, which is held out of the patients' sight, or by asking them to state how many fingers are between two being touched by the examiner while the patients' eyes are closed. Gerstmann syndrome reliably indicates the presence of a left angular gyrus lesion when all elements of the syndrome are simultaneously present. Individually, the components of the syndrome can be seen with lesions of other brain regions and do not imply the presence of a lesion of the angular gyrus.

Angular gyrus syndrome occurs with lesions of the left angular gyrus; the lesions are generally larger than those that produce Gerstmann syndrome. Angular gyrus syndrome includes all elements of Gerstmann syndrome plus a constructional disturbance, alexia, anomia, parietal-type ideomotor apraxia, and verbal memory disturbance. The syndrome may be mistaken for Alzheimer's disease because it involves multiple cognitive abnormalities and no motor deficits.

■ DISCONNECTION SYNDROMES

Alexia without agraphia is an example of a *disconnection syndrome*: the right occipital lobe perceives the information to be read, but the signal cannot be transferred to the left hemisphere because of the lesion of the corpus callosum. The left and right hemispheres are disconnected. Conduction aphasia (discussed earlier in this chapter) and sympathetic and callosal apraxias are other examples of disconnection syndromes.

■ REFERENCES

Altshuler LL, Cummings JL, Mills MJ: Mutism: review, differential diagnosis, and report of 22 cases. Am J Psychiatry 143(11):1409–1414, 1986

Ardila A: A proposed reinterpretation of Gerstmann's syndrome. Arch Clin Neuropsychol 29(8):828–833, 2014 25377466

Ardila A, Rosselli M: Spatial agraphia. Brain Cogn 22(2):137–147, 1993 8373568

Arnts H, van Erp WS, Lavrijsen JCM, et al: On the pathophysiology and treatment of akinetic mutism. Neurosci Biobehav Rev 112:270–278, 2020

Benavides-Varela S, Piva D, Burgio F, et al: Re-assessing acalculia: distinguishing spatial and purely arithmetical deficits in right-hemisphere damaged patients. Cortex 88:151–164, 2017

Blonder LX, Bowers D, Heilman KM: The role of the right hemisphere in emotional communication. Brain 114(Pt 3):1115–1127, 1991 2065243

Cancelliere AE, Kertesz A: Lesion localization in acquired deficits of emotional expression and comprehension. Brain Cogn 13(2):133–147, 1990 1697174

Caplan D: Aphasic syndromes, in Clinical Neuropsychology, 5th Edition. Edited by Heilman KM, Valenstein E. New York, Oxford University Press, 2012, pp 22–41

Cappelletti M, Cipolotti L: The neuropsychology of acquired calculation disorders, in The Handbook of Clinical Neuropsychology, 2nd Edition. Edited by Gurd J, Kischka U, Marshall J. New York, Oxford University Press, 2010, pp 401–417

Chawal J, Epstein N: Apraxia in Neurologic Differential Diagnosis, A Case Based Approach. Edited by Ettinger AB, Weisbrot DM. Cambridge, UK, Cambridge University Press, 2014, pp 41–44

Damasio AR, Damasio H: Aphasia and the neural basis of language, in Principles of Behavioral and Cognitive Neurology, 2nd Edition. Edited by Mesulam M-M. New York, Oxford University Press, 2000, pp 294–315

Darley FL, Aronson AE, Brown JR: Motor Speech Disorders. Philadelphia, PA, WB Saunders, 1975

de Smet HJ, Engelborghs S, Paquier PF, et al: Cerebellar-induced apraxic agraphia: a review and three new cases. Brain Cogn 76:424–434, 2011

Enderby P: Disorders of communication: dysarthria. Handb Clin Neurol 110:273–281, 2013 23312647

Fridriksson J, den Ouden DB, Hillis AE, et al: Anatomy of aphasia revisited. Brain 141:848–862, 2018

Gardner H, Winner E, Rehak A: Artistry and aphasia, in Acquired Aphasia, 2nd Edition. Edited by Sarno MT. New York, Academic Press, 1991, pp 373–404

Goodglass H, Kaplan E, Barresi B: The Assessment of Aphasia and Related Disorders, 3rd Edition. Philadelphia, PA, Lippincott Williams and Williams, 2001

Graff-Radford NR, Welsh K, Godersky J: Callosal apraxia. Neurology 37(1):100–105, 1987 3796825

Grandjean D: Brain networks of emotional prosody processing. Emotion Review 13:34–43, 2021

Heilman KM: Apraxia. Continuum (Minneap Minn) 16(4):86–98, 2010

Kang EK, Sohn HM, Han MK, Paik NJ: Subcortical aphasia after stroke. Ann Rehabil Med 41:725–733, 2017

Kertesz A, Ferro JM. Lesion size and location in ideomotor apraxia. Brain 107(pt 3):921–933, 1984 6206911

Klein GE, Micic D: Aphasia, in Neurologic Differential Diagnosis: A Case-Based Approach. Edited by Ettinger AB, Weisbrot DM. Cambridge, UK, Cambridge University Press, 2014, pp 34–40

Leff A, Starrfelt R: Alexia: Diagnosis, Treatment and Theory. London, Springer-Verlag, 2014

Leon SA, Rodriguez AD, Rosenbek JC: Right hemisphere damage and prosody, in The Oxford Handbook of Aphasia and Language Disorders. Edited by Raymer AM, Gonzalez Rothi LJ. New York, Oxford University Press, 2017, pp 277–289

McPherson SE, Kuratani JD, Cummings JL, et al: Creutzfeldt-Jakob disease with mixed transcortical aphasia: insights into echolalia. Behav Neurol 7(3):197–203, 1994 24487337

Norbury C, Paul R: Disorders of speech, language, and communication, in Rutter's Child and Adolescent Psychiatry, 6th Edition. Edited by Thaper A, Pine DS, Leckman FJ, et al. Hoboken, NJ, John Wiley and Sons, 2015, pp 683–701

Oggioni GD, Espay AJ: Mutism, in Neurologic Differential Diagnosis: A Case-Based Approach. Edited by Ettinger AB, Weisbrot DM. Cambridge, UK, Cambridge University Press, 2014, pp 266–269

Park JE: Apraxia: review and update. J Clin Neurol 13(4):317–324, 2017

Ross ED: Affective prosody and the aprosodias, in Principles of Behavioral and Cognitive Neurology, 2nd Edition. Edited by Mesulam M-M. New York, Oxford University Press, 2000, pp 316–331

Rosselli M, Ardila A: Calculation deficits in patients with right and left hemisphere damage. Neuropsychologia 27(5):607–617, 1989 2739887

Rusconi E: Gerstmann syndrome: historic and current perspectives. Handb Clin Neurol 151:395–411, 2018 29519471

Sandson J, Albert ML: Perseveration in behavioral neurology. Neurology 37(11):1736–1741, 1987 3670611

Starkstein SE, Fedoroff JP, Price TR, et al: Catastrophic reaction after cerebrovascular lesions: frequency, correlates, and validation of a scale. J Neuropsychiatry Clin Neurosci 5(2):189–194, 1993 8508037

Starrfelt R, Behrmann M: Number reading in pure alexia: a review. Neuropsychologia 49(9):2283–2298, 2011 21554892

Tippett DC, Ross E: Prosody and the aprosodias, in The Handbook of Language Disorders. Edited by Hillis AE. New York, Psychology Press, 2015, pp 518–529

Vandenborre D, van Dun K, Engelborghs S, Marien P: Apraxic agraphia following thalamic damage: three new cases. Brain Lang 150:153–165, 2015 26460984

Wallesch CW, Johannsen-Horbach H, Blanken G: The assessment of acquired spoken language disorders, in The Handbook of Clinical Neuropsychology, 2nd Edition. Edited by Gurd J, Kischka U, Marshall J. New York, Oxford University Press, 2010, pp 235–250

Willmes K: Acalculia. Handb Clin Neurol 88:339–358, 2008 18631700

7

VISUAL, VISUOSPATIAL, AND RIGHT-BRAIN DISORDERS

Lauren Drag, Ph.D.

The ability to understand and interact with the complex visual environment around us relies on a range of critical processes, including visual perception; recognition of places, objects, and people; visuospatial memory and construction; processing of visuospatial patterns; and spatial orientation and navigation. Processing of visuospatial information relies heavily on the right hemisphere, and right-hemisphere injury also causes various neuropsychiatric symptoms. This chapter discusses the principal visuospatial disorders and their associated lesions or causative disorders.

■ VISUOPERCEPTUAL DISORDERS

Visual connections begin with photo and color receptors in the retina and travel the optic nerve. Fibers mediating vision from the medial region of each retina cross in the optic chiasm. Crossed and uncrossed fibers travel the optic tract to the lateral geniculate body, where fibers synapse with geniculocalcarine fibers projecting to the occipital cortex. Fibers carrying visual data from the superior visual fields sweep anteriorly through the temporal lobe to the inferior sulcus of the occipital lobe. Fibers carrying information from the inferior visual fields project posteriorly through the parietal lobe to the superior sulcus of the occipital lobe.

Perception refers to the ability to sense a stimulus regardless of whether it is recognized. Recognition of a stimulus is a sequential process that begins with perception and progresses through stages of increasing refinement. Visuospatial processing is often separated into two complementary streams. A ventral stream extends from the primary visual cortex into the temporal cortex, subserving recognition and the discrimination of objects

120

TABLE 7–1.	Visuoperceptual disorders
Achromatopsia	Central color blindness
Balint's syndrome	Optic ataxia, sticky fixation (difficulty volitionally redirecting gaze), and simultanagnosia
Cortical blindness	Vision loss due to bilateral lesions of geniculolocalcarine radiations or occipital cortex
Homonymous hemianopsia	Bilateral visual field loss in two halves of visual field
Monocular blindness	Total or partial blindness of involved eye
Simultanagnosia	Failure to perceive one of two objects presented simultaneously, typically associated with bilateral parietal lesions

(i.e., the "what" stream). There is also a dorsal stream that extends from the primary visual cortex into the parietal cortex and has traditionally been associated with visually guided reaching and other spatial-based behaviors (i.e., the "where" stream). It has been proposed that this dorsal stream involves multiple complex pathways involving the prefrontal, premotor, and medial temporal cortices to support visually guided executive of actions and spatial behaviors. The dorsal stream has been associated with top-down attentional control (e.g., deploying goal-directed spatial behaviors), which is in contrast to the bottom-up nature of the ventral stream (e.g., recognizing and directing attention to environmental stimuli).

Interruption of the perceptual process at different stages results in different types of clinical deficits (Table 7–1). Lesions of the eye or optic nerve produce ipsilateral blindness (partial or total); lesions behind the optic chiasm result in homonymous visual field defects; pathological changes in the inferior calcarine cortex produce achromatopsia (central color blindness); medial occipitotemporal lesions of the right hemisphere are associated with prosopagnosia (inability to recognize familiar faces) and environmental agnosia (impaired recognition of familiar places); and bilateral lesions of the medial occipitotemporal cortex or inferior longitudinal fasciculi cause visual object agnosia.

Monocular Blindness

Ocular disorders—including diseases of the lens (cataracts), retina, or macula—produce total or partial blindness of the in-

TABLE 7–2. Characteristics of blindness of different etiologies

Characteristic	Prechiasmal lesion	Cortical blindness	As a conversion symptom
Consensual pupillary reaction	Present*	Present	Present
Direct pupillary reaction	Absent	Present	Present
Optokinetic nystagmus	Absent	Absent	Present
Visual evoked response	Abnormal	Abnormal	Normal

*A consensual pupillary response is present in blindness with prechiasmal lesions when the blindness is unilateral; bilateral prechiasmal blindness would eliminate the consensual response.

volved eye. Likewise, diseases of the optic nerve (e.g., glaucoma affecting the nerve head, ischemic optic neuritis, and optic neuritis) produce unilateral blindness ipsilateral to the lesion. Pupillary responses are usually compromised in diseases of the eye and optic nerve because there is diminished light conduction, and this sign may help distinguish blindness as a manifestation of ocular or neurological disease from feigned blindness or from blindness as a manifestation of a conversion reaction. In addition, patients with conversion disorders or who are malingering have intact optokinetic nystagmus (i.e., nystagmus normally induced by passing a striped cloth in front of the eyes of a sighted person). Table 7–2 presents characteristics that aid in distinguishing among different types of blindness.

Acute optic neuritis may produce edema of the nerve head; this can be identified by ophthalmoscopy and must be distinguished from papilledema associated with raised intracranial pressure. Visual acuity is compromised in the former and spared in the latter.

Long-standing bilateral blindness may result in pendular nystagmus with spontaneous to-and-fro movements of the eyes. Visual hallucinations ("release" hallucinations) are not uncommon in patients with ocular disorders and may be either formed or unformed. Phosphenes (sudden flashes of light) often accompany retinal or optic nerve disease, and some patients may experience synesthesia characterized by phosphenes occurring in response to loud sounds or noises.

Visual evoked responses are slowed in patients with optic nerve disease; they offer a means of documenting the presence of disease in patients with normal fundoscopic examinations. Visual evoked potentials may be slowed even when visual acuity is measurably normal and may be useful in establishing the presence of optic nerve disease in patients with suspected multiple sclerosis or other conditions affecting the optic nerves.

Homonymous Hemianopsia

Lesions of the optic tract, optic chiasm, geniculate nucleus of the thalamus, or geniculocalcarine radiations produce homonymous visual field defects. Temporal lobe lesions are associated with asymmetric (incongruent) field defects, and occipital lesions cause symmetric (congruent) defects. Lesions involving the entire radiation produce homonymous hemianopsias (usually with sparing of the central few degrees of vision), whereas lesions affecting only some of the fiber tracts produce quadrantanopsias or other incomplete field defects. Pupillary responses are intact in patients with homonymous visual-field defects, and visual acuity is normal. Hallucinations are common in the period immediately following an injury to the geniculocalcarine radiations (e.g., in the first few days after a stroke) and may be unformed (lights), semiformed (tire track or herringbone patterns), or formed (complex scenes, animals, or people). The hallucinations are usually confined to the area of the visual field defect.

Achromatopsia

Achromatopsia refers to central color blindness. Patients lose the ability to distinguish color in the contralateral visual field. The associated lesions involve the cortex inferior to the calcarine fissure of the medial occipital lobe. There is often an associated partial hemianopsia. The color blindness is difficult to demonstrate except when it is bilateral. Color blindness is assessed with color-naming tests, tests requiring sorting of colors by shades, and Ishihara pseudoisochromatic plates.

Cortical Blindness

Cortical or cerebral blindness occurs when bilateral lesions of the geniculocalcarine radiations or occipital cortex deprive patients of all vision. They may be totally blinded or have sufficient residual vision to distinguish light from darkness and to be able to count fingers. If central vision is spared, patients may be able to see minimally by moving their heads to allow exploration of the environment via a tiny retained central visual field. They may see very small objects better than large objects; their reduced visual field allows them to see small objects as a whole, but they must scan larger objects. Pupillary responses are intact, but optokinetic nystagmus is lost. Some individuals may experience blindsight, in which they are able to respond to visual stimuli despite an inability to consciously perceive these stimuli.

The most common cause of cortical blindness is occlusion of both posterior cerebral arteries with bilateral medial occipital infarction. The lesions may be observed on CT or MRI. Cortical blindness has occurred with diffuse cortical injuries, such as anoxic insults.

Anton's syndrome is blindness with denial of blindness. Patients claim to see and even describe what they think they see but are inaccurate in the descriptions and can be shown to be blind. Anton's syndrome occurs most commonly in patients with cortical blindness but may also occur in patients with other types of blindness when they are in acute confusional states or have dementia. Many patients with blindness due to bilateral posterior cerebral lesions are severely agitated even if they are unaware of their blindness.

Simultanagnosia

Simultanagnosia is a misnamed exception. In this disorder, when patients are shown two objects simultaneously, they fail to perceive one of them. For example, when shown a figure consisting of a circle and a cross, patients see the circle or the cross but not both; when shown a number drawn by juxtaposing many small numbers (e.g., a number 2 drawn using many little number 3s), they see either the number 2 or the number 3s but not both. The neurophysiological basis of this mysterious condition has not been determined, but it is most likely attributable to an abnormality of visual attention and typically occurs in patients with bilateral parietal lobe lesions.

Simultanagnosia is frequently observed as part of *Balint's syndrome*. The latter consists of optic ataxia (the inability to touch objects accurately using visual guidance), sticky fixation (difficulty volitionally redirecting gaze), and simultanagnosia.

■ VISUAL DISCRIMINATION DEFICITS

Impaired visual discrimination takes many forms, and each can be demonstrated with a specific discrimination task. Discrimination abnormalities include difficulties with matching the orientation and angles of lines, matching unfamiliar faces (e.g., similar faces with different emotional expressions or faces of the same person viewed from different angles), discriminating between overlapping or embedded figures, and matching complex visual patterns. These disorders are more common with lesions of the posterior aspect of the right hemisphere than with lesions elsewhere in the brain.

■ VISUAL RECOGNITION DISORDERS

Agnosias are disorders of visual recognition and perception with spared basic vision. Most agnosias are associated with bilateral involvement of the occipital, occipitoparietal, and occipitotemporal areas (Table 7–3).

Color Agnosia

Color agnosia is present in some individuals with alexia without agraphia (see Chapter 6, "Aphasia and Related Syndromes"). This is a deficit neither of naming nor of perception. Patients do not have abnormalities of color naming and can name the colors as appropriate to specific settings (e.g., a banana is yellow, a fire engine is red); they also can sort and match colors. They do not have color blindness. However, they cannot point to named colors or name colors pointed to by the examiner. These patients have lesions of the left or bilateral occipitotemporal region.

Environmental Agnosia

Environmental agnosia is a clinical syndrome characterized by the inability to recognize familiar places. Patients see normally and are able to describe their surroundings but have no sense of familiarity. Patients frequently adopt verbal strategies in order to compensate for the deficit; for example, they may find their homes using the street signs and house numbers. Environmental agnosia and prosopagnosia often coexist. The causative lesion is in the medial occipitotemporal region of the right hemisphere.

TABLE 7–3.	Visual recognition disorders
Color agnosia	Inability to point to named colors or to name colors pointed to by the examiner; associated with lesions of the medial left occipital cortex and the splenium of the corpus callosum
Environmental agnosia	Inability to recognize familiar places, associated with right medial occipitotemporal lesions
Finger agnosia	Inability to name, localize, or discriminate among fingers, a characteristic of Gerstmann syndrome
Prosopagnosia	Inability to recognize familiar faces, associated with right or bilateral medial occipital lesions
Visual object agnosia	Apperceptive (inability to recognize objects due to perceptual processing impairments) vs. associative (inability to recognize objects despite intact perception)

Finger Agnosia

Finger agnosia, the disorder accompanying Gerstmann syndrome, is characterized by an inability to name, localize, or discriminate among fingers (the patient's own fingers and the fingers of others). This can be assessed by asking patients to follow a series of commands involving specific fingers (e.g., "Touch your middle finger to my thumb"). Other aspects of Gerstmann syndrome include agraphia, acalculia, and right-left disorientation.

Prosopagnosia

Prosopagnosia refers to the inability to recognize familiar faces. Visual perception is intact; patients see normally and can describe unrecognized faces in detail. However, familiar faces, such as those of family members and famous people, cannot be recognized, and patients cannot deduce the person's identity without the aid of nonvisual clues. They are also unable to learn new faces. In some cases, specific facial features (e.g., moustache, glasses of a specific type) are used to facilitate recognition, but patients are easily fooled if someone with similar characteristics appears. This impairment is specific to visual information; when the person's voice is heard, recognition is usually immediate, demonstrating that nonvisual means of recognition and naming are intact. Despite these conscious deficits in facial recognition, individuals with prosopagnosia may show above-chance performance when asked to recognize familiar faces, suggesting some degree of retained implicit knowledge. Tests of visual discrimination (e.g., matching faces photographed from two different angles and matching different faces with similar emotional expressions) are not necessarily compromised; facial recognition and facial discrimination are different neuropsychological capacities mediated by different processes and affected by lesions in different locations.

Bilateral occipitotemporal lesions are present in many reported patients with prosopagnosia, but right unilateral regions appear to be sufficient to produce the syndrome.

Visual Object Agnosia

Two principal types of visual object agnosia have been identified: apperceptive agnosia and associative agnosia. These syndromes reflect disruption of different stages of complex visual information processing, and variations of the syndromes are common. *Apperceptive visual agnosia* is characterized by the failure to recognize a stimulus due to an inability to integrate individual components despite an intact ability to perceive these components. This reflects disturbance of perception. Patients can distinguish shades of light intensity, identify colors, determine line orientation, exhibit depth perception, see movement, and distinguish thin from thick lines. They can negotiate their surroundings but cannot recognize, describe, or match perceived objects. They cannot draw objects they see and cannot point to objects named by the examiner. The agnosia involves all visual stimuli, including faces, the environment, and objects. Apperceptive agnosia may occur as a phase of recovery from cortical blindness following anoxia, carbon monoxide poisoning, or bilateral posterior hemispheric strokes.

Associative visual agnosia involves the impaired retrieval of knowledge about an object despite intact elementary perception and preserved ability to describe, draw, and match visual stimuli. This reflects a disturbance of memory. For example, when shown an object (e.g., shoe, toothbrush), patients can draw the object and match it with an identical one from a group of objects, but they cannot recognize the object or describe its use. When allowed to touch the object or hear any sounds it may make (e.g., a bell or ring), patients immediately recognize the object and can describe it or demonstrate its use. Object recognition and naming by touch indicates that patients are not anomic and that the agnosia is modality specific, limited to the visual domain. Agnosia for faces, letters, and colors usually but not invariably accompanies visual object recognition defect. Visual-field defects, particularly a right homonymous hemianopsia, may be present. Most patients with associative visual agnosia have diffuse cortical injury or bilateral medial occipitotemporal lesions involving the cortex or the inferior longitudinal fasciculi.

■ DISTURBANCES OF VISUOSPATIAL ATTENTION

Insult to various regions of the brain can cause disorders of visuospatial inattention, resulting in difficulty directing attention to locations or stimuli in space (Table 7–4). Deficits in visuospatial attention can be lateralized (e.g., the left side of space) or more generalized in nature (e.g., poor attention to visual detail).

Unilateral Neglect

The right hemisphere is dominant for spatial attention, and right-hemisphere dysfunction can result in diminished awareness of information, particularly that presented to the left side. *Unilateral* (or *hemispatial*) *neglect* refers to a lack of attention to events and actions in one half of space. Neglect may involve all sensory modalities—visual, auditory, and somatosensory—as well as motor acts and motivation. *Unilateral visual neglect* is the most commonly observed form of hemispatial neglect. In its most subtle form, patients ignore the stimulus presented in the neglected hemifield. This type of neglect can be demonstrated by facing patients and holding one's hands in equivalent portions of each visual field, quickly moving the fingers of each hand, and asking patients to point to the hand whose fingers moved (the technique of double simultaneous stimulation). Patients will perceive movement only in the nonneglected visual field. This test requires that patients not have a field defect.

In its more obvious form, unilateral visual neglect may be evidenced by failure to copy one-half of model objects, read one-half of words, dress one-half of the body, or shave one-half of the face. A common test for visual neglect is line bisection, in which patients are given a sheet of paper with randomly distributed lines and asked to cross each line in the middle; only those lines in the nonneglected field will be crossed, and the patients' bisection will be biased toward the nonneglected side of the line. Visual neglect can also be evident on tasks requiring visual scanning and search. For example, the Bells Test requires patients to scan and cross out a target item; objects are scattered on the page in a nonlinear fashion, requiring that patients implement a search strategy. Patients

128

TABLE 7–4. Disturbances of visuospatial attention

Neglect syndromes and anosognosia	
Unilateral neglect	Lack of attention to events and actions in one half of space
Anosognosia and anosognosic syndromes	Denial of illness, typically associated with right parietal lesions
Symbol or figure-cancellation abnormalities	Nonlateralized inattention can occur with frontal lobe lesions or more diffuse cerebral disorders

with left neglect will be prone to omitting targets on the left side of the page (with omissions occurring closer to the middle of the page indicating more severe neglect). Constructional tasks, such as asking patients to copy a figure (Figure 7–1) or draw a clock, often reveal the neglect: they copy or draw only the nonneglected portion of the figure. Clock-drawing tests can be misleading in patients with frontal lobe syndromes and poor planning because these patients fail to properly space the figures on the clock face and may include most of the digits on one part of the clock, thus producing a drawing that superficially resembles figures produced by patients with true unilateral neglect.

Neglect may occur in the absence of a homonymous hemianopia, and patients with homonymous field defects may learn to compensate for their visual impairment if they do not have a neglect syndrome. Neglect and visual-field defects have no obligatory relationship and must be assessed separately.

In severe forms of neglect, all types of stimuli in the affected hemiuniverse are neglected. *Somesthetic neglect* is established by touching patients simultaneously on both sides of the body and asking them where they were touched; patients perceive only the touch on the nonneglected side of the body. *Auditory neglect* is assessed by standing behind patients, snapping one's fingers on either or both sides of the head, and asking them to point toward the side on which a stimulus was heard. Patients point only toward the nonneglected side during double simultaneous auditory stimulation.

Sensory neglect is most severe and enduring after damage to the right parietal region, but it may occur with left parietal and subcortical lesions. Hemispatial neglect is contralateral to the side of the lesion.

Motor neglect syndromes involve action-intention disorders affecting the half of space that is contralateral to the frontal lobe

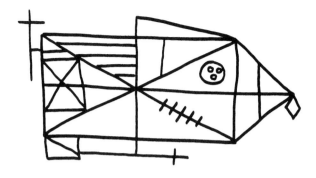

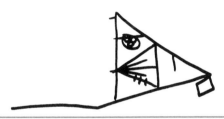

FIGURE 7–1. Rey-Osterreith Complex Figure (*top*) and a copy of the figure made by a patient with a right parietal lobe lesion (*bottom*).

The copy demonstrates neglect of the left half of the figure.

or basal ganglia lesions. Patients are aware of stimuli in the neglected hemispace (no sensory neglect is present) but produce no motor response in the neglected area. They may appear to have a hemiparesis because the limb with action-intention neglect is unused, but when tested, their strength and coordination are found to be normal. The abnormality may be most evident when patients are asked to perform movements with both arms, such as extending or drawing circles in the air with them: the limb with action-intention neglect fails to perform normally.

Anosognosia and Anosognosic Syndromes

Anosognosia is a clinical syndrome characterized by denial of hemiparesis. It classically occurs in patients with right-parietal lesions and left-unilateral neglect who deny their left hemiparesis. The extended syndrome of denial of illness may involve other types of disability, such as blindness and aphasia. Risk factors for persistent anosognosia include large right-sided lesions, severe left-sided neglect, cognitive and memory deficits, apathy, and cerebral atrophy.

Variants of anosognosia include *somatoparaphrenia* (denial of ownership of the paralyzed limbs), *anosodiaphoria* (minimization of and unconcern about the weakness without complete denial), *misoplegia* (hatred of the paralyzed or weak limb), *personification* (naming the limb and giving it an identity), and *supernumerary limbs* (reduplication of limbs on the neglected side). Patients with anosognosia or its variants typically have other evidence of neglect, such as extinguishing stimuli on the paretic side during double simultaneous stimulation or failing to reproduce elements on the neglected side when asked to copy model figures.

Symbol- or Figure-Cancellation Abnormalities

In addition to lateralized neglect contralateral to a hemispheric lesion, some patients may have nonlateralized visual attention disturbances. These disturbances occur with frontal lobe lesions, right-hemisphere injuries, or more diffuse cerebral disorders (extensive white matter alterations) and can be seen on cancellation tests in which patients are asked to survey a page with multiple letters or symbols and to circle or cross out a specific target. Targets are most likely to be neglected on the side contralateral to the lesion but may be missed in any part of space.

■ BODY-SPATIAL DISORIENTATION

Disturbances can arise in individuals' ability to orient to parts of the body, the position of the body in space, and to general spatial awareness (Table 7–5).

Dressing Disturbances

Although frequently called dressing "apraxia," these abnormalities are typically associated with difficulty with orientation and positioning of clothing and body parts and are best regarded as special cases of visuospatial disorders. They are constructional and visual synthesis abnormalities and are not solely due to primary motor, sensory, or general cognitive deficits. Three types of dressing disturbances are seen in clinical practice. *Body-garment*

TABLE 7–5. Body-spatial disorientation

Dressing disturbances

  Body-garment disorientation: Right parietal lesions, inability to orient body parts with respect to clothing

  Unilateral neglect: Results in dressing or attending to only one side of the body

  Excessive layering: Can be associated with more generalized cognitive impairment

Impaired map reading

Impaired route finding when map is not used

Impaired visual determination of vertical when one's body is not vertical

disorientation occurs almost exclusively with right parietal-lobe lesions and consists of an inability to properly orient the limbs and trunk with respect to clothing. Patients may put on a shirt or blouse inside out or even try to put a leg into a sleeve. The task is made particularly difficult by giving the patients a garment that is turned inside out and asking them to correct it and put it on. Lesions to the left parietal lobe typically impact dressing due to generalized difficulty with planning and sequencing of movements of limbs (akin to an ideational apraxia). *Unilateral neglect* may be manifest by dressing only one-half of the body. Patients may put only one arm (the nonneglected side) into a shirt or may comb the hair on only one-half of the head. A third type of dressing disturbance, *excessive layering* of clothes, occurs in patients with dementia and schizophrenia and in this instance can be associated with more generalized confusion and cognitive impairment.

Other Body-Spatial Disturbances

Other disorders of orientation of the body within space include impaired map reading, impaired route finding when no map is utilized, and impaired visual determination of vertical when one's body is not vertical.

■ CONSTRUCTIONAL DISORDERS

Constructional apraxia is broadly defined as an inability to assemble individual elements into a whole (i.e., impairment in part-to-whole relationships) (Table 7–6); this can involve build-

132

TABLE 7–6.	Constructional disorders
Copying deficits	Associated with both perceptual and executive difficulties and lesions to occipital, parietal, or frontal regions
Drawing abnormalities	Can be more impacted by frontal compared with parietal lesions

ing or assembling objects but is most often assessed with copying or drawing tasks. This constructional deficit cannot solely be attributed to impairment in motor output, although individuals with motor apraxia will nevertheless have significant difficulties in copying and drawing. Constructional tasks are one of the best means of assessing visuospatial function in the clinic or at the bedside, and copying and drawing tests should be part of every mental status examination. A series of constructions of graded difficulty is used to assess copying skills. Begin by having patients draw a circle; this helps them understand the test, experience some initial success, and engage the task. Then have the patients copy more complicated figures, such as a diamond, overlapping rectangles, or a cube or more demanding models such as the Rey-Osterreith or Taylor Complex figures (Figure 7–2). Drawing abilities can be evaluated by asking patients to draw a clock, a flower, and a house. Copying and drawing of figures can be disrupted by a range of factors, including failure to perceive a gestalt, inattention or neglect, spatial deficits, and difficulty with planning a systematic approach to the task.

Copying tests assess both perception and executive visuomotor abilities and may be affected by occipital, parietal, or frontal lobe dysfunction of either hemisphere. Temporal lobe lesions have little effect on copying tests. Unilateral neglect implies the presence of a lesion of the contralateral hemisphere; other lesion effects are less discriminating. Occipitoparietal lesions disturb perception and figure recognition and tend to produce more profound constructional changes. Left-hemisphere lesions tend to have a greater effect on patients' ability to reproduce the internal detail of an object, while leaving the ability to reproduce the external, holistic configuration intact. Right-sided lesions have the opposite effect; they adversely affect patients' ability to perceive the object as a whole despite intact ability to execute internal details (i.e., missing the proverbial forest for the trees). Thus, the left hemisphere is superior for processing details whereas the right hemisphere is superior for processing in-

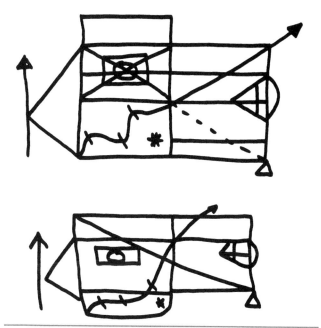

FIGURE 7–2. Taylor Complex Figure (*top*) and a copy of the figure made by a patient with a dementia syndrome and visuospatial dysfunction (*bottom*).

The copy demonstrates distortions and omissions.

formation as a whole (i.e., the gestalt). Frontal lobe lesions affect the planning and strategy patients use to accomplish the copying task; these patients usually take a fragmented approach to the task, copying individual subsegments of the figure without an organized approach, perseverating on certain details, and over-developing portions of the figure that attract their attention.

Patients with parietal lobe lesions may do better on spontaneous drawing tasks (for which they have less dependence on reproducing a model figure) than on copying tasks (for which they must accurately perceive and reproduce the figure). Individuals with frontal lobe disorders have equal difficulty with drawing and copying or may exhibit environmental dependency and slavishly copy the presented figure while having more difficulty with spontaneous drawing. Patients with right-hemisphere lesions can demonstrate left-sided neglect, but there is some indication that, in general, spontaneous drawing is impacted more by left-hemisphere than right-hemisphere lesions. Spontaneous drawing can also be affected by a loss of semantic knowledge (e.g., in semantic dementia) and in these cases, drawings will be simplified.

■ VISUOSPATIAL COGNITION AND MEMORY DISORDERS

In addition to the visual and visuospatial deficits described, a variety of other cognitive and memory disturbances have been described that primarily affect processing of nonverbal information (i.e., information that cannot be readily described verbally). This can include, for example, difficulties performing arithmetic calculations requiring spatial organization, difficulty navigating even in familiar surroundings, and reduced attention span and recall of visual information.

Detection of most of these disturbances depends on the use of structured neuropsychological tests, and most are more common after lesions of the right hemisphere than after lesions of the left hemisphere. However, neuropsychological tests do not always localize well to the right hemisphere, and many tasks assess multiple cognitive domains that rely on bilateral processes. Even measures putatively visuospatial in nature (e.g., visual memory) are not always specific to right-hemisphere dysfunction, given that multiple processes can be involved (e.g., planning and organization). Furthermore, even visual-based tasks without words can still be verbalized in some way, which introduces potential involvement of the left hemisphere.

Design fluency (see Chapter 5, "Frontal Lobe Syndromes," Figure 5–1) assesses patients' ability to generate novel designs using four lines of equal length that touch at least one other line. This task can recruit both right- and left-frontal processes. The ability to synthesize fragments of objects into a whole and properly identify them is evaluated by tests such as the Hooper Visual Organization Test. Commonly associated with the right parietal lobe, Judgment of Line Orientation is a measure of visuospatial perception that requires patients to match the angle and orientation of arrays of lines. In mental rotation tests, patients are asked to imagine what a specific complex figure would look like if rotated and then choose the answer from among several similar-appearing alternatives. Mental rotation is also typically localized to the right parietal lobe. *Visual search* is the ability to scan a visual environment for a particular object. Like visual neglect, the organization and efficiency of visual search can be measured with cancellation tasks that require identification of target stimuli from among distractors. Visual search is thought to involve the right or bilateral posterior regions. Finally, right-sided posterior injuries can impact the organization and sequencing of visual information, such as understanding temporal ordering and relationships (e.g., sequencing pictures into a story).

Revisualization refers to the ability to produce and describe an "internal" image of a named object (e.g., flag, bicycle, elephant). Patients with bilateral parietal lobe lesions may have deficits in recalling imagery (i.e., internal revisualization) and in imagining or describing a named object. This can also result in a loss of dreams (Charcot-Wilbrand syndrome).

Visual memory disturbances are best identified by showing patients figures that cannot be easily verbalized or named (e.g., tangled lines, line drawings, symbols) and asking them to draw the figures from memory or choose the figures from a multiple-choice array after a delay. Right temporal lobe lesions have the greatest effect on visual memory.

Reduplicative paramnesia is a syndrome in which patients claim they are simultaneously in two or more locations; it occurs in patients with lesions of both frontal lobes and the right temporal lobes (see Chapter 8, "Memory and Its Disorders").

Although language capabilities are typically ascribed to the left hemisphere, right-hemisphere injuries can affect language processing in more subtle ways. Right-hemisphere dysfunction can result in fluent (and possibly overly verbose) but illogical and aprosodic speech. Language comprehension can also be impacted by a failure to organize and a loss of the gist and gestalt of information.

■ NEUROPSYCHIATRIC SYNDROMES ASSOCIATED WITH RIGHT-BRAIN DYSFUNCTION

The disturbances addressed in this chapter are seen more often with right-hemisphere dysfunction than with left-brain disorders; thus, they may coexist with neuropsychiatric syndromes that occur with right-brain lesions. The principal neuropsychiatric syndromes occurring in patients with right-brain dysfunction and their anatomic correlates are presented in Table 7–7. A contrasting set of syndromes occurring with left-brain lesions is provided in Table 7–8.

Mania occurs with lesions of the right hemisphere affecting the orbitofrontal, caudate, perithalamic, or temporobasal region.

TABLE 7–7. Neuropsychiatric syndromes reported in patients with right-brain lesions

Syndrome	Lesion location
Amusia	Temporal lobe
Anosognosia	Parietal lobe
Anxiety	Temporal lobe (especially medially)
Delusions	Temporal lobe, temporoparietal region
Depression	Posterior hemispheric cortex
Dressing disturbance	Parietal lobe
Environmental recognition	Medial occipitotemporal region defects
Executive aprosodia	Frontal lobe
Facial discrimination defects	Parietal lobe
Hyposexuality	Temporal lobe
Left spatial neglect	Parietal lobe
Mania	Orbitofrontal cortex, caudate nucleus, thalamus, temporobasal region
Nonverbal amnesia	Temporal lobe
Palinopsia	Occipital cortex
Prosopagnosia	Medial occipitotemporal region
Receptive aprosodia	Temporal lobe
Schizoid behavior	Posterior hemispheric cortex (especially if sustained early in life)
Visual hallucinations	Geniculocalcarine radiations, occipital cortex, temporal lobe
Visuospatial deficits	Parietal lobe
Voice discrimination deficits	Parietal lobe, temporal lobe
Voice recognition deficits	Parietal lobe

In patients with right-brain lesions, depression is most often associated with right posterior lesions, and anxiety is associated with right temporal lobe dysfunction. Delusions occur with lesions of the right temporal lobe or temporoparietal junction regions. Misidentification syndromes, such as *Capgras syndrome* (i.e., delusion that someone has been replaced by an identical-appearing impostor), are more common with right-sided lesions than with left-sided lesions. Patients with psychotic disorders accompanying right-brain lesions often have marked visual hallucinations with their delusions. Visual hallucinations without delusions may occur with right hemisphere lesions affecting the

TABLE 7–8. Neuropsychiatric syndromes associated with left-brain lesions

Syndrome	Lesion location
Aphasia	Temporal lobe, inferior parietal region, frontal lobe
Apraxia	Parietal lobe, frontal lobe, corpus callosum
Denial of language deficit	Temporoparietal region
Depression	Frontal lobe, temporal lobe, caudate nucleus
Depression with anxiety	Frontal cortex
Primary acalculia	Parietal lobe
Psychosis	Temporal lobe
Right spatial neglect	Parietal lobe
Verbal amnesia	Temporal lobe
Visual hallucinations	Geniculocalcarine radiations, occipital cortex, temporal lobe

geniculocalcarine radiations, occipital cortex, or temporal lobes. Visual hallucinations also are common with lesions affecting the anterior visual structures (either right or left side) and compromising vision. *Palinopsia* is a syndrome of visual perseveration characterized by abnormal persistence or recurrence of visual images; it is most common with right posterior lesions. Schizoid behavior has been reported in patients who sustained right-brain lesions as children. Hyposexuality has been found to be more common after right-hemisphere than left-hemisphere lesions; hypersexuality may occur with the manic syndromes associated with right-brain lesions. Right-hemisphere lesions can result in impaired emotion recognition (e.g., understanding intonation, facial expressions, nonverbal cues) or inappropriate or blunted emotional reactions. Right-hemisphere injuries are also associated with impaired self-awareness; patients may be unaware or indifferent to their difficulties and more apathetic.

■ REFERENCES

Aimola Davies AM, White RC, Davies M: The assessment of anosognosia for motor impairments, in The Handbook of Clinical Neuropsychology, 2nd Edition. Edited by Gurd J, Kischka U, Marshall J. New York, Oxford University Press, 2010, pp 436–470

Aldrich MS, Alessi AG, Beck RW, Gilman S: Cortical blindness: etiology, diagnosis, and prognosis. Ann Neurol 21(2):149–158, 1987 3827223

Bartolomeo P, de Schotten MT, Chica AB: Brain networks of visuospatial attention and their disruption in visual neglect. Front Hum Neurosci 6:110, 2012

Bauer RM, Demery JA: Agnosia, in Clinical Neuropsychology, 5th Edition. Edited by Heilman KM, Valenstein E. New York, Oxford University Press, 2012, pp 238–295

Chechlacz M, Rotshtein P, Hansen PC, et al: The neural underpinings of simultanagnosia: disconnecting the visuospatial attention network. J Cogn Neurosci 24(3):718–735, 2012 22066584

Cutting J: Study of anosognosia. J Neurol Neurosurg Psychiatry 41(6):548–555, 1978 671066

Cutting J: The Right Cerebral Hemisphere and Psychiatric Disorders. New York, Oxford University Press, 1990

Damasio A, Yamada T, Damasio H, et al: Central achromatopsia: behavioral, anatomic, and physiologic aspects. Neurology 30(10):1064–1071, 1980 6968419

Damasio AR, Damasio H, Van Hoesen GW: Prosopagnosia: anatomic basis and behavioral mechanisms. Neurology 32(4):331–341, 1982 7199655

Damasio AR, Tranel D, Rizzo M: Disorders of complex visual processing, in Principles of Behavioral and Cognitive Neurology. Edited by Mesulam M-M. New York, Oxford University Press, 2000, pp 332–372

Eknoyan D, Hurley RA, Taber KH: The clock drawing task: common errors and functional neuroanatomy. J Neuropsychiatry Clin Neurosci 24(3):260–265, 2012 23037640

Farah MJ, Epstein RA: Disorders of visual-spatial perception and cognition, in Clinical Neuropsychology, 5th Edition. Edited by Heilman KM, Valenstein E. New York, Oxford University Press, 2012, pp 152–168

Ffytche DH, Blom JD, Catani M: Disorders of visual perception. J Neurol Neurosurg Psychiatry 81(11):1280–1287, 2010 20972204

Goldenberg G: Apraxia and the parietal lobes. Neuropsychologia 47(6):1449–1459, 2009 18692079

Heilman KM, Watson RT, Valenstein E: Neglect and related disorders, in Clinical Neuropsychology, 5th Edition. Edited by Heilman KM, Valenstein E. New York, Oxford University Press, 2012, pp 296–348

Kravitz DJ, Saleem KS, Baker CI, Mishkin M: A new neural framework for visuospatial processing. Nat Rev Neurosci 12(4):217–230, 2011 21415848

Landis T, Cummings JL, Benson DF, Palmer EP: Loss of topographic familiarity: an environmental agnosia. Arch Neurol 43(2):132–136, 1986 3947250

Mendez MF: Visuoperceptual function in visual agnosia. Neurology 38(11):1754–1759, 1988 3185910

Mesulam M-M: Attentional networks, confusional states and neglect - syndromes, in Principles of Behavioral and Cognitive Neurology, 2nd Edition. Edited by Mesulam M-M. New York, Oxford University Press, 2000, pp 174–256

Pearson J, Naselaris T, Holmes EA, Kosslyn SM: Mental imagery: functional mechanisms and clinical applications. Trends Cogn Sci 19(10):590–602, 2015 26412097

Rizzo M, Smith V, Pokorny J, Damasio AR: Color perception profiles in central achromatopsia. Neurology 43(5):995–1001, 1993 8492959

Robinson RG, Starkstein SE: Current research in affective disorders following stroke. J Neuropsychiatry Clin Neurosci 2(1):1–14, 1990 2136055

Rosen HJ: Anosognosia in neurodegenerative disease. Neurocase 17(3):231–241, 2011 21667396

Shelton PA, Bowers D, Duara R, Heilman KM: Apperceptive visual agnosia: a case study. Brain Cogn 25(1):1–23, 1994 8043261

Swindell CS, Holland AL, Fromm D, Greenhouse JB: Characteristics of recovery of drawing ability in left and right brain-damaged patients. Brain Cogn 7(1):16–30, 1988 3345266

Van Lancker D: Personal relevance and the human right hemisphere. Brain Cogn 17(1):64–92, 1991 1781982

Vuilleumier P: Anosognosia, in Behavior and Mood Disorders in Focal Brain Lesions. Edited by Bogousslavsky J, Cummings JL. Cambridge, UK, Cambridge University Press, 2000, pp 465–519

8

MEMORY AND ITS DISORDERS

Jagan Pillai, M.D., Ph.D.

Several memory systems have been defined. However, overlapping clinical signs and terminologies often make diagnosis challenging. A suggested scheme is outlined in Table 8–1. Most agree that an immediate memory buffer holds information until it is discarded or stored. This buffer is sometimes called *working memory*.

Delayed recall or *short-term memory* (STM) refers to memory traces encoded by the hippocampal system that can be retrieved even after a short interval that is usually tested from 5 to 30 minutes afterward.

In contrast, *long-term memory* (LTM) or *secondary memory* is, essentially, all that is not STM. There is good evidence that LTM is a separate system from STM. A classification system for LTM is shown in Figure 8–1.

Retrograde amnesia (RA) refers to the period of time for which patients' memories are obliterated prior to the amnesia-producing event. *Posttraumatic amnesia* (PTA) is the length of time for which memories are lost following a trauma, usually a cerebral injury. It is judged by the time it takes for a continuous stream of ongoing memory to return. Many patients report islands of memory after a head injury, which may reflect reality or be a part of a posttraumatic confusional state. These are not included in the determination of the length of PTA or the return of memory function. Amnesia caused by the sedative and anesthetic agents the patient may have received during early intensive treatment must be considered a factor obscuring the PTA.

RA and PTA are both reflections of the severity of a cerebral injury. It is probably true that any trauma that leads to a clearly identifiable PTA of longer than 1 hour will be associated with a loss of some cerebral neurons and that a PTA of 24 hours or longer represents a severe injury (see Chapter 14, "Brain Tumors"). An isolated PTA is frequent, but isolated RA virtually

TABLE 8–1. Memory tasks

System	Characteristics
Immediate recall	Memory immediately after presentation without an intervening distractor
	Limited capacity
	Rapid decay
	Tested by digit span (capacity) or working memory tasks (duration)
Delayed recall	
Retrieval	Activation of long-term memory traces
	Depends on frontal-subcortical circuits
Recognition	Ability to identify previously learned information
	Depends on initial information storage and hippocampal-hypothalamic-thalamic system
	Unlimited capacity; slow rate of forgetting
Long-term memory	
Declarative memory	Memory for facts (knowing that…)
	Accessible to consciousness (can be declared)
Semantic	Memory of general knowledge, world events (also called reference memory)
Episodic	Memory for ongoing autobiographical events (related to working memory, which in some classifications is a form of short-term memory)
Procedural memory	Memory for skills or modifiable cognitive operations (knowing how…), in some classifications is a form of implicit memory
	Spared in amnesia
	Includes classical conditioning
Implicit memory	Variation of procedural memory, demonstrated by completion of tasks that do not require conscious processing (e.g., completing word fragments)
Explicit memory	Variation of declarative memory, in some classifications is same as declarative memory
	Conscious recollection of recent events

Note. The classification of memory is confusing, and here an amalgam is given.

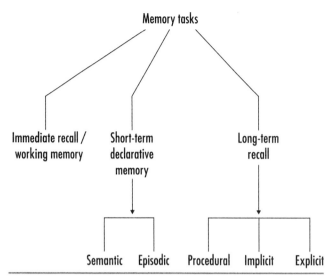

FIGURE 8–1. Classification of memory tasks relating to clinical phenomenology.

All tests described in Table 8–4 test this system.

never occurs. Usually the PTA is longer than the RA, and a long RA in the presence of a short PTA suggests a conversion disorder. RA can become smaller as injury resolves.

Anterograde amnesia refers to impairment in retaining everyday information. It overlaps with PTA and can persist long after resolution of the PTA if patients have a severe memory disorder after cerebral injury. Persistent anterograde amnesia is always associated with the presence of some RA and PTA.

Confabulation is often observed in patients with memory disorders. These patients give completely erroneous answers to questions elaborate on those answers with apparent conviction. Confabulation is most commonly seen soon after the onset of a memory disorder.

■ ANATOMY OF MEMORY

The underlying anatomy of memory has been defined by studying patients with a variety of memory disorders as well as animal models. Crucial anatomical sites are listed in Table 8–2. The

TABLE 8-2. Some causes of the amnestic syndrome

Etiology	Lesion site	Associated features
Alcoholism	Mammillary bodies or thalamus	Vitamin deficiency
Anoxia	Hippocampus	Anoxic episode
Epilepsy surgery	Hippocampus	Bilateral disease
Head trauma	Hippocampus	History of trauma
Herpes simplex encephalitis	Hippocampus	Seizures, aphasia, Klüver-Bucy syndrome
Hypoglycemia	Hippocampus	Diabetes and insulin
Neoplasms, especially around third ventricle	Thalamus	Headache, papilledema
Stroke, posterior cerebral artery	Hippocampus	Homonymous hemianopsia
Thiamine deficiency	Mammillary bodies or thalamus	Alcoholism or starvation
Tuberculous meningitis	Hippocampus	Tuberculoma; vascular occlusion

limbic system is central, but there are also extralimbic mechanisms. These are related to habit and skill learning because procedural memory requires the function of the basal ganglia. STM depends on intact attentional mechanisms. The ability to repeat digits, which is a common test of STM, depends on intact linguistic processes.

The amygdala and the hippocampus, especially the CA1 and CA3 subfields, and the entorhinal and perirhinal cortices are involved in laying down memory traces and in anterograde amnesia. The hypothalamic and diencephalic structures most implicated are the mammillary bodies and the mediodorsal and anterior nuclei of the thalamus. The amygdala is involved in the formation of LTM, notably in emotionally influenced memories, and in reinforcement.

The frontal lobes are also important in memory function. Patients with frontal lesions have impaired memory, especially for sequencing and ordering of events and retrieval of stored information. In some studies, retrograde memory impairment correlates with frontal impairments, and frontal lesions are often associated with confabulation. It has been suggested that patients with frontal lesions have a specific type of memory problem referred to as "forgetting to remember."

Acetylcholine is the main neurotransmitter identified with memory. Cholinergic blockade disrupts memory, whereas choline agonists may improve memory in some patients with dementia (see Chapter 11, "Dementia"). The forebrain cholinergic system, which ascends from the nucleus basalis of Meynert to the cortex and from the septal nuclei to the hippocampus, is crucial for memory function; patients with lesions at these sites have anterograde amnesias.

■ MEMORY DISORDERS IN CLINICAL PRACTICE

Memory is impaired secondarily in many states—for example, in anxiety and depression. Memory impairment is an integral aspect of conditions such as head injury and the dementias. There are also primary memory disorders. *Amnesia* is an acquired disturbance of memory in which new information is not stored by any LTM system. There are several well-recognized etiologies (see Table 8–2). It is still unclear, from a psychological point of view, whether there is only one amnestic syndrome with several etiologies or there are several different syndromes.

The best-known amnestic syndrome is *Korsakoff's syndrome*. It usually develops secondary to *Wernicke's encephalopathy*, which is due to thiamine deficiency. The latter presents with nystagmus, ophthalmoplegia, ataxia, peripheral neuropathy, and clouding of consciousness. After recovering from the acute state, patients may be left with severe anterograde memory disturbance, confabulation, lack of insight, and a mood disturbance. They may have intact STM, but Korsakoff's syndrome is evident if there is a delay, or interference, between the presentation of a stimulus to be recalled and the recording of a response.

Transient global amnesia is defined as a sudden global amnesia sometimes associated with minor clouding of consciousness that ends with recovery. It is more common among males ages 50–70 years. During the attack, personal identity is retained, significant persons are recognized, and motor skills are unimpaired. It lasts up to 24 hours, and when memory returns, there is amnesia for the duration of the episode. There may be associated RA, which may be extensive but which quickly shrinks on recovery. Usually patients have only one attack, but multiple episodes have been reported in some cases. The etiology of transient global amnesia is unclear, although epilepsy, migraine, and transient ischemia have been implicated in some patients. Pre-cipitating events can sometimes be identified, including stress, physical activity, and sexual intercourse. The electroencephalo-gram is often abnormal during the attack.

Many neurological disorders involve parts of the anatom-ical circuit for memory (see Table 8–2). The dementias are de-scribed in Chapter 11, epilepsy in Chapter 9, and head trauma in Chapter 16. In all of these conditions, the medial temporal ar-eas often bear the brunt of the pathology, and complaints of dis-turbed memory are common.

Because the major blood supply of the hippocampus is from the posterior cerebral artery, occlusion of this vessel may lead to amnesia. This damage is often associated with a homonymous hemianopsia and sometimes with hemiplegia. In many cases, bi-lateral disease is present, but cases are described with unilateral infarction. Damage to the anterior cerebral artery and the ante-rior communicating artery leads to frontal lobe impairment and has been reported to lead to memory problems associated with confabulation. These problems probably result from damage to basal forebrain nuclei. Strokes of the thalamus may lead to am-nesia; if bilateral, they may provoke a syndrome of amnesia and confusion. If the adjacent rostral brain stem is involved, there will be associated eye movement abnormalities.

Encephalitis sometimes selectively affects the limbic struc-tures. The main virus involved is herpes simplex type 1, which causes acute necrotizing hemorrhagic encephalitis. The pre-sentation is usually with focal neurological signs and seizures, but long-term sequelae are, in addition to seizures, usually be-havioral. Amnesia is inevitable, and various manifestations of Klüver-Bucy syndrome may be seen (see Chapter 9, "Epilepsy and Limbic System Disorders").

Memory impairment that is secondary to cerebral tumors is greatest when those tumors involve subcortical structures, especially in and around the third ventricle, the thalamus, and the hippocampus.

A number of neuropsychiatric treatments have been associ-ated with transient amnesia. These include the benzodiazepines, electroconvulsive therapy, and anticholinergic drugs.

Often the concerns regarding memory difficulties in clinic patients are related more to impairments in working memory (due to poor sleep, sleep apnea, depression, or medication side effects) or to poor memory retrieval from stored traces (due to

TABLE 8–3.	Varieties of psychogenic amnesia

Situational

PTSD[b]

Ganser syndrome[a]

Psychogenic fugue

Hysterical dementia

Depressive dementia

Dissociative identity disorder[a]

Histrionic personality disorder[b]

[a]The nosological validity of these syndromes is least certain.
[b]Amnesia is commonly but not invariably present.

cerebrovascular disease or depression) than to any hippocampal changes.

■ PSYCHOGENIC AMNESIAS

Psychogenic amnesia is currently classified as *dissociative amnesia*, which is an episodic autobiographical memory loss inconsistent with normal forgetfulness. The abilities to comprehend environmental information and to perform complex learned skills are preserved. Psychogenic amnesia is a variation of dissociative disorder, and dissociation and repression are common underlying mechanisms. Psychogenic amnesia frequently occurs in the setting of neurological illness. Table 8–3 lists varieties of psychogenic amnesias in their approximate order of episode duration.

Situational amnesia may occur in isolation, in association with a psychologically significant or traumatic event, or as part of PTSD. *Fugues* are episodes of wandering with amnesia. Patients remain in good contact with their surroundings, and when they emerge from the fugue, they may emerge with an amnesic gap, especially with loss of their personal identity, and sometimes with amnesia for their entire life.

Ganser syndrome is a complex of hallucinations, cognitive disorientation, conversion disorder, and the symptom of approximate answers (*Vorbeireden*). It has been described in numerous settings and associated with head injury, depression, epilepsy, schizophrenia, chronic neurological disorders, and malingering. *Vorbeireden* is the inability to answer simple questions correctly. Although the nature of the questions is known, only approximate answers are given, and the absurd nature of the answers is striking.

Pseudodementia is a term that was previously used for conditions such as the cognitive and memory impairments of depression (see Chapter 11), Ganser syndrome, and hysterical dementia; this term is no longer employed. Patients with hysterical dementia have a bizarre memory loss that is associated with variable results on psychological testing and often with other conversion phenomena. The memory loss may be acute or chronic and may be precipitated by head injury. Episodes of Ganser syndrome may be brief, whereas hysterical dementia may be chronic and relapsing.

■ DYSMNESIC STATES

In dysmnesic states, patients' memory is not so much lost as distorted. These conditions are usually associated with a diagnosis of some underlying neurological impairment or schizophrenia. The *delusional misidentification syndromes* include the *Capgras syndrome* and the *Fregoli syndrome*. In the former, patients insist that a person, usually a close relative or friend, has been replaced by an impostor. In the Fregoli syndrome, patients falsely identify a familiar person, often a persecutor, in strangers. Good evidence links misidentification syndromes to the dysfunction of the right hemisphere and to frontal lobe disorders, and they are often seen in dementia with Lewy bodies (see Chapter 11). *Déjà vu* and *jamais vu* are described in Chapter 1, "Neuropsychiatric Assessment."

Reduplicative paramnesia is a related syndrome in which patients are certain that a familiar place, person, object, or body part has been duplicated. It commonly presents when a patient insists that a familiar place (e.g., the hospital room) exists in an impossible location (e.g., the patient's house).

■ TESTS OF MEMORY FUNCTION

In practice, several tests are used in the clinic and more formal neuropsychological settings. Some of the most common tests are listed in Table 8–4.

TABLE 8–4.	Memory tests

Digit span (auditory-verbal short-term memory)**

Corsi Blocks (visuospatial short-term memory)

General knowledge

Memory for word lists

Memory for stories**

Memory for nonverbal material**

Rey-Osterreith Complex Figure Test (recall of a figure)

Rey Auditory Verbal Learning Test

Recognition memory tasks—visual and verbal (patients are shown words*, faces,* objects, or shapes or are given word lists; after an interval, the same process is repeated with distractors, and those items already seen are to be identified)

Hidden Objects Task (hide objects in view of patient)

Brown-Peterson Task (Test of short-term memory duration; patients are given items to remember, followed by a distraction task, and then a recall)

Wechsler Memory Scale–Revised (12 separate subtests, including tests above marked by double asterisks [**])

Photographs of famous faces

Photographs of famous landmarks

Word completion

Warrington Recognition Memory Test (includes tests above marked by single asterisk [*])

Autobiographical Memory Interview

■ REFERENCES

American Psychiatric Association: Diagnostic and Statistical Manual of Mental Disorders, 5th Edition. Arlington, VA, American Psychiatric Association, 2013

Cummings JL, Mega MS: Memory Disorders in Neuropsychiatry and Behavioral Neuroscience. New York, Oxford University Press, 2003

Damasio AR, Graff-Radford NR, Eslinger PJ, et al: Amnesia following basal forebrain lesions. Arch Neurol 42(3):263–271, 1985 3977657

Hodges JR, Ward CD: Observations during transient global amnesia: a behavioural and neuropsychological study of five cases. Brain 112(Pt 3):595–620, 1989 2731023

Kapur N, Ellison D, Smith MP, et al: Focal retrograde amnesia following bilateral temporal lobe pathology: a neuropsychological and magnetic resonance study. Brain 115(pt 1):73–85, 1992 1559164

150

Kopelman MD, Stevens TG, Foli S, Grasby P: PET activation of the medial temporal lobe in learning. Brain 121(pt 5):875–887, 1998 9619191

Kopelman MD, Stanhope N, Kingsley D: Retrograde amnesia in patients with diencephalic, temporal lobe or frontal lesions. Neuropsychologia 37(8):939–958, 1999 10426519

Lewis SW: Brain imaging in a case of Capgras' syndrome. Br J Psychiatry 150:117–121, 1987 3651660

Mace CJ, Trimble MR: Psychogenic amnesia, in Memory Disorders: Research and Clinical Practice. Edited by Yanagihara T, Petersen RC. New York, Marcel Dekker, 1991, pp 429–457

Squire LR: Memory and the Brain. New York, Oxford University Press, 1987

Stuss DT, Alexander MP, Lieberman A, Levine H: An extraordinary form of confabulation. Neurology 28(11):1166–1172, 1978 568737

Warrington EK: Recognition Memory Test. Windsor, UK, NFER-Nelson, 1984

Yudofsky SC, Hales RE: The neuropsychiatry of memory, in American Psychiatric Press Review of Psychiatry, Vol 12. Edited by Oldham JM, Riba MB, Tasman A. Washington, DC, American Psychiatric Press, 1993, pp 661–833

Zola-Morgan S, Squire LR, Amaral DG: Human amnesia and the medial temporal region: enduring memory impairment following a bilateral lesion limited to field CA1 of the hippocampus. J Neurosci 6(10):2950–2967, 1986 3760943

9

EPILEPSY AND LIMBIC SYSTEM DISORDERS

Juliana Lockman, M.D.
John J. Barry, M.D.

The lifetime risk of a person developing a single seizure is estimated at 8%–10%. Epilepsy is a cerebral disorder in which patients have a predisposition to recurrent unprovoked seizures. Epilepsy is one of the most common neurological disorders, affecting approximately 50 million people around the world. In the United States, active epilepsy affects 1.2% of the population. Table 9–1 shows the classification of seizures.

Focal seizures are those in which clinical and electroencephalographic changes suggest a localized onset. Further classification depends on whether consciousness is impaired during the attack, along with motor features and secondary generalization (i.e., focal to bilateral tonic-clonic). *Automatisms* refer to automatic motor acts carried out in a state of altered consciousness during or after seizures, for which there is usually amnesia. They may be featured in both focal and generalized seizure types. *Cursive seizures* are characterized by running, and *gelastic seizures* feature "mirthless laughter."

Generalized seizures are those in which the first clinical and electroencephalographic changes suggest bilateral abnormalities with widespread disturbance in both hemispheres. *Absence seizures* are nonmotor generalized seizures with behavioral arrest and impaired awareness. *Tonic-clonic seizures* are classic convulsive episodes with either focal or generalized electrographic onset. *Myoclonic seizures* are sudden, brief, jerklike contractions that may be focal or generalized. *Atonic seizures* may present as drop attacks due to abrupt onset of loss of bodily tone.

In *status epilepticus*, recurrent seizures occur continuously or without full return of consciousness between attacks. It is characterized by the International League Against Epilepsy (ILAE) as the failure of a seizure to cease within a predefined time pe-

152

TABLE 9–1.   Classification of seizures

---

1. Focal onset seizures

    Focal aware seizure (formerly "simple partial")

    Focal impaired awareness seizure (formerly "complex partial")

    Focal to bilateral tonic-clonic seizure

    Motor/Nonmotor onset

2. Generalized onset seizures

    Motor (includes tonic-clonic, myoclonic, atonic, and others)

    Nonmotor (absence)

3. Unknown onset seizures

    Motor (includes tonic-clonic and epileptic spasms)

    Nonmotor (includes behavior arrest)

Source.   Adapted from Fisher 2017.

riod (T1) and the potential for long-term cerebral damage to occur beyond a second predefined time period (T2). T1 and T2 vary by seizure type, but for generalized convulsive status epilepticus T1 is 5 minutes and T2 is 30 minutes.

Status epilepticus is further classified as convulsive or nonconvulsive, and both types require emergent medical care. In the nonconvulsive type, patients present with prolonged episodes of abnormal behavior due to continuous seizures of either the focal impaired awareness or absence type. Focal status epilepticus with retained awareness is otherwise known as *epilepsia partialis continua*. *Rasmussen's syndrome* refers to a viral encephalitis that presents as persistent focal seizures with slowly progressive neurological deterioration. There is often evidence of lateralized focal brain atrophy.

Although not formally included in ILAE epilepsy classification, recognizing epilepsy syndromes is important for guiding treatment. The classification of epilepsy type designated by the ILAE is shown in Table 9–2. There is no formal classification by the ILAE for epilepsy syndromes, which are typically defined by the patient's age at presentation, clinical symptoms, and electroencephalographic and neuroimaging data. Syndromes are not typically based on etiology or may even have more than one etiology.

Focal epilepsy syndromes include *benign epilepsy with centrotemporal spikes* and the occipital epilepsies of childhood, which include the Panayiotopoulos and Gastaut syndromes. Be-

5

TABLE 9–2.   Epilepsy syndromes

1. Focal epilepsies (formerly known as "localization-related" or "partial" epilepsy): examples include benign epilepsy with centrotemporal spikes and occipital epilepsies of childhood, including the Panayiotopoulos and Gastaut syndromes

2. Generalized epilepsies: examples include childhood absence epilepsy, juvenile absence epilepsy, juvenile myoclonic epilepsy, generalized tonic-clonic seizures alone, and developmental and epileptic encephalopathies

3. Combined generalized and focal epilepsies

4. Unknown

Source.   Adapted from Fisher 2017.

nign epilepsy with centrotemporal spikes, also known as *Rolandic epilepsy*, is the most common focal epilepsy of childhood, typically affecting school-age children between the ages of 5 and 10 years. It is characterized by nocturnal motor seizures involving the face, drooling, and vocalizations. It typically does not require anticonvulsants and resolves with age. Panayiotopoulos and Gastaut syndromes feature visual symptoms in the context of occipital abnormalities on electroencephalogram (EEG).

Common generalized epilepsy syndromes that affect developmentally normal individuals include *childhood absence epilepsy* and *juvenile myoclonic epilepsy*. Childhood absence epilepsy presents with absence seizures in association with 3-Hz spike wave activity on EEG. Juvenile myoclonic epilepsy, also known as Janz syndrome, presents in adolescence and may feature absence, tonic-clonic, and myoclonic seizure types. The EEG typically shows 4–5 Hz polyspike wave activity.

Progressive myoclonic epilepsy syndromes, such as Lafora disease and Baltic myoclonus, are rare and afflict neurotypical individuals. As seizure types such as tonic-clonic and myoclonic develop, progressive decline in cognitive function and balance ensues. A genetic etiology for these syndromes has been established.

The "developmental and epileptic encephalopathies" include syndromes that feature static encephalopathy referable to persistent underlying seizure activity. Examples include *West's syndrome*, diagnosed in the first year of life; the clinical triad includes infantile spasms, developmental delay, and an electroencephalographic pattern called hypsarrhythmia. Hypsarrhythmia features high-amplitude slow waves at frequencies of 1–7 Hz,

154

TABLE 9–3.	Principal etiologies of epilepsy
Structural	Tumor, traumatic brain injury, stroke, mesial temporal sclerosis, demyelinating disease, Sturge-Weber syndrome, tuberous sclerosis, cortical dysplasias, Rasmussen syndrome, hypoxic ischemic injury
Genetic	Benign familial neonatal epilepsy, childhood absence epilepsy, juvenile myoclonic epilepsy, Dravet syndrome
Infectious	Neurocysticercosis, HIV, tuberculosis, toxoplasmosis, cytomegalovirus, neurosyphilis
Metabolic	Amino acid disorders, pyridoxine-dependent seizures, porphyria, lysosomal storage diseases
Immune	Anti-NMDA receptor encephalitis, anti-leucine-rich glioma-inactivated 1 encephalitis
Unknown	

mixed with sharp waves and spikes of varying amplitude, morphology, duration, and site. The *Lennox-Gastaut syndrome* occurs in children up to about 8 years of age and presents with multiple seizure types, a slow spike wave pattern on EEG, and mental disability.

In the *reflex epilepsies*, seizures are provoked by cognitive, emotional, sensory, or motor events.

The principal etiologies of epilepsy are shown in Table 9–3. In the most recent ILAE classification, etiology is subgrouped into six categories: structural, genetic, infectious, metabolic, immune, and unknown. Some epilepsies may span more than one category. Examples include tuberous sclerosis and cortical dysplasias, which are structural conditions with genetic bases.

■ PSYCHIATRIC DISORDERS OF EPILEPSY

Psychiatric conditions occur in an estimated 20%–30% of patients with epilepsy. In patients with intractable focal unaware seizures, rates approach 70%. Research supports a two-way relationship between mental health and epilepsy. Observations supporting an overlap in neurobiological mechanism include the presence of psychiatric conditions often preceding the onset of seizures and vice versa.

Population-based studies in Canada and the United Kingdom report the prevalence of psychiatric diagnoses in patients with epilepsy compared to the general population (Table 9–4).

TABLE 9–4. Prevalence of psychiatric diagnoses among patients with epilepsy

Condition	The Canadian Community Health Survey, 2007 Prevalence, %	Adult Psychiatric Morbidity Survey (United Kingdom), 2012 Prevalence, %
Any mental health condition	35.5 EP, 1.7 times higher than GP (lifetime)	Not reported
Anxiety disorder	22.8 EP, 2 times higher than GP (lifetime)	12.5 EP, 2.6 times higher than the GP when adjusted for demographics (for GAD)
Depression	17.4 EP, 1.6 times higher than GP (for lifetime MDD)	9.6 EP, 2.7 times higher than GP when adjusted for demographics (types of depression not specified)
Panic disorder	6.6 EP, 1.8 times higher than GP (lifetime)	Not reported
Psychotic disorder	Not reported	1.1 EP, 1.7 times higher than GP when adjusted for demographics
Suicidal ideation	25.0 EP, 1.8 times higher than GP (lifetime)	26.5 EP, 2 times higher than GP when adjusted for demographics (lifetime)

EP = epilepsy population; GAD = generalized anxiety disorder; GP = general population; MDD = major depressive disorder.

Lifetime prevalence of epilepsy in these studies was 0.6% and 1.2%, respectively. In both surveys, diagnostic interviews were employed in an effort to promote reliable and standardized results. The most common psychiatric comorbidities in epilepsy are mood and anxiety disorders and psychosis.

In addition to optimizing seizure control, identifying and treating mental illness improves quality of life. The symptomatology of neuropsychiatric conditions may elude the standard DSM-5 classifications. The biopsychosocial model can be a useful framework for understanding factors that contribute to mental illness. Special considerations include whether symptoms are adverse medication effects (discussed later in the chapter) or are temporally related to seizures or seizure remission.

TABLE 9–5. Classification of psychiatric symptoms in people with epilepsy

Peri-ictal	
Preictal	Symptoms preceding seizures by minutes to days; 13% express dysphoria hours to days before ictus
Ictal	Symptoms occurring during seizures, including auras; very brief, stereotyped with fear more common than depression followed by psychosis
Postictal (two types)	1) Occurring immediately after seizures (e.g., delirium associated with a slow, disorganized electroencephalogram)
	2) Occurring after a lucid interval of 12–120 hours (e.g., in postictal psychosis)
	13.9% of patients with epilepsy and postictal psychosis go on to interictal psychosis
Paraictal	
Alternative psychosis	Symptoms arise with the cessation of seizures
Forced normalization	Symptoms arise with electroencephalographic normalization
Interictal	
Affective disorders, interictal dysphoric disorder	
Anxiety states	
Paranoid states	
Personality features	
Schizophrenia-like psychoses	

A classification of behavioral disorders encountered in patients with epilepsy is shown in Table 9–5. The distinction between *ictal* and *interictal* syndromes is not always clear. In some patients, prolonged postictal psychotic states may occur, merging into interictal psychoses in the setting of clear consciousness.

Personality Features

Interictal personality syndrome (Gastaut-Geschwind syndrome) is characterized by hyperreligiosity, disordered sexual function (often hyposexuality), hypergraphia, irritability, and viscosity. Aggression is not a specific component. The Bear-Fedio Inventory was designed in the 1970s to assess the presence of these and other personality features in people with epilepsy. Initial testing supported these personality features as prevalent in patients with temporal lobe epilepsy. However, subsequent investigation found them to be nonspecific and present in a range of conditions. However, epilepsy may affect behavior and result in an aberration from the expected mean.

Mood Disorders

Depression is the most common psychiatric comorbidity and often predates seizures. In a study evaluating 174 patients with epilepsy that utsed the Structured Clinical Interview for DSM-IV module for depression, 21.2% had current major depressive disorder and 17.2% had dysthymia. There is a fairly linear relationship between depression and seizure frequency. However, even patients who are seizure-free while off anticonvulsants have a higher rate of depression than the average population. The suicide rate in people with epilepsy is up to 10 times higher than that of the general population. Mania occurs at a higher rate in epilepsy but may be attributed to postictal phenomena.

Research has revealed biological parallels between mood disorders and epilepsy. Common neurotransmitter concentration patterns have been identified. PET scans have shown lower serotonin (5-HT$_{1A}$) in the hippocampi in both depression and temporal lobe epilepsy without depression. Lower cerebrospinal fluid and cortical GABA concentrations on magnetic resonance spectroscopy have been observed in both depression and epilepsy. The reverse is seen with glutamate levels in the cerebrospinal fluid and on magnetic resonance spectroscopy.

Overlapping inflammatory mechanisms are suggested by findings of increased interleukin-β in both depression and epilepsy. Finally, atrophy of the orbitofrontal cortex, cingulate gyrus, and amygdala have been observed in both uncontrolled mood disorders and epilepsy. Altogether, evidence of common biological processes helps explain the close relationship between epilepsy and comorbid mood disorders.

Unfortunately, mood disorders are underrecognized and undertreated in patients with epilepsy. As part of its quality measurement initiative, the American Academy of Neurology recommends screening for mental health conditions at each encounter. Screening may include well-validated measures such

158

TABLE 9–6.	The Neurological Disorders Depression Inventory for Epilepsy			
	Always/ Often	Sometimes	Rarely	Never
Everything I do is a struggle	4	3	2	1
Nothing I do is right	4	3	2	1
Feel guilty	4	3	2	1
I'd be better off dead	4	3	2	1
Frustrated	4	3	2	1
Difficulty in finding pleasure	4	3	2	1

Source. Adapted from Sheehan DV, Lecrubier Y, Sheehan KH, et al.: "The Mini International Neuropsychiatric Interview (MINI): The Development and Validation of a Structured Diagnostic Psychiatric Interview for DSM-IV and ICD-10." *Journal of Clinical Psychiatry* 59(suppl 20):22–23, 1998.

as the Neurological Disorders Depression Inventory, shown in Table 9–6. This measure controls for symptoms that may be attributed to medication side effects, with scores >15 considered positive for a possible depressive disorder. The American Epilepsy Society also provides screening algorithms among their clinical practice tools.

Treatment includes optimizing seizure control and assessing for iatrogenic causes, such as anticonvulsant therapy. In addition, any recent discontinuation of antiepileptic drugs with positive psychotropic effects should be investigated. Consideration should then address the possibility of adding cognitive-behavioral therapy, which has been shown to be effective for depression in patients with epilepsy.

Antidepressants, including the selective serotonin reuptake inhibitors (SSRIs) and serotonin-norepinephrine reuptake inhibitors (SNRIs), are first-line treatments when appropriate. Keep in mind that these medications can sometimes exacerbate anxiety initially, and venlafaxine can increase blood pressure. In addition, before starting an antidepressant, the presence of bipolar affective disorder should be determined because antidepressants are not generally effective in this condition and may induce a switch to mania. This is discussed in detail in Chapter 22, "Treatments in Neuropsychiatry."

Caution is also needed when SSRIs, SNRIs, or tricyclic antidepressants are combined with enzyme-inducing antiepileptic drugs, such as carbamazepine, phenobarbital, or phenytoin, because serum levels of the antidepressant may be negatively affected and thus will require a dosage adjustment of 20%–30%. Conversely, although some controversy exists, fluoxetine (and, to a lesser extent, paroxetine) may affect the 2D6 isoenzyme, causing an increase in the serum levels of carbamazepine and phenytoin. The aim of therapy is symptom remission because anything less can be associated with relapse. Commonly used psychometric questionnaires can be utilized validly in patients with epilepsy.

Anxiety Disorders

Anxiety is highly prevalent among patients with both poorly and well-controlled epilepsy. In the aforementioned study evaluating for current psychopathology, patients with epilepsy had anxiety disorders at a frequency of 52.1%. The fear of having a seizure and the loss of independence are among the contributing factors. Well-validated screening tools include the Generalized Anxiety Disorder–7. When assessing patients who have transient anxiety symptoms, it is important to distinguish between panic attacks and temporal-origin seizures, of which anxiety is a symptom. Elucidating characteristics such as the duration (e.g., seizures often lasting <90 seconds, panic attacks lasting 10–15 minutes) and provoking factors may be helpful.

Medication management with SSRIs is first-line, with additional consideration for agents such as gabapentin and pregabalin that have both anticonvulsant and anxiolytic properties. Epilepsy type may guide whether the latter narrow-spectrum anticonvulsant options are appropriate. Psychotherapy and behavioral activation are also mainstays in treatment.

Psychotic Disorders

Psychosis occurs at a higher rate in patients with epilepsy, with a frequency of 5.9% reported in one study. Positive symptoms such as hallucinations and delusions are most prevalent. Negative symptoms such as apathy, alogia, and affective blunting are relatively lacking. Assessing the relationship with seizure timing and anticonvulsant therapy is key for guiding treatment. Psychosis may occur during or after seizures or be interictal.

Forced normalization is an interictal condition originally associated with psychosis emerging with electroencephalographic normalization. The clinical parallel is known as *alternative psychosis*, in which psychiatric symptoms appear with the cessation of clinical seizures. The mechanism for this phenomenon remains unclear but is speculated to be associated with central increases of dopamine. Forced normalization has been seen associated with antiepileptic drugs, vagus nerve stimulation, and postepilepsy surgery, coupled with seizure cessation. Criteria include behavioral dysfunction that begins abruptly and may manifest as either depression or mania or psychotic, mood, anxiety, or conversion disorders. It occurs in adult patients with epilepsy at a frequency of approximately 7.8% but is less frequent in the pediatric population.

Postictal psychosis occurs in approximately 7% of patients with epilepsy evaluated in video-EEG settings and in approximately 25% of those with epilepsy and psychotic symptoms. It is often associated with intractable temporal lobe epilepsy with bilateral independent seizure origins. Patients commonly present with a cluster of convulsive seizures followed by a period of 24 hours to 1 week of lucidity, after which psychosis begins. Aggression, if it occurs as a result of seizure activity, is most common in the postictal period. The duration of psychosis may span days to months. Untreated, postictal psychosis may assume a pattern of chronic or stable psychosis, which has minimal fluctuation with seizures and resembles paranoid-type schizophrenia. Screening may involve asking about unusual thoughts and sleep disturbance. The treatment for acute postictal psychosis includes antipsychotics, such as risperidone 1–2 mg once or twice daily, and benzodiazepines as needed. The regimen is administered on a scheduled basis and titrated to effect. Once the patient is stabilized, the drug can be tapered for use as needed.

■ ANTICONVULSANTS AND PSYCHIATRIC RISK

Anticonvulsants may affect psychiatric conditions differently. A brief overview of such effects is provided in Table 9–7. All have the potential to influence mood. In 2008, the FDA issued a black box warning for all anticonvulsants for their potential increased risk for suicidality. Methodological issues with these data have subsequently been cited. However, due to increased suicide risk in general, screening for suicidal ideation is an important part of caring for patients with epilepsy. Side effects of anticonvulsants are listed in the table. Emergence of psychosis, irritability, and mood symptoms has been noted to be particularly associated with levetiracetam and zonisamide.

■ PSYCHIATRIC TREATMENTS AND SEIZURE RISK

When selecting medication, the potential for side effects, drug interactions, and changes in seizure threshold must be consid-

161

Psychiatric effects	Anticonvulsant or device
Antidepressant effects	Lamotrigine and vagus nerve stimulation
Anxiolytic effects	Gabapentin, pregabalin, and tiagabine
Iatrogenic depression potential	Phenobarbital, primidone, vigabatrin, levetiracetam, felbamate, topiramate
Mood and anxiety neutral	Lacosamide
Mood-stabilizing effects	Carbamazepine, oxcarbazepine, valproate, lamotrigine*
Psychotic potential	Topiramate, levetiracetam, zonisamide

*Depression can occur after discontinuation of any of these medications.

ered. In general, first-line antidepressants such as SSRIs and SNRIs are safe when used within therapeutic dosing range. Researchers have determined that some may actually have some antiepileptic properties. Doxepin, trazodone, and fluvoxamine also appear to have a low risk. Medications to avoid due to the potential to lower seizure threshold include bupropion (at dosages >300 mg/day), clomipramine, maprotiline, amoxapine, and monoamine oxidase inhibitors (see Chapter 22).

The antipsychotic medication found in studies to have the lowest risk in patients with epilepsy is risperidone. Higher-risk medications include quetiapine, clozapine, olanzapine, and haloperidol. Clozapine carries the most risk and decreases seizure threshold in a dosage-dependent fashion. One study indicated that a dosage of 300–600 mg/day resulted in a seizure incidence of 1.8%. Both clozapine and olanzapine can cause electroencephalographic changes (see Chapter 22).

Biological therapies such as electroconvulsive therapy (ECT) have demonstrated safety in patients with epilepsy. Anticonvulsants increase the seizure threshold, so dosage reduction may be needed in order to allow ECT charge to be titrated to effect. Transcranial magnetic stimulation (TMS) carries a low risk of provoking seizures and requires caution when considered for patients with epilepsy. Consensus guidelines have been developed for safe use of TMS in patients who have increased risk of seizures.

■ TREATMENT OF EPILEPSY

Pharmacological treatments for epilepsy are discussed in Chapter 22. In cases of medication-resistant epilepsy, treatments include cerebral resective surgery (via craniotomy or stereotactic laser), vagus nerve stimulation (VNS), deep brain stimulation (DBS), and responsive neurostimulation (RNS).

Cerebral surgery is the most common type of surgery in adults with epilepsy. Focal resective surgery may be indicated for lesions such as tumors, cortical dysplasias, or regions of damage from traumatic brain injury that contain an epileptogenic focus. Anterior temporal lobectomy is a surgery in which the anterior temporal pole, hippocampus, and a portion of the amygdala on the side of seizure origin are removed (Table 9–8). This procedure is often used for patients with medication-resistant mesial temporal sclerosis in whom a seizure focus is well-defined.

Before cerebral surgery, ensure that the remaining temporal lobe can sustain memory. The *Wada test* involves anesthetizing first one and then the other hemisphere with intracarotid amobarbital sodium (Amytal) to determine patients' language laterality and the ability of their opposite-side hippocampus to sustain memory. Functional MRI has also been demonstrated to be a valid tool for lateralizing language and verbal memory and for defining eloquent motor areas prior to surgery.

Presurgical psychiatric assessment helps identify mental health risks with surgery and optimize surgery candidacy. Most psychiatric conditions improve post-surgery, particularly when seizure freedom is attained. Mood lability may occur acutely following surgery and is often self-limited. De novo depression or anxiety affects approximately one-third of surgery patients and typically remits within 1 year. Worsened depression may occur in approximately 15% of patients. Postictal and interictal psychosis are not contraindications for surgery, and symptoms may potentially improve. De novo psychosis post-surgery is unusual.

Long-term prognosis is very good in patients who are good candidates, particularly those with unilateral lesions as determined with MRI and video EEG and those deemed to have a low risk of neurological deficits from the area of planned resection.

Neuromodulation may be an option for patients with medication-resistant epilepsy who are not candidates for resective surgery by craniotomy or stereotactic laser. VNS was approved by the FDA for the treatment of epilepsy in 1997 and for depression in 2005. It involves surgically implanting a wire coil on a cervical segment of the vagus nerve, with stimulation provided by a subcutaneous generator. DBS and RNS are the most recent to be FDA-approved for treatment in epilepsy. RNS requires the surgical placement of intracranial electrodes in the brain near

TABLE 9–8. Indications for anterior temporal lobectomy

Failure of seizures to respond to medication

Evidence of a unilateral focus, preferably by magnetic resonance, video electroencephalogram, and clinical semiology; may require other measures such as PET imaging

Evidence that memory function can be sustained based on baseline neuropsychological function, functional MRI, and sometimes amobarbital sodium (Amytal or Wada) test

Patient wants the operation

the location of seizure onset to detect, prevent, and interrupt seizure propagation. Neurologists are able to interrogate the RNS device to obtain seizure activity data and to optimize programming to manage seizures. DBS requires a device be implanted in the anterior nucleus of the thalamus and delivers intermittent stimulation to modulate brain activity and reduce seizure frequency. Compared with RNS, it is useful when the epileptic focus cannot be localized or is multifocal.

■ OTHER TEMPORAL LOBE DISORDERS

Although temporal lobe epilepsy is the most common temporal lobe syndrome seen in neuropsychiatry, other pathologies also have a predilection for damaging the limbic system. Head injury is discussed in Chapter 16, "Head Injury and Its Sequelae." Three viruses that frequently affect this region of the brain are those that cause rabies, encephalitis lethargica, and herpes encephalitis. The latter is caused by the herpes simplex virus and has a high mortality rate. Survivors often display psychopathology. Part or all of the Klüver-Bucy syndrome may be present, manifested by hyperorality, hyperphagia, hypersexuality, docility, and visual agnosia and often includes severe amnesia, irritability, distractibility, and dysphoria with apathy.

Cerebral tumors include gliomas and hamartomas. Hamartomas may occur anywhere in the brain but seem to be more commonly associated with psychopathology, especially psychosis, when they occur in the temporolimbic areas (see Chapter 14, "Brain Tumors").

Limbic encephalitides such as anti-NMDA receptor encephalitis and leucine-rich glioma inactivated 1 encephalitis are associated with acute-onset seizures, cognitive disturbance, and

behavioral changes. The former is associated with systemic carcinoma (see Chapter 20, "Limbic Encephalitis").

■ REFERENCES

Adachi N, Kanemoto K, de Toffol B, et al: Basic treatment principles for
 psychotic disorders in patients with epilepsy. Epilepsia 54(suppl
 1):19–33, 2013 23458463

Adelöw C, Andersson T, Ahlbom A, Tomson T: Hospitalization for
 psychiatric disorders before and after onset of unprovoked sei-
 zures/epilepsy. Neurology 78(6):396–401, 2012 22282649

Alper K, Schwartz KA, Kolts RL, Khan A: Seizure incidence in psychopharmacological clinical trials: an analysis of Food and Drug Administration (FDA) summary basis of approval reports. Biol
 Psychiatry 62(4):345–354, 2007 17223086

American Epilepsy Society: Practice Tools (online). Aesnet.org, 2022.
 Available at: https://www.aesnet.org/clinical-care/running-
 your-practice/practice-tools. Accessed January 31, 2022.

American Psychiatric Association: Diagnostic and Statistical Manual
 of Mental Disorders, 5th Edition. Arlington, VA, American Psychiatric Association, 2013

Barry JJ, Lembke A, Huynh N: Affective disorders in epilepsy, in Psy-
 chiatric Issues in Epilepsy: A Practical Guide to Diagnosis and
 Treatment. Edited by Ettinger AB, Kanner AM. Philadelphia, PA,
 Lippincott Williams and Wilkins, 2001, pp 45–73

Bear DM, Fedio P: Quantitative analysis of interictal behavior in temporal lobe epilepsy. Arch Neurol 34(8):454–467, 1977 889477

Binder JR: Functional MRI is a valid noninvasive alternative to Wada
 testing. Epilepsy Behav 20(2):214–222, 2011 20850386

de Toffol B, Trimble M, Hesdorffer DC, et al: Pharmacotherapy in patients with epilepsy and psychosis. Epilepsy Behav 88:54–60, 2018

Fisher RS: The new classification of seizures by the International League
 Against Epilepsy 2017. Curr Neurol Neurosci Rep 17(6):48, 2017

Fountain NB, Van Ness PC, Swain-Eng R, et al: Quality improvement
 in neurology: AAN epilepsy quality measures: report of the Quality Measurement and Reporting Subcommittee of the American
 Academy of Neurology. Neurology 76(1):94–99, 2011 21205698

Gandy M, Sharpe L, Perry KN, et al: Rates of DSM-IV mood, anxiety
 disorders, and suicidality in Australian adult epilepsy outpatients:
 a comparison of well-controlled versus refractory epilepsy. Epilepsy Behav 26(1):29–35, 2013 23201610

Gilliam FG, Barry JJ, Hermann BP, et al: Rapid detection of major depression in epilepsy: a multicentre study. Lancet Neurol 5(5):399–
 405, 2006 16632310

Gilliam FG, Black KJ, Carter J, et al: A trial of sertraline or cognitive behavior therapy for depression in epilepsy. Ann Neurol 86(4):552–
 560, 2019 31359460

Hesdorffer DC, Ishihara L, Mynepalli L, et al: Epilepsy, suicidality, and psychiatric disorders: a bidirectional association. Ann Neurol 72(2):184–191, 2012 22887468

Hilger E, Zimprich F, Pataraia E, et al: Psychoses in epilepsy: a comparison of postictal and interictal psychoses. Epilepsy Behav 60:58–62, 2016 27179193

Jacoby A, Baker GA, Steen N, et al: The clinical course of epilepsy and its psychosocial correlates: findings from a U.K. Community study. Epilepsia 37(2):148–161, 1996 8635425

Jones JE, Hermann BP, Barry JJ, et al: Clinical assessment of Axis I psychiatric morbidity in chronic epilepsy: a multicenter investigation. J Neuropsychiatry Clin Neurosci 17(2):172–179, 2005 15939970

Kanemoto K, Tadokoro Y, Oshima T: Violence and postictal psychosis: a comparison of postictal psychosis, interictal psychosis, and postictal confusion. Epilepsy Behav 19(2):162–166, 2010

Kanner AM: Depression in epilepsy: prevalence, clinical semiology, pathogenic mechanisms, and treatment. Biol Psychiatry 54(3):388–398, 2003

Kanner AM: Hippocampal atrophy: another common pathogenic mechanism of depressive disorders and epilepsy? Epilepsy Curr 11(5):149–150, 2011 22020737

Kanner AM: The treatment of depressive disorders in epilepsy: what all neurologists should know. Epilepsia 54(suppl 1):3–12, 2013 23458461

Kanner AM, Stagno S, Kotagal P, Morris HH: Postictal psychiatric events during prolonged video-electroencephalographic monitoring studies. Arch Neurol 53(3):258–263, 1996 8651879

Kawakami Y, Itoh Y: Forced normalization: antagonism between epilepsy and psychosis. Pediatr Neurol 70:16–19, 2017 28460793

Mazarati AM, Pineda E, Shin D, et al: Comorbidity between epilepsy and depression: role of hippocampal interleukin-1beta. Neurobiol Dis 37(2):461–467, 2010 19900553

Mula M, Monaco F: Ictal and peri-ictal psychopathology. Behav Neurol 24(1):21–25, 2011 21447894

Mula M, Schmitz B, Jauch R, et al: On the prevalence of bipolar disorder in epilepsy. Epilepsy Behav 13(4):658–661, 2008

Rai D, Kerr MP, McManus S, et al: Epilepsy and psychiatric comorbidity: a nationally representative population-based study. Epilepsia 53(6):1095–1103, 2012 22578079

Ristic AJ, Pjevalica J, Trajkovic G, et al: Validation of the Neurological Disorders Depression Inventory for epilepsy (NDDI-E) Serbian version. Epilepsy Behav 57(pt A):1–4, 2016

Ritaccio AL, Devinski O: Personality disorders, in Psychiatric Issues in Epilepsy: A Practical Guide to Diagnosis and Treatment. Edited by Ettinger AB, Kanner AM. Philadelphia, PA, Lippincott Williams and Wilkins, 2001, pp 147–162

Sanacora G, Mason GF, Rothman DL, et al: Reduced cortical gamma-aminobutyric acid levels in depressed patients determined by proton magnetic resonance spectroscopy. Arch Gen Psychiatry 56(11):1043–1047, 1999 10565505

Sanacora G, Treccani G, Popoli M: Towards a glutamate hypothesis of depression: an emerging frontier of neuropsychopharmacology for mood disorders. Neuropharmacology 62(1):63–77, 2012 21827775

Scheffer IE, Berkovic S, Capovilla G, et al: ILAE classification of the epilepsies: Position paper of the ILAE Commission for Classification and Terminology. Epilepsia 58(4):512–521, 2017 28276062

Shannon MW, Borron SW, Burns M: Haddad and Winchester's Clinical Management of Poisoning and Drug Overdose, 4th Edition. London, WB Saunders, 2007

Spitzer RL, Kroenke K, Williams JBW, Löwe B: A brief measure for assessing generalized anxiety disorder: the GAD-7. Arch Intern Med 166(10):1092–1097, 2006 16717171

Stephen LJ, Wishart A, Brodie MJ: Psychiatric side effects and antiepileptic drugs: observations from prospective audits. Epilepsy Behav 71(pt A):73–78, 2017 28551500

Tellez-Zenteno JF, Patten SB, Jetté N, et al: Psychiatric comorbidity in epilepsy: a population-based analysis. Epilepsia 48(12):2336–2344, 2007 17662062

Theodore WH, Hasler G, Giovacchini G, et al: Reduced hippocampal 5HT1A PET receptor binding and depression in temporal lobe epilepsy. Epilepsia 48(8):1526–1530, 2007 17442003

Torta R, Keller R: Behavioral, psychotic, and anxiety disorders in epilepsy: etiology, clinical features, and therapeutic implications. Epilepsia 40(suppl 10):S2–S20, 1999 10609602

Tucker GJ: Seizure disorders presenting with psychiatric symptomatology. Psychiatr Clin North Am 21(3):625–635, vi, 1998 9774800

U.S. Food and Drug Administration: Statistical Review and Evaluation: Antiepileptic Drugs and Suicidality (online). Silver Spring, MD, U.S. Food and Drug Administration, May 23, 2008. Available at: https://www.fda.gov/files/drugs/published/Statistical-Review-and-Evaluation--Antiepileptic-Drugs-and-Suicidality.pdf. Accessed December 9, 2020.

Vuilleumier P, Jallon P: [Epilepsy and psychiatric disorders: epidemiological data]. Rev Neurol (Paris) 154(4):305–317, 1998 9773058

Wassermann EM: Risk and safety of repetitive transcranial magnetic stimulation: report and suggested guidelines from the International Workshop on the Safety of Repetitive Transcranial Magnetic Stimulation, June 5–7, 1996. Electroencephalogr Clin Neurophysiol 108(1):1–16, 1998

DELIRIUM

Yelizaveta Sher, M.D.

■ WHAT IS DELIRIUM?

Delirium is an acute or subacute neuropsychiatric condition primarily characterized by disturbance in attention and awareness and representing a change in mental status. Additional symptoms include deficits in memory, visuospatial awareness, language, perception, and sleep-wake cycle and changes in mood and psychomotor activity. Delirium occurs in the context of an underlying medical or neurological condition or as an effect of a substance. Classically, arousal and symptoms of delirium fluctuate. Although delirium traditionally has been thought to be fully reversible, we now know that in some cases it can be persistent, with many patients having residual cognitive deficits.

Delirium is common in hospitalized patients. On average, in a large general hospital, one in five patients shows signs of a delirium. Some studies estimate that delirium occurs in ≤50% of elderly inpatients. The rate is even higher in the intensive care unit (ICU), where 82% of intubated patients will be affected at some point during their hospital stay. Delirium is distressing to patients, their families, and caregivers and is associated with worse medical outcomes, longer hospital stays, and increased mortality. It also contributes to increased rates of cognitive impairment.

There are several motoric types of delirium: hyperactive, hypoactive, and mixed. The *hyperactive* type is characterized by psychomotor agitation, often coupled with psychotic symptoms. This is a less common type of delirium, but it presents with more dramatic manifestations. Patients who present as more overtly dangerous to self and others are common.

The *hypoactive* type of delirium is characterized by apathy, lethargy, withdrawal, and quiet confusion and is often missed by providers, although it is more clinically prevalent. Patients with hypoactive delirium can present with avolition, anhedonia, and low mood and may even endorse suicidal ideation. Hypoactive delirium is frequently misidentified as depression.

A *mixed* type of delirium is characterized by fluctuating hyperactive and hypoactive episodes. Among older, medically ill patients presenting with delirium, the hypoactive type is prevalent in 65% as compared with the hyperactive (25%) or mixed (10%) types. In addition, researchers highlight a presyndromal delirium that, if missed clinically, can profoundly affect patient outcome, with one-third of patients experiencing cognitive dysfunction for more than 3 months after discharge.

■ MENTAL STATUS AND NEUROLOGICAL EXAMINATION

Mental Status

Patients' disturbed cognitive state may manifest in several ways. It may first appears as impairment of attention characterized by inability to focus, sustain, or appropriately shift attention. Second, it may involve disturbance of arousal that varies from somnolence with poor attention to hypervigilance associated with a prominent startle response. Attention can be tested by asking patients to recite the days of the week or the months of the year backward or to perform a serial-A task in which they raise their hand or squeeze the examiner's hand each time the examiner reads the letter A; examiners present the letters at a rate of one per second over a 30-second period. This test is particularly useful for patients who are not able to communicate verbally.

Patients' orientation to place, date, situation, and even their own person might be impaired. However, intact orientation does not rule out the presence of a delirium. Short-term memory might be compromised and coherence of thought processes may be affected, leading to incoherent speech output and rapid shifting from one topic to another. Patients might have illusions when they misperceive visual stimuli (e.g., mistake an electrical cord for a snake) or have frank audio, visual, or tactile hallucinations consisting of persecutory or paranoid delusions.

Anomia and nonaphasic misnaming, for example, calling a stethoscope a wrench, are linguistic changes that may accompany delirium. Agraphia may be prominent; patients make errors of omission and repetition when writing words, phrases, and sentences. A variety of memory abnormalities may occur.

Patients may be so inattentive that information is not registered, both recall and recognition may be disturbed, or registration may occur but recall is unpredictable, with patients showing impaired recall but preserved recognition. Constructional apraxia and dysgraphia are present and characterized by poor organization and omission of details. A clock drawing test may be an easy method to follow patients' clinical progress. Neuropsychological abilities such as calculation and executive functions are highly vulnerable to attentional disturbances, and performances requiring these skills are error ridden in patients with delirium.

Neuropsychiatric examination is not only helpful in the diagnosis of delirium but also in monitoring its resolution. For example, deficits and hopefully incremental improvements in constructional apraxia such as with the clock drawing test can help to follow patients' progress.

Neurological Examination

Several features should be focused on during the neurological examination for delirium. Patients can have myoclonic jerks or tremors on direct observation. Those who present with delirium due to a particular etiology, such as hepatic or uremic encephalopathy, may display asterixis. Patients might also have dysarthria with slurring of speech.

It might be helpful to evaluate for the presence of the frontal release or primitive signs (resulting from the disinhibition of usually extinguished or suppressed primitive reflexes; refer to Chapter 1, "Neuropsychiatric Assessment"), including the grasp, palmomental, glabellar, routing, and snout reflexes. These signs indicate global dysfunction of the cortex and, in particular, the frontal lobes. However, they are not specific to delirium; patients with a frontal tumor or dementia might also have them. Frontal release signs might be helpful with the diagnosis of milder cases or hypoactive delirium. This may be important, especially when it is imperative to distinguish delirium from other psychiatric conditions, such as depression. The presence or absence of these signs may also help with monitoring for resolution of delirium.

■ PATHOPHYSIOLOGY OF DELIRIUM

Predisposing and precipitating factors may catalyze the development of a delirium. *Predisposing* risk factors include advanced age, underlying cognitive impairment, dementia, visual or hearing impairment, severity of the underlying medical condition, presence of certain underlying psychiatric comorbidities (e.g., schizophrenia), or substance use. *Precipitating* factors (see Table 10–1) include inciting events, such as surgery; certain medications (e.g., benzodiazepines) or substances (e.g., alcohol), or withdrawal from these substances; metabolic derangements; infection; major organ dysfunction; and sleep deprivation. The etiology of delirium usually is multifactorial, with several precipitating factors in a person with preexisting risk factors.

These systemic disturbances are hypothesized to lead to transient disruption of normal brain neuronal activity resulting in neurotransmitter dysfunction. Variability in the integration and appropriate processing of sensory information and motor responses also results in a breakdown in cerebral network connectivity. It is postulated that most altered neurotransmitters are excess of dopamine and low acetylcholine levels with additional alterations in glutamate, serotonin, GABA, and melatonin. A bi-directional relationship exists between delirium and dementia, with the presence of either factor predisposing to the other.

■ DIAGNOSIS

DSM-5 provides criteria for the diagnosis of delirium. However, several screening tools are available to increase the recognition and diagnosis of delirium, including the Confusion Assessment Tool, Confusion Assessment Tool for ICU, Delirium Rating Scale–Revised-98, Intensive Care Delirium Screening Checklist, and Stanford Proxy Test for Delirium. Each of these tools has unique characteristics, strengths, and weaknesses.

A full underlying medical workup must be performed to evaluate for underlying and precipitating factors in delirium, including a review of any recent medication additions or dosage changes. Laboratory abnormalities may reflect the underlying etiology of the delirium. Serum or urine drug assays, blood gases, and serum chemistry may identify intoxications, hypoxic states, and electrolyte or glucose disturbances responsible for the delirium. Urinalysis, chest X-ray, and stool cultures might be needed for assessment of an underlying infectious process. Diagnosis of more unusual causes of delirium may require specialized testing. The electroencephalogram (EEG) is nearly always abnormal in patients with toxic and metabolic disorders and might help distinguish delirium from other neuropsychiatric disorders. The EEG is typically normal in patients with depres-

TABLE 10–1. Causes of delirium/Precipitating factors

Cardiopulmonary disease
  Asthma with respiratory compromise
  Chronic obstructive pulmonary disease
  Congestive heart failure
  Myocardial infarction
  Pneumonia
Dehydration
Gastrointestinal disturbances
  Constipation/Ileus
  Hepatic encephalopathy
  Pancreatitis
Genitourinary abnormalities
  Renal failure/ uremic encephalopathy
  Urinary tract infection
Hypo- or hyperglycemia
Hypo- or hyperkalemia
Hypo- or hypernatremia
Hypo- or hyperthyroidism
Intoxication and Withdrawal
  Alcohol
  Illicit drugs
  Over-the-counter agents (e.g., sleeping aids)
  Prescribed medications (e.g., benzodiazepines, opioids, steroids, anticholinergics)
Metabolic/Endocrinopathies
Neurological disorders
  Bilateral occipital lesions
  Encephalitis
  Limbic encephalitis/ paraneoplastic syndrome
  Meningitis
  Nonconvulsive seizures
  Normal pressure hydrocephalus
  Right temporal-parietal lesions
  Stroke
Pain, poorly controlled
Postoperative
Sepsis
Sleep deprivation
Systemic

sion, schizophrenia, and early degenerative dementias, whereas marked generalized slowing is characteristic of toxic-metabolic encephalopathies. Lumbar puncture may be needed to assess for encephalitis, meningitis, or a limbic encephalitis (to send for a cerebrospinal fluid paraneoplastic panel; refer to Chapter 19, "Evaluation and Treatment of Endocrine Disorders With Neuropsychiatric Symptoms (Thyroid and Adrenal)"). Brain imaging may be necessary to detect strokes or other structural lesions.

Several helpful mnemonics are available to help clinicians be thorough in their workup for delirium etiologies. One such mnemonic is I WATCH DEATH (Table 10–2).

■ PREVENTION AND TREATMENT

Prevention is the best strategy to minimize the harms of delirium. High-risk patients must be identified. Nonpharmacological interventions conducted by staff and family members can be helpful. The Hospital Elder Life Program, a set of multicomponent nonpharmacological interventions pioneered by Dr. Sharon Inouye and colleagues, includes a multidisciplinary team focused on delirium prevention; reorientation and cognitive stimulation of patients; provision of sensory aids (e.g., glasses, hearing aids); prevention of malnutrition, dehydration, aspiration, and constipation; early mobilization; nonpharmacological sleep enhancement; and other components.

If delirium is suspected or diagnosed, a medical workup focused on identification of contributing factors or etiologies should be undertaken. Treatment of delirium includes treating the underlying cause, such as dehydration, infection (e.g., antibiotics), or uremic encephalopathy (e.g., dialysis). Medications that can contribute to delirium should be stopped or tapered (with caution to avoid withdrawal). Behavioral interventions are often interventions of choice. Medications can also be used to treat distressing symptoms and when patients are of risk to themselves or others. If antipsychotics are used, patients' QTc should be monitored. No FDA recommendations are available for use of these medications for this purpose. Other medications used for treatment of delirium include α_2 agonists (e.g., dexmedetomidine in the ICU, clonidine, guanfacine), melatonin and ramelteon, NMDA antagonists (e.g., amantadine for hypoactive and valproic acid for hyperactive and mixed types). Differentiating delirium from dementia may be difficult; contrasting features are listed in Table 10–3.

TABLE 10–2. I WATCH DEATH mnemonic for diagnosis of delirium causes

Cause	Differential
Infectious	Urinary tract infection, pneumonia, sepsis, encephalitis, meningitis, abscess, HIV, syphilis
Withdrawal	Alcohol, benzodiazepines, barbiturates, opiates, sedative-hypnotics
Acute metabolic	Acidosis, alkalosis, electrolyte disturbances, renal or hepatic failure, other metabolic disturbances (e.g., glucose, calcium, magnesium)
Trauma	Head trauma, burns, postoperative
CNS disease	Stroke, hemorrhage, vasculitis, tumors, seizures, autoimmune encephalitis
Hypoxia	Acute hypoxia, hypotension, chronic lung disease, heart failure
Deficiencies	Vitamin B_{12}, thiamine, folate, niacin
Environmental/ Endocrine	Hypothermia, hyperthermia, endocrinopathies (e.g., thyroid, adrenal, diabetes)
Acute vascular	Hypertensive emergency, subarachnoid hemorrhage, sagittal vein thrombosis
Toxins, drugs	Medications (e.g., anticholinergics, benzodiazepines, opiates, psychotropics), street drugs, industrial toxins (e.g., carbon monoxide, pesticides, solvents)
Heavy metals	Lead, mercury

Source. Adapted from Wise MG, Brandt GT: Delirium, in *American Psychiatric Press Textbook of Neuropsychiatry*, 2nd Edition. Edited by Yudofsky SC, Hales RE. Washington, DC, American Psychiatric Press, 1992, pp 291–308

Case Example

A psychiatrist is consulted for treatment of depression in a 72-year-old woman with a prior history of hypertension and no past psychiatric history who was hospitalized after elective knee replacement surgery. She has been in the hospital for 3 days, and the surgeons noticed that in the preoperative setting she was a lively and happy woman, but since her surgery she has been withdrawn and quiet. She has not been participating in physical therapy, sleeps for most of the day (but has difficulty sleeping at night), and refuses some of her medications.

On neuropsychiatric evaluation, the patient is drowsy and frequently dozes off. She is able to state her name and why she is in the hospital but is not able to state her location or date. She is not able to recite the days of the week backward. She reports a vague sensation that she is not safe in the hospital. She

TABLE 10–3. Contrasting features of dementia and delirium

Feature	Delirium	Dementia
Onset	Acute or subacute	Insidious
Course	Fluctuating	Persistent
Duration	Limited	Chronic
Attention	Impaired	Intact until advanced stages
Language	Incoherent	More coherent until late
Speech	Slurred dysarthria	Dysarthria uncommon
Visual hallucinations	Common	Uncommon
Tremor	Common	Uncommon
Myoclonus	Common	Occurs in only a few types
Electroencephalogram	Prominent abnormalities	Mild changes

also reports feeling down. She is able to follow simple commands of closing and opening her eyes but not complex three-step commands. On neurological evaluation, the patient has prominent bilateral palmomental and grasp reflexes.

Review of her recent medical history and hospital course reveals aggressive pain management with opiates and slightly increased white count. To help with her sleep, the team has also been scheduling diphenhydramine 25 mg at bedtime. Of note, she has had her urine catheter since her surgery.

The psychiatrist asks to repeat the patient's blood work and to conduct a urinalysis and chest X-ray. These laboratory investigations reveal a urinary infection. She is diagnosed with delirium of hypoactive subtype with the following likely contributors: postoperative status, urinary tract infection, opiates, and anticholinergics. The psychiatrist recommends stopping the diphenhydramine, decreasing the opiates, treating the infection, starting melatonin for her sleep-wake cycle, and initiating aggressive nonpharmacological measures. With these interventions, she improves within the next 3 days, with a re-equilibrated sleep-wake cycle and improved attention, wakefulness, and mood.

■ CONCLUSION

Delirium is an acute or subacute neuropsychiatric condition primarily characterized by a disturbance in attention and awareness that arises within hours or days, represents a change from the individual's baseline, and is due to medical, neurological, or substance-related causes. Although common, it is often under- and misdiagnosed in hospital patients. The most common motoric subtype of delirium is hypoactive, which is often missed. Delirium is diagnosed with a neuropsychiatric evaluation focused on patients' attention, awareness, cognition, language, mood, perceptual disturbances, and psychomotor changes. Neurological examination, such as evaluation of primitive reflexes, is also helpful. Mnemonics such as I WATCH DEATH can be helpful in investigation of contributing etiologies.

It is best to prevent delirium utilizing nonpharmacological measures. When delirium is diagnosed, clinicians should identify and treat contributing factors, implement nonpharmacological interventions, and consider psychotropic medications to address distressing symptoms or prevent harm to the patient or staff. No medications have been FDA-approved for treatment of delirium.

■ REFERENCES

American Psychiatric Association: Diagnostic and Statistical Manual of Mental Disorders, 5th Edition. Arlington, VA, American Psychiatric Association, 2013

Baranowski SL, Patten SB: The predictive value of dysgraphia and constructional apraxia for delirium in psychiatric inpatients. Can J Psychiatry 45(1):75–78, 2000 10696493

Ely EW, Margolin R, Francis J, et al: Evaluation of delirium in critically ill patients: validation of the Confusion Assessment Method for the Intensive Care Unit (CAM-ICU). Crit Care Med 29(7):1370–1379, 2001 11445689

Ely EW, Shintani A, Truman B, et al: Delirium as a predictor of mortality in mechanically ventilated patients in the intensive care unit. JAMA 291(14):1753–1762, 2004 15082703

Hshieh TT, Yang T, Gartaganis SL, et al: Hospital Elder Life Program: systematic review and meta-analysis of effectiveness. Am J Geriatr Psychiatry 26(10):1015–1033, 2018 30076080

Inouye SK: Delirium in older persons. N Engl J Med 354(11):1157–1165, 2006 16540616

Jiang S, Czuma R, Cohen-Oram A, et al: Guanfacine for hyperactive delirium: a case series. J Acad Consult Liaison Psychiatry 62(1):83–88, 2021 33272699

Lipowski ZJ: Delirium: Acute Confusional States. New York, Oxford University Press, 1990

Liptzin B, Levkoff SE: An empirical study of delirium subtypes. Br J Psychiatry 161:843–845, 1992 1483173

Maldonado JR: Acute brain failure: pathophysiology, diagnosis, management, and sequelae of delirium. Crit Care Clin 33(3):461–519, 2017 28601132

Maldonado JR: Delirium pathophysiology: an updated hypothesis of the etiology of acute brain failure. Int J Geriatr Psychiatry 33(11):1428–1457, 2018 29278283

Maldonado JR, Sher YI, Benitez-Lopez MA, et al: A study of the psychometric properties of the "Stanford Proxy Test for Delirium" (S-PTD): a new screening tool for the detection of delirium. Psychosomatics 61(2):116–126, 2020 31926650

Oldham MA, Flanagan NM, Khan A, et al: Responding to ten common delirium misconceptions with the best evidence: an educational review for clinicians. J Neuropsychiatry Clin Neurosci 30(1):51–57, 2018 28876970

Pandharipande PP, Girard TD, Ely EW: Long-term cognitive impairment after critical illness. N Engl J Med 370(2):185–186, 2014 24401069

Sher Y, Miller Cramer AC, Ament A, et al: Valproic acid for treatment of hyperactive or mixed delirium: rationale and literature review. Psychosomatics 56(6):615–625, 2015 26674479

Trzepacz PT, Mittal D, Torres R, et al: Validation of the Delirium Rating Scale-Revised-98: comparison with the delirium rating scale and the cognitive test for delirium. J Neuropsychiatry Clin Neurosci 13(2):229–242, 2001 11449030

van Eijk MM, van Marum RJ, Klijn IA, et al: Comparison of delirium assessment tools in a mixed intensive care unit. Crit Care Med 37(6):1881–1885, 2009 19384206

Wise MG, Brandt GT: Delirium, in American Psychiatric Press Textbook of Neuropsychiatry, 2nd Edition. Edited by Yudofsky SC, Hales RE. Washington, DC, American Psychiatric Press, 1992, pp 291–308

11

DEMENTIA

Jeffrey L. Cummings, M.D., Sc.D.

Dementia is a clinical syndrome characterized by cognitive impairment that is sufficiently severe to cause functional impairment. The cognitive and behavioral changes represent a decline from a previous level of function, are not better explained by delirium or a psychiatric disorder, are well-documented by neuropsychological assessments, and have at least two of the following features: memory impairment, impaired reasoning and complex thinking, impaired visual-spatial abilities, impaired language, or changes in personality, behavior, or comportment. Dementia is not an etiological diagnosis; it is a syndrome that accompanies many neurological disorders, including neurodegenerative disorders, cerebrovascular disease, traumatic brain injury, multiple sclerosis, infectious and inflammatory disorders, metabolic disorders, subdural hematomas, hydrocephalus, and neoplastic disorders. Dementia is often progressive, as observed in neurodegenerative disorders, but it may be acute, after stroke or traumatic brain injury. Dementia is also called *major neurocognitive disorder*, and *mild cognitive impairment* (MCI) is called *mild neurocognitive disorder* in some nomenclature systems.

This chapter focuses on clinically important information applicable in daily practice and emphasizes the neuropsychiatric aspects of dementia syndromes. It begins by discussing the assessment of patients presenting with dementia, then describes the differential diagnosis of dementia. This is followed by discussion of the most common forms of dementia, including Alzheimer's disease (AD), frontotemporal dementia (FTD) and its spectrum disorders, chronic traumatic encephalopathy (CTE), dementia with Lewy bodies (DLB), Parkinson's disease dementia (PDD), multiple system atrophy (MSA), vascular cognitive disorders (VCD) and vascular dementia (VaD). Disorder and syndrome-specific treatments are discussed with each disease. Best practices for the use of psychotropics and management of neuropsychiatric syndromes across dementias are presented in the final portion of the chapter.

■ ASSESSMENT OF PATIENTS WITH DEMENTIA SYNDROMES

Dementia is a syndrome that results from many types of brain dysfunction. The specific etiology of the dementia syndrome is determined by a thorough assessment (Table 11–1). A carefully taken history builds a relationship with patients and their caregivers and guides selection of the tests to be used in the evaluation. The history includes the onset and evolution of cognitive and behavioral changes; review of past medical illnesses, current medical symptoms, and medications and over-the-counter treatments taken; review of sleep and appetite changes; discussion of any family history of neurological illnesses; and a review of risk factors for cognitive decline. Mental status testing refines the diagnostic hypothesis generated by the history and interview and informs the use of laboratory testing, brain imaging, and elective assessments. Neurological examination may identify parkinsonism consistent with DLB, PDD, MSA, and some forms of FTD or focal neurological signs indicative of VCD/VaD and other focal brain lesions.

A neuropsychological assessment can provide important diagnostic and differential diagnostic information. Patients in the early stages of symptomatic disease can be difficult to distinguish from cognitively normal older adults. Neuropsychological assessments have age- and education-matched norms that allow more refined judgments regarding cognitive function; the profile of tests scores can assist in distinguishing dementia types. A comprehensive neuropsychological evaluation assesses attention, language, memory, visuospatial skills, and executive function. Psychomotor speed is assessed with timed tests.

Basic laboratory tests are collected on all patients, and optional tests are chosen based on the history, clinical presentation, and physical and neurological examination. MRI or CT are obtained on all patients to exclude brain tumor, subdural hematoma and other focal lesions, hydrocephalus, and evidence of stroke or ischemic brain injury. Fluorodeoxyglucose (FDG) PET imaging is particularly useful in identifying stroke (focal hypometabolic regions) and in distinguishing AD (bilateral parietal and posterior medial hypometabolism) from FTD (bilateral usually asymmetric hypometabolism). Amyloid PET identifies

TABLE 11–1. **Assessment of patients with dementia**

Clinical assessment	History of onset, progression, and major features of the cognitive syndrome, including cognitive, emotional, and behavioral changes
	Review of risk factors for cerebrovascular disease (diabetes, hypertension, obesity, cigarette smoking), acute events (stroke, head trauma), educational level, nutrition and dietary habits, physical exercise, recent changes in medical status or medications
	Review of family history of neurological disorders
Clinical examination	Mental status examination
	Physical and cardiovascular examination
	Neurological examination
	Neuropsychological evaluation
Laboratory evaluation	Complete blood count
	Electrolytes, blood sugar, blood urea nitrogen, cholesterol and triglycerides, liver functions
	Thyroid-stimulating hormone
	Vitamin B_{12} level
Genetic testing	Not recommended for most patients
	APOE ε4 alleles present in 60%–70% of patients with late-onset Alzheimer's disease; autosomal dominant mutations (*PSEN1*, *PSEN2*, *APP*) may be present in early-onset cases (onset typically before 60 years of age)
	Genes most commonly implicated in frontotemporal dementia include *MAPT*, *GRN*, *C9orf72*
Optional informative laboratory tests	Vitamin D, homocysteine, c-reactive protein, erythrocyte sedimentation rate, testosterone (males), HgbA1c, antiphospholipid antibodies, serum or urine levels of prescribed medications or illegal drugs, HIV test
Brain imaging	MRI or CT
Optional informative imaging	Fluorodeoxyglucose PET, amyloid PET

TABLE 11–1.	Assessment of patients with dementia *(continued)*
Elective assessments	Lumbar puncture
	Amyloid, phosphorylated tau, total tau
	White cell counts and evidence of infectious meningitis tests (e.g., cryptococcus, histoplasmosis, cysticercosis, toxoplasmosis, tuberculosis, syphilis, Lyme disease, viral meningitis)
	14-3-3 protein if Creutzfeldt-Jakob disease suspected
	Electroencephalography
	Electromyography
	Nerve conduction studies
	Carotid doppler studies

the presence of fibrillar/plaque amyloid. A negative amyloid PET scan essentially excludes AD as the cause of any cognitive impairment; a positive scan is supportive of a diagnosis of AD but may also occur in DLB and amyloid angiopathy. Amyloid PET is not commonly used in routine clinical practice but may be required for the use of anti-amyloid therapies in the future. Lumbar puncture and cerebrospinal fluid (CSF) studies are required if meningitis is suspected. Decreased CSF amyloid (amyloid β [Aβ] protein 42) and elevated CSF phosphorylated-tau (p-tau) and total tau are characteristic of AD. Electrophysiological studies (electroencephalogram [EEG], electromyogram [EMG], and nerve conduction studies) are employed to explore specific diagnostic hypotheses.

The results of the assessment are synthesized with the historical, family history, and risk factor information to develop a working diagnosis that will guide interventions and be constantly reassessed as new information and treatment response observations accrue.

■ DIFFERENTIAL DIAGNOSIS OF DEMENTIA

Table 11–2 shows how data collected during the dementia assessment as outlined in Table 11–1 are synthesized to differentiate the multiple potential causes of dementia, especially as they present in older adults. Combinations of cognitive, behavioral, and motor disturbances are synthesized into phenotypes. These disease-related phenotypes reflect the regional vulnerability of

TABLE 11–2. Differential diagnosis of dementia

Disorder	Cognitive features	Behavioral features	Motor features
Alzheimer's disease	Amnestic onset followed by language and visuospatial deterioration	Agitation, apathy, depression, sleep disorders most common; psychosis observed in some	Normal until advanced phases; rigidity and paratonia in severe phase of dementia
FTD behavioral variant	Executive dysfunction (may be mild)	Disinhibition, socially inappropriate behavior; compulsions and repetitive behaviors in some	Normal or parkinsonism
FTD with motor neuron disease	Executive dysfunction (may be mild)	Disinhibition, socially inappropriate behavior	Fasciculations; EMG features consistent with motor neuron disease
Nonfluent variant PPA	Nonfluent aphasia with progressive mutism	Apathy, depression, irritability	Normal or rigidity; may develop PSP-like phenotype
Semantic variant PPA	Fluent semantic-type aphasia with visual agnosia	Disinhibition, poor judgment	Normal until advanced phases
Progressive supranuclear palsy	Executive dysfunction; some cases have progressive nonfluent aphasia	Apathy common; disinhibition in some	Progressive axial rigidity; freezing of gait; falls; pseudobulbar palsy
Corticobasal degeneration	Visuospatial dysfunction prominent; some cases have progressive nonfluent aphasia	Depression common	Asymmetric limb rigidity; alien limb phenomena; limb myoclonus

TABLE 11–2. Differential diagnosis of dementia (*continued*)

Disorder	Cognitive features	Behavioral features	Motor features
Traumatic encephalopathy syndrome	Executive dysfunction; episodic memory impairment	Neurobehavioral dysregulation with explosiveness and impulsiveness	Parkinsonism; ataxia; dysarthria
Dementia with Lewy bodies	Fluctuating cognitive changes; executive and visuospatial dysfunction more prominent than memory loss (parkinsonism follows onset of cognitive changes)	Visual hallucinations; delusions; depression; REM sleep behavioral disturbance	Parkinsonism
Parkinson's disease dementia	Fluctuating cognitive changes; executive and visuospatial dysfunction more prominent than memory loss (parkinsonism precedes onset of cognitive changes)	Visual hallucinations; delusions; depression; REM sleep behavioral disturbance	Parkinsonism
Multiple system atrophy	Executive dysfunction and psychomotor retardation	Apathy, depression	Parkinsonism; ataxia; pyramidal tract signs; dysarthria
Vascular cognitive disorder/Vascular dementia	Executive dysfunction	Depression, apathy common	Focal neurological signs; pyramidal signs (brisk reflexes); "lower half parkinsonism" with gait abnormalities

EMG=electromyogram; FTD=frontotemporal dementia; PPA=primary progressive aphasia; PSP=progressive supranuclear palsy; REM=rapid eye movement.

brain regions or functional systems to accumulation of specific types of protein in the neurodegenerative disorders, leading to local brain dysfunction and the ensuing phenotype. Accurate diagnosis based on the phenotype reflects the disease-specific pathology and related regional abnormalities of function.

None of the disorders presented in Table 11–2 has a diagnostic blood test, although a plasma ratio of Aβ protein 42/40 and of p-tau promise to emerge as supportive of the diagnosis of AD, and abnormally low plasma progranulin levels predict the presence of progranulin gene mutation in patients with this rare form of FTD.

Clinically, episodic recent memory impairment is the most common presentation of AD. A variety of neuropsychiatric syndromes may occur, including apathy, depression, agitation, and sleep disturbances. FTD may present as a disinhibited socially inappropriate syndrome (behavioral variant, bvFTD) or as a primary progressive aphasia (PPA) of the nonfluent (nfPPA) or semantic (loss of word meaning; svPPA) type. Two disorders on the FTD spectrum include progressive supranuclear palsy (PSP) and corticobasal degeneration (CBD). The former features bradykinesia, axial rigidity, pseudobulbar palsy, cognitive impairment and prominent apathy. CBD presents with unilateral limb apraxia and action myoclonus with frequent depression. CTE occurs in athletes and others with repetitive head injury and is characterized by cognitive impairment and personality changes and may manifest as parkinsonism. DLB features dementia, visual hallucinations, delusions, depression, and rapid eye movement (REM) sleep behavioral disorder. Parkinsonism commonly follows onset of dementia. PDD resembles dementia of DLB, but the parkinsonism precedes dementia onset. MSA is a rapidly progressive form of parkinsonism with marked autonomic dysfunction and motoric disability. VCD/VaD occurs in patients with vascular risk factors, usually has a sudden onset with stepwise decline, and features prominent executive dysfunction with apathy and depression. Focal neurological findings or pyramidal track signs are often present.

■ ALZHEIMER'S DISEASE

AD is the most common of the late-onset dementias, accounting for 60%–70% of dementias in older adults. AD may occur in individuals age 50 or younger; early-onset cases are more likely to be familial, with autosomal dominant genetic mutations or apolipoprotein ε4 alleles that determine or contribute to disease pathogenesis.

The AD continuum extends from preclinical AD to prodromal AD to AD dementia. Preclinical AD is characterized by normal cognition in individuals with positive amyloid biomarkers (positive amyloid PET or CSF biomarkers consistent with AD). The preclinical phase is present for 15 years prior to the onset of symptoms and for 20 years prior to onset of dementia in most cases. Prodromal AD features mild cognitive symptoms, no or very mild impairment of daily function, and positive biomarkers for AD. AD dementia is characterized by impaired cognition, impaired activities of daily living, and positive biomarkers for AD. It progresses through mild, moderate, and severe phases and to death, which is usually due to aspiration pneumonia or other disability-related cause unless cardiovascular, neoplastic, or another illness supervenes to shorten the course.

Risk factors of AD include age, family history and genetic influences, head injury, diabetes, hypertension, obesity, sleep disturbances, smoking, stress, and depression. Protective factors include physical exercise, higher educational levels, mental fitness, connectedness and sense of purpose, and good nutrition with a high content of antioxidant foods.

AD typically presents as a gradually progressive amnestic syndrome with episodic recent memory impairment manifested in repeating questions and forgetfulness about recent events. Clinically, this is recognized as MCI. Approximately 50% of patients with MCI have prodromal AD; others are in the very early stages of non-AD dementias, may have nonprogressive forms of MCI, or may even revert to normal on subsequent examinations. As the AD progresses, there is increasing deterioration of memory, language, visuospatial function, and executive abilities. Dependency on caregivers increases as cognition declines. The neurological examination remains normal until late in the illness when rigidity and paratonia emerge. Seizures are not common in AD but may occur in younger patients during the later stages of the disease.

Atypical presentations include a frontal-type AD that must be distinguished from FTD; an aphasic type of AD with logopenic aphasia (characterized by progressive loss of word retrieval and repetitions with errors in spontaneous speech) that must be differentiated from other types of PPA; and a posterior cortical atrophy variant that features prominent visuospatial impairment and relative preservation of memory.

AD is characterized by amyloid plaques, neurofibrillary tangles, and neurodegeneration with loss of neurons and synapses (Table 11–3). This is recognized in the amyloid, tau, neurodegeneration (ATN) framework for the biological diagnosis of AD. Amyloid is generated from amyloid precursor protein and progresses through increasingly complex aggregations from monomers, to oligomers, to protofibrils, and then to the fibrillar amyloid that composes the plaques. Neurofibrillary tangles form from p-tau protein, which spreads through networks of connected neurons in a prion-like manner. Neuroinflammation, microglial activation, astrogliosis, mitochondrial dysfunction, and accumulation of other types of proteins (e.g., α-synuclein, transactive response DNA-binding protein 43 [TDP-43]) are present in the brains of most patients at autopsy. There is marked cholinergic deficit in the brain produced by neurodegeneration of the cholinergic source neurons in the nucleus basalis of Meynert of the basal forebrain.

Plasma and CSF biomarkers reflect this ongoing central pathology: plasma $A\beta_{42/40}$ ratios and CSF $A\beta_{42}$ measures decline as amyloid is increasingly deposited in the brain; total tau in the CSF rises with cell death; p-tau increases in the CSF and blood as a marker of decreased clearance and discharge of p-tau from injured neurons in the brain. Amyloid PET and tau PET detect the accumulation of neuritic plaques and neurofibrillary tangles, respectively, in the brain (Table 11–4).

Treatment of AD builds upon a foundation of accurate diagnosis and includes aducanumab for patients with mild cognitive impairment of mild dementia due to AD; cholinesterase inhibitors for mild, moderate, and severe AD; memantine for moderate and severe AD; nonpharmacological interventions and psychotropic medications (discussed later) for neuropsychiatric syndromes; and caregiver support. Table 11–5 outlines the drugs available for treatment of AD, the specific indications for which each agent is approved, available dosages, administration regimens, and principal side effects. Aducanumab is initiated in mildly affected patients with confirmed brain amyloid. Following that, a cholinesterase inhibitor is initiated and the dosage optimized; in some cases, intolerable side effects will require switching to a different cholinergic agent. Once the cholinesterase inhibitor is optimized, memantine is added and this combination therapy is continued as long as patients have an acceptable quality of life. Therapy with these agents improves cognition above baseline in approximately 25% of treated pa-

TABLE 11–3. Major pathological and neurochemical changes of the neurodegenerative disorders

Disorder	Principal pathology	Neurochemical abnormalities
Alzheimer's disease	Amyloid plaques, neurofibrillary tangles, neuronal loss	Cholinergic deficit
FTD behavioral variant	Tau protein or TDP-43 protein aggregation in most patients; white matter changes common	Serotoninergic deficit
FTD with motor neuron disease	TDP-43 protein aggregation in brain and spinal cord	Serotonergic deficit
Nonfluent variant PPA	Tau protein aggregation most common	No specific transmitter deficit
Semantic variant PPA	TDP-43 protein aggregation most common	No specific transmitter deficit
Progressive supranuclear palsy	Tau protein aggregation	Dopamine deficit
Corticobasal degeneration	Tau protein aggregation	No specific transmitter deficit
Chronic traumatic encephalopathy	Tau protein aggregation	Dopamine deficit in those with parkinsonism
Dementia with Lewy bodies	α-Synuclein protein aggregation in neurons; amyloid plaques in approximately 70% of patients	Cholinergic deficit; dopamine deficit
Parkinson's disease dementia	α-Synuclein protein aggregation in neurons	Cholinergic deficit; dopamine deficit
Multiple system atrophy	α-Synuclein protein aggregation in oligodendrocytes	Dopaminergic deficit
Vascular cognitive disorder/Vascular dementia	White matter ischemic injury and lacunar infarctions; cortical microinfarcts in some	Mixed moderate transmitter deficits

FTD=frontotemporal dementia; PPA=primary progressive aphasia; TDP-43=transactive response DNA-binding protein 43.

TABLE 11–4. Brain imaging findings in patients with major dementia syndromes

Disorder	Brain imaging
Alzheimer's disease	MRI: generalized and hippocampal atrophy
	FDG PET: decreased medial posterior (cuneus) and bilateral parietal metabolism
	Amyloid PET: positive
FTD behavioral variant	MRI: frontotemporal atrophy (often more severe on the right)
FTD with motor neuron disease	Frontotemporal atrophy
Nonfluent variant PPA	MRI: frontotemporal atrophy (left frontal predominant)
	FDG PET: left frontal-opercular hypometabolism
Semantic variant PPA	MRI: frontotemporal atrophy (left posterior predominant)
	FDG PET: left anterior temporal hypometabolism
Progressive supranuclear palsy	MRI: brain stem atrophy with "morning glory sign" in transaxial views and "hummingbird sign" in sagittal views
	FDG PET: brain stem and medial frontal hypometabolism
	DAT SPECT or PET: reduced dopamine transporter update
Corticobasal degeneration	MRI: generalized atrophy, often asymmetric
Traumatic encephalopathy syndrome	MRI: atrophy with disproportionate frontal ventricular enlargement
	FDG PET: bilateral dorsolateral and orbitofrontal hypometabolism
Dementia with Lewy bodies	MRI: generalized atrophy; mild hippocampal atrophy
	FDG PET: posterior parietal and occipital hypometabolism with precuneus "island sign"
	DAT SPECT or PET: reduced dopamine transporter update

188

Disorder	Brain imaging
Parkinson's disease dementia	MRI: generalized atrophy; mild hippocampal atrophy
	FDG PET: cortical hypometabolism with relative increase in basal ganglia metabolism
	DAT SPECT or PET: reduced dopamine transporter update
Multiple system atrophy	MRI: posterior putaminal hypointensity, hyperintense lateral putaminal rim, and "hot cross bun sign"; brain stem and cerebellar atrophy
	FDG PET: brain stem and cerebellar hypometabolism
	DAT SPECT or PET: diminished DAT activity in the striatum
Vascular cognitive disorder/vascular dementia	Cortical infarctions; lacunar infarctions; periventricular and deep white matter ischemic injury

TABLE 11–4. Brain imaging findings in patients with major dementia syndromes *(continued)*

DAT=dopamine transporter; FDG=fluorodeoxyglucose; FTD=frontotemporal dementia; PPA=primary progressive aphasia; SPECT=single-photon emission computed tomography.

tients and delays decline by 6–9 months in 80% of these patients. Disease progression is eventually observed; patients who are receiving therapy continue to function better than those who are untreated throughout the disease course. Agitation, apathy, psychosis, depression, anxiety, and sleep disturbances are treatment targets for pharmacology if patients are unresponsive to nonpharmacological interventions (Table 11–6). Levetiracetam is the anticonvulsant most often used for seizures in AD.

Pharmacotherapy should be combined with recommendations for a brain-healthy lifestyle for patients and their families. Lifestyle recommendations include daily physical exercise, socialization, mental fitness (e.g., games, puzzles), sleep optimization, healthy diet, and control of vascular risk factors (e.g., hypertension, elevated cholesterol). Caregivers are at increased risk for depression, substance and alcohol use, and physical illness. Clinicians must build an alliance with the caregivers and be vigilant about their health and wellness; referrals to support groups, community resources, or professional services may be required.

TABLE 11–5. Treatments for Alzheimer's disease (AD)

Treatment (brand)	Indication	Dosages	Regimen	Side effects
Aducanumab (Aduhelm)	MCI, mild AD, dementia	Target is 10 mg/kg	Titrate from 1 mg/kg to 3 mg/kg, 6 mg/kg, and 10 mg/kg at 2-month intervals	Amyloid-related imaging abnormalities
Donepezil (Aricept)	Mild, moderate, severe AD	1 mg, 10 mg, 23 mg	Titrate from 5 mg/day for 1 month to 10 mg/day given qam; increase to 23 mg/day (or 10 mg bid) if warranted	Diarrhea, anorexia, muscle cramps, unpleasant dreams
Galantamine (Razadyne ER)	Mild, moderate AD	8 mg, 16 mg, 24 mg	Begin with 8 mg/day and titrate to 16 mg/day and then to 24 mg/day	Nausea and vomiting, anorexia
Memantine (Namenda)	Moderate, severe AD	5 mg, 10 mg, 28 mg	Begin at 5 mg/day and titrate in 5-mg increments to 10 mg bid; 28 mg/day may be substituted for 10 mg bid	Dizziness, headache, drowsiness
Namzaric	Moderate, severe AD	Fixed dosage of donepezil 10 mg and memantine 28 mg	Switch to Namzaric if desired for patients taking donepezil 10 mg and memantine 28 mg or donepezil 10 mg and memantine 10 mg bid	Diarrhea, muscle cramps, unpleasant dreams, dizziness, headache, drowsiness
Rivastigmine* (Exelon Patch)	Mild, moderate, severe AD; PDD	4.6 mg, 9.4 mg, 14.4 mg	One new patch each day applied to a new upper body location; previous day's patch is removed	Nausea and vomiting, skin irritation from patch

ER=extended release; MCI=mild cognitive impairment; PDD=Parkinson's disease dementia.
*Rivastigmine is approved for use in PDD.

TABLE 11–6. Psychotropic drugs for neuropsychiatric syndromes in dementia

Neuropsychiatric syndrome	Agent	Daily dosage	Side effects
Agitation	Brexpiprazole	0.25–4 mg	Weight gain, akathisia
	Citalopram	10–20 mg	QT prolongation
	Quetiapine	25–200 mg	Somnolence, dry mouth, dizziness, constipation, postural hypotension
	Risperidone	0.5–1 mg	Parkinsonism, akathisia, dystonia, tremor, sedation, dizziness, nausea, vomiting, dry mouth, increased appetite, increased weight
Apathy	Methylphenidate	10–20 mg	Insomnia, appetite suppression, hypertension, dependency
	Modafinil	200 mg	Headache, nausea, diarrhea, dry mouth, anorexia
Depression	Citalopram	10–40 mg	QT prolongation, nausea, dry mouth, somnolence
	Duloxetine	20–60 mg	Nausea, dry mouth, insomnia, sexual dysfunction (males)
Disinhibition	Citalopram	10–40 mg	QT prolongation, nausea, dry mouth, somnolence
	Dextromethorphan/ quinidine	20/10 mg bid	Diarrhea, dizziness, cough, vomiting, asthenia, peripheral edema, urinary tract infection, influenza, increased γ-glutamyltransferase, flatulence
Psychosis	Olanzapine	2.5–20 mg	Postural hypotension, constipation, weight gain, dizziness, akathisia, parkinsonism
	Pimavanserin	34 mg	Peripheral edema, confusion
	Quetiapine	25–200 mg	Somnolence, dry mouth, dizziness, constipation, postural hypotension

TABLE 11–6. Psychotropic drugs for neuropsychiatric syndromes in dementia *(continued)*

Neuropsychiatric syndrome	Agent	Daily dosage	Side effects
Repetitive behavior	Citalopram	10–40 mg	QT prolongation, nausea, dry mouth, somnolence
	Sertraline	25–200 mg	Nausea, diarrhea/loose stool, tremor, dyspepsia, decreased appetite, hyperhidrosis, ejaculation failure, decreased libido
Sleep disturbances	Suvorexant	5–20 mg	Somnolence
	Trazodone	25–100 mg	Edema, blurred vision, syncope, drowsiness, fatigue, diarrhea, nasal congestion, weight loss
	Zolpidem	5 mg	Drowsiness, diarrhea, dizziness

Note. Only the most commonly used first-line treatments are presented. All prescribing for behavioral disorders in dementia is off-label; no therapies are FDA approved for behavioral changes in patients with dementia.

■ FRONTOTEMPORAL DEMENTIA AND SPECTRUM DISORDERS

There are four presentations of FTD: bvFTD, bvFTD with motor neuron disease, nfPPA, and svPPA. There are two related FTD spectrum disorders: PSP and CBD.

Behavioral Variant Frontotemporal Dementia

bvFTD is one of the most dramatic clinical disorders presenting to neuropsychiatrists and behavioral neurologists. Patients exhibit behavioral disinhibition characterized by socially inappropriate behavior; loss of manners or impulsivity; apathy and inertia; loss of sympathy or empathy; stereotyped, perseverative, or compulsive/ritualistic behavior; and hyperorality and dietary changes. On cognitive assessment, patients display deficits in executive function with relative sparing of memory and visuospatial function. Some patients exhibit parkinsonian features. MRI shows frontal or anterior temporal atrophy (often asymmetric) and FDG PET shows frontal or anterior temporal hypometabolism.

Repetitive behaviors and rituals may improve with serotonergic drugs such as citalopram (Celexa) or sertraline (Zoloft). Disinhibition may improve with anticonvulsant agents or dextromethorphan/quinidine (Nuedexta). Parkinsonism may respond to treatment with dopaminergic agents.

Three pathology types account for the biology of FTD. Most cases have a tau or TDP-43-type pathology; very few have fused in sarcoma–related pathology. White matter pathology is often prominent (see Chapter 12, "Movement Disorders").

Frontotemporal Dementia With Motor Neuron Disease

FTD with motor neuron disease is usually characterized by behavioral changes, including disinhibition and loss of empathy, with an amyotrophic lateral sclerosis–type disorder reflecting progressive motor neuron disease. Electromyography reveals fasciculations consistent with motor neuron disease. TDP-43 is the most common underlying pathology. Riluzole and edaravone may be helpful in the management of the motor neuron disorder.

Nonfluent Variant of Primary Progressive Aphasia

nfPPA features agrammatism in language production; effortful, halting speech; and impaired comprehension of syntactically complex sentences. Output is usually decreased, without dysarthria or orofacial dyspraxia. Mutism may occur, whereas other cognitive functions remain largely intact. Word comprehension and object knowledge (e.g., name-object matching) are spared. MRI demonstrates left-predominant posterior frontoinsular atrophy, and FDG PET shows left posterior frontoinsular hypometabolism. The most common accompanying pathology is tau aggregation, but some cases have TDP-43 protein aggregation or AD at autopsy.

Semantic Variant of Primary Progressive Aphasia

svPPA is characterized by anomia; impairments in naming, single word comprehension (e.g., cannot decipher what the sound of individual words means), and object knowledge (e.g., visual agnosia for uncommon items); and dyslexia or dysgraphia. Output is fluent, with paraphasia and circumlocutions. Repetition of language and speech production are spared throughout most of the illness course. MRI shows anterior temporal lobe atrophy, and FDG PET reveals anterior temporal hypometabolism. TDP-43 inclusions are the most common pathology found at autopsy.

Progressive Supranuclear Palsy

PSP is an FTD spectrum disorder; tau protein inclusions are found in the brain at autopsy. The clinical phenotype includes dementia, pseudobulbar pathology and prominent dysarthria, axial rigidity with progressive postural extension, and vertical supranuclear gaze palsy. Progressive freezing of gait and falls are common. Apathy is prominent, and some patients exhibit disinhibition or depression. Brain imaging may show a "morning glory sign" on axial brain stem imaging and a "hummingbird sign" on sagittal images of the upper brain stem. These may not occur until late in the illness. Pathologically, PSP is characterized by tau inclusions forming neurofibrillary tangles in neurons and glial cells Parkinsonian features may improve with dopaminergics. Neuropsychiatric and behavioral aspects may respond to psychotropics (see Table 11–6).

Corticobasal Degeneration

CBD is a 4R tauopathy that features asymmetric limb rigidity, akinesia, or dystonic limb posturing; limb myoclonus; orofacial or limb apraxia; and alien limb phenomena (e.g., the sense that one's limb has autonomous activity). Apraxia with an inability to follow complex commands despite sufficiently intact motor and sensory function is present in many of these cases. Eye movements are often abnormal, with increased latency to initiate saccades and jerky pursuit movements. Brain imaging findings are asymmetric but nonspecific. Neuronal and glia tau inclusions are evident at autopsy (see Chapter 12).

■ CHRONIC TRAUMATIC ENCEPHALOPATHY

Repetitive head injuries in athletes (e.g., boxing, American football, soccer, hockey), in soldiers experiencing repetitive blast injuries, and in others with a similar exposure history are characterized clinically as traumatic encephalopathy syndrome. This comprises a progressive dementing disorder that includes deficits in executive function and episodic memory accompanied by neurobehavioral dysregulation featuring explosiveness, impulsivity, rage, and aggressive outbursts. Parkinsonism with bradykinesia, gait changes, and rest tremor are commonly present, and many patients have dysarthria and ataxia. Motor neuron disease with fasciculations may occur. In addition to neurobehavioral dysregulation, other neuropsychiatric symptoms are common, including apathy, anxiety, depression, and paranoid thinking. Certainty of diagnosis for predicting the pathology of CTE increases when more cognitive and behavioral changes are present and the number of head injuries is greater (e.g., diagnosis is most certain in those with athletic exposures to injury for more than 10 years).

Structural MRI demonstrates cerebral atrophy with disproportionate enlargement of the frontal ventricular horns. FDG PET shows reduced metabolism in the bilateral prefrontal and orbitofrontal regions. Research imaging with tau PET shows the subtle accumulation of tau protein. Pathologically, CTE is diagnosed by the presence of tau pathology around vessels and in the depths of the cerebral sulci. Amyloid plaques characteristic of AD are not typically found in CTE.

■ DEMENTIA WITH LEWY BODIES AND PARKINSON'S DEMENTIA

Dementia With Lewy Bodies

Core features of DLB include fluctuating cognition, REM sleep behavior disorder, recurrent formed visual hallucinations, and parkinsonism. Indicative biomarkers include reduced dopamine transporter uptake in the basal ganglia, as seen with PET imaging or single-photon emission tomography, abnormal (low uptake) [123]iodine-metaiodobenzylguanidine (MIBG) myocardial scintigraphy, and polysomnographic confirmation of REM sleep without atonia. A diagnosis of probable DLB is made based on the presence of two core features or one core feature and one indicative biomarker. Supportive features occurring in many individuals with DLB include the relative preservation of medial temporal lobe structures on CT/MRI scans and generalized low uptake on FDG PET metabolism scan with reduced occipital activity, sometimes with the "cingulate island sign." There is prominent posterior slow-wave activity on electroencephalography, with periodic fluctuations in the pre-alpha/theta range. Delusions are common, and misidentification delusions such as Capgras syndrome (the belief that someone has been replaced by an imposter), television sign (people on the television are in the house), and belief that the house is not one's home are especially common in DLB. REM sleep behavior disorder may be dangerous to the bed partner because of dream-related striking out, pushing, and kicking behavior.

Atrophy of the cortical and subcortical structures is evident. Hippocampal atrophy is less severe than observed in AD, but there is substantial overlap in the atrophy severity. Dopamine transporter imaging demonstrates diminished binding in the caudate and posterior putamen. FDG PET shows diminished parietal and occipital hypometabolism. Electroencephalography reveals slowing of the normal background rhythms, intermittent delta activity, transient temporal slow waves, and epoch-by-epoch fluctuations.

The pathology of DLB includes accumulation of intraneuronal α-synuclein in the form of Lewy bodies and Lewy neurites that occur in the brain stem, amygdala, limbic/paralimbic regions, and neocortex. Approximately 70% of patients have extracellular amyloid deposits similar to AD. There is atrophy of the basal forebrain and a marked cholinergic deficit. The basal ganglia exhibit a deficit in dopamine.

DLB typically has a more robust response to cholinesterase inhibitors than is typical of AD. Cholinergic agents may reduce apathy and hallucinations and improve cognition. REM sleep behavior disorder may respond to clonazepam (Klonopin) or to dual orexin receptor antagonists such as suvorexant (Belsomra). Delusions and hallucinations may respond to treatment with pimavanserin (Nuplazid) or quetiapine (Seroquel). Extrapyramidal side effects are frequently severe in DLB in response to treatment with dopamine-blocking antipsychotics. The parkinsonism of DLB may respond to dopaminergic agents. Depression is treated with citalopram or duloxetine (Cymbalta) (see Table 11–5 and Chapter 12).

Parkinson's Disease With Dementia

Dementia occurs in at least 80% of adults with Parkinson's disease as it progresses. PDD is similar to DLB; it is distinguished by the onset of motor signs prior to onset of dementia. Mental status changes include attention fluctuations, impairment of executive function, deterioration of visuospatial function, impairment of recall with relative preservation of recognition memory, and preservation of language functions. Apathy, delusions, hallucinations, REM sleep behavioral disturbances, and excessive daytime sleepiness are the most common behavioral features. Parkinson's disease motor features include bradykinesia, rest tremor, rigidity, and gait disturbance with falls. Dementia is more common in the Parkinson's disease subtype that has predominant postural instability and gait disturbances and is less common in the subtype with predominant tremors.

Structural brain imaging shows cortical and hippocampal atrophy that is less severe than the atrophy seen in AD. There is also subcortical atrophy. FDG PET shows decreased parietal and temporal metabolism similar to AD, often accompanied by frontal hypometabolism. Dopamine transporter imaging demonstrates diminished markers in caudate and anterior and posterior putamen; these changes are often asymmetric.

The pathology of PDD is similar to that of DLB with intraneuronal Lewy bodies, Lewy neurites, cell loss, and deficits of acetylcholine and dopamine (see Table 11–3). Parkinsonian features respond to treatment with anti-parkinsonism agents, including levodopa and dopamine agonists. Pimavanserin is approved for treatment of Parkinson's disease psychosis and quetiapine and clozapine are useful alternatives. Parkinson's disease and PDD have a cholinergic deficit, and cognitive impairment may respond to treatment with cholinesterase inhibitors (rivastigmine is approved for this indication).

■ MULTIPLE SYSTEM ATROPHY

The dementia of MSA is characterized by executive dysfunction with poor abstraction, set switching, and perseveration. Psychomotor retardation is evident. Parkinsonism is the most common motor manifestation; cerebellar signs, pyramidal tract signs, dystonia, and dysarthria are often seen. Autonomic dysfunction with orthostatic hypotension, bladder control abnormalities, constipation, impotence, and loss of sweating (anhidrosis) are present in nearly all cases.

MRI shows posterior putaminal hypointensity, hyperintense lateral putaminal rim, and the "hot cross bun sign" with brain stem and cerebellar atrophy. FDG PET shows brain stem and cerebellar hypometabolism. Dopamine transporter imaging reveals diminished activity in the striatum.

Pathologically, olivopontocerebellar degeneration and striatonigral degeneration correspond to the cerebellar and parkinsonian forms of the disease, respectively. Neuronal loss and axonal degeneration are evident in these systems. The hallmark histological change is the accumulation of α-synuclein inclusions in oligodendrocytes.

Parkinsonism in MSA is treated with dopaminergic agents, and dystonia may be managed with botulinum toxin injections. Orthostatic hypotension requires attention and may improve with nonpharmacological interventions, such as elastic support stockings and a high-salt diet. Pharmacological management with midodrine (Orvaten, Proamatine), fludrocortisone (Florinef), or droxidopa (Northera) is often required to control orthostatic changes and prevent syncope (see Chapter 12).

■ VASCULAR COGNITIVE DISORDERS

VCDs are characterized by clinical and brain imaging findings. Clinically, the cognitive changes begin after a cerebrovascular event and exhibit a stepwise or fluctuating course. Patients have focal neurological signs (e.g., hemiparesis, Babinski sign, sensory deficit, visual field defect, pseudobulbar palsy). Cognitive alterations feature predominant slowing of information processing and abnormalities of frontal-executive functioning. Gait abnormalities, urinary incontinence, and personality changes are common. Apathy, depression, and irritability/lability are common neuropsychiatric features. Neuroimaging findings in VCDs include large vessel infarctions, single strategically located infarctions (e.g., thalamic infarction, posterior inferior left parietal [angular gyrus] region), multiple lacunar infarctions, extensive confluent white matter lesions, intracerebral hemorrhage, or combinations of these lesions (see Table 11–3).

Some individuals with small vessel disease and white matter ischemic injury (leukoaraiosis) may have a gradually progressive decline that resembles a degenerative disorder. Many patients who meet the criteria for VCD also have AD when assessed with amyloid imaging or with CSF measures of amyloid and tau.

Treatment approaches for VCD include treatment of underlying vascular disease (e.g., aspirin, other anticoagulants) and of vascular risk factors (e.g., hypertension, hypercholesterolemia). Some patients may respond to cholinesterase inhibitor or memantine using dosages and regimens like those used in AD (see Table 11–4). Psychotropics may be needed for depression, apathy, or other neuropsychiatric symptoms (see Table 11–6). Dextromethorphan/Quinidine is approved for pseudobulbar affect and may reduce the number of episodes.

■ OTHER DEMENTIAS

Normal Pressure Hydrocephalus

Normal pressure hydrocephalus presents with the triad of dementia, gait disturbance, and incontinence. This triad is nonspecific and present in VCD and other neurological disorders. Recognition of the clinical syndrome is followed by neuroimaging studies and, if indicated, studies of CSF dynamics. MRI demonstrates enlarged ventricles with disproportionately enlarged frontal horns, "flattened" cortical sulci, and increased periventricular signal from transudation of CSF. Useful tests to support the diagnosis include a lumbar puncture with large-volume (30–50 mL) CSF removal to determine the effect on gait changes; CSF drainage for 72 hours with neuropsychological testing and gait testing following the drainage; and intracranial pressure monitoring (abnormal pressure waves are present in normal pressure hydrocephalus). The predictive value of these assessments for benefit from shunting is imperfect. Shunting is most likely to improve gait and least likely to improve cognitive impairment.

Creutzfeldt-Jakob Disease

Creutzfeldt-Jakob disease (CJD) is a transmissible prion disease that commonly presents as a rapidly progressive dementia (progression to profound disability or death within 12 months) with myoclonus. Cortical blindness, impaired judgment, neuropsychiatric symptoms (psychosis, depression, anxiety), ataxia, chorea, and eventual akinetic mutism may be seen. Startle myoclonus may be dramatic, with marked myoclonus in response to unexpected acoustic, tactile, or visual stimuli. Supportive lab findings include basal ganglia hyperintensities (i.e., "pulvinar sign") on diffusion weighted imaging or fluid-attenuated inversion recovery sequences of MRI; periodic sharp wave complexes on EEG; and presence of 14-3-3 protein in the CSF. Total tau protein is elevated in the CSF.

Management of CJD is symptomatic; currently, no specific intervention is available to halt its rapid progression and fatal outcome. Clonazepam may reduce myoclonus. Psychopharmacological intervention may aid management of the neuropsychiatric and behavioral aspects of the disorder (see Table 11–6).

Other Dementias

There are numerous other causes of dementia. Some are common, such as traumatic brain injury; others are associated with recognized neurological diseases such as multiple sclerosis, HIV; or brain tumors. Inflammatory disorders, including systemic lupus erythematosus, can produce dementia when they affect the CNS. Multiple types of infection—bacterial, viral, fungal—can cause dementia associated with chronic meningitis. Metabolic conditions have been associated with dementia, including renal failure, liver failure, chronic anemia, hypothyroidism, vitamin B_{12} deficiency, vitamin D deficiency, and other systemic disorders. White matter disorders with dementia represent a less common cause of cognitive impairment, and the onset may be earlier in life, including in childhood. Table 11–7 lists the most common white matter disorders that may manifest dementia.

■ TREATMENT OF NEUROPSYCHIATRIC DISORDERS IN DEMENTIAS

Neuropsychiatric symptoms are common in dementia syndromes, and the pattern of behavioral changes often assists in diagnosis and differential diagnosis (Table 11–2). In the absence of any disease-modifying therapies and with limited cognitive-enhancing treatments, management of the behavioral changes is one of the most important aspects of dementia care (see Table 11–6). Neuropsychiatric symptoms have a devastating impact

TABLE 11–7. White matter disorders with dementia

Class	Specific disorder
Degenerative disorders	Alzheimer's disease with amyloid angiopathy
	Frontotemporal dementia
Demyelinating	Balo's concentric sclerosis
	Marburg's disease
	Multiple sclerosis
	Schilder's disease
Genetic	Adrenoleukodystrophy
	Alexander's disease
	Aminoacidurias
	Fragile X tremor ataxia syndrome
	Globoid cell leukodystrophy
	Metachromatic leukodystrophy
	Mitochondrial encephalopathy with lactic acid and stroke (MELAS)
	Mucopolysaccharidoses
	Muscular dystrophy
	Phakomatoses (e.g., neurofibromatosis)
	Polycystic lipomembranous osteodysplasia with sclerosing leukoencephalopathy
	Vanishing white matter disease
Hydrocephalus	Childhood hydrocephalus
	Normal pressure hydrocephalus
Infectious	Cytomegalovirus encephalitis
	HIV and AIDS dementia complex
	Lyme encephalopathy
	Progressive multifocal leukoencephalopathy
	Progressive rubella panencephalitis
	Subacute sclerosing panencephalitis
	Varicella zoster encephalitis
Inflammatory	Behcet's syndrome
	Sarcoidosis
	Scleroderma
	Sjogren's syndrome
	Systemic lupus erythematosus
	Temporal arteritis
	Wegener's granulomatosis
Metabolic	Central pontine myelinolysis
	Cobalamin deficiency
	High altitude cerebral edema
	Hypertensive encephalopathy/eclampsia
	Hypoxic-ischemic injury

TABLE 11–7. White matter disorders with dementia *(continued)*	
Class	**Specific disorder**
Neoplastic	Focal white matter tumors
	Gliomatosis cerebri
	Primary CNS lymphoma
Toxic	Alcohol, Marchiafava-Bignami disease
	Amyloid-related imaging abnormalities
	Arsenic
	Carbon monoxide
	Carbon tetrachloride
	Chemotherapy: cyclosporine, tacrolimus
	Cranial irradiation
	Drug of abuse: toluene, heroin, cocaine, psilocybin, NMDA
Traumatic	Multifocal traumatic injury
	Shaken baby syndrome
	Traumatic brain injury with diffuse axonal injury
Vascular	Binswanger's disease
	CADASIL
	Cerebral amyloid angiopathy
	Intravascular lymphoma

CADASIL=Cerebral autosomal dominant arteriopathy with subcortical infarcts and leukoencephalopathy.

on caregivers, and control of behavioral symptoms is a key aspect of assisting caregivers and reducing their burden.

Cholinesterase inhibitors are used for cognitive enhancement in AD, DLB, PDD, and VCD/VaD. These agents often have benefits for apathy, depression, and hallucinations. Memantine is standard therapy for AD and is associated with reduced agitation.

Agitation is one of the most common of behavioral changes in dementia and is especially common in AD; up to 70% of patients may exhibit agitation at some point in the illness. Agitation is characterized by verbal aggression, physical aggression, or motor hyperactivity. Kicking, shouting, shoving, and active resistance to care are common. Nonpharmacological interventions such as reassurance, diversion, and avoiding confrontation are useful. Some patients will require pharmacological management. The antipsychotics quetiapine, risperidone (Risperdal), and brexpiprazole (Rexulti) have all been used for treatment of agitation, and the antidepressant citalopram has been shown to reduce mild to moderate agitation. Common side effects of these medications are shown in Table 11–6.

Psychosis is a common manifestation of dementia, especially DLB. Pimavanserin is approved for treatment of psychosis in Parkinson's disease, and pimavanserin, quetiapine, and olanzapine (Zyprexa) are often used for psychosis in other neurodegenerative disorders (see Table 11–5). Patients with neurological disorders are vulnerable to extrapyramidal side effects from dopamine-blocking antipsychotic agents, and lower dosages than those used in schizophrenia are usually sufficient for symptoms reduction or control.

Depression is commonly associated with dementias. The selective serotonin reuptake inhibitor (SSRI) citalopram is one of the more commonly used antidepressants. The selective serotonin-norepinephrine reuptake inhibitor duloxetine is a useful second-line agent.

Apathy is common across neurological disorders and can be disabling for patients and distressing for caregivers. Methylphenidate (Ritalin) reliably diminishes apathy, and modafinil is a useful alternative (see Table 11–6).

Repetitive behaviors in bvFTD and occasionally in other dementias may respond to treatment with SSRIs (citalopram, sertraline). Disinhibition may improve with valproic acid, dextromethorphan/quinidine), or citalopram.

Sleep disturbances are common in dementia and become more so as the disease progress. Wakefulness in patients usually results in wakefulness and exhaustion in caregivers. Dual orexin antagonists such as suvorexant have been shown useful in AD and are used in other neurodegenerative disorders. Hypnotics such as zolpidem (Ambien) can be useful for some patients; increased daytime confusion and drowsiness must be monitored. Trazodone (Desyrel) is a common alternative agent in patients with insomnia and nighttime behavioral changes.

■ REFERENCES

Armstrong MJ, Litvan I, Lang AE, et al: Criteria for the diagnosis of corticobasal degeneration. Neurology 80(5):496–503, 2013 23359374

Begali VL: Neuropsychology and the dementia spectrum: differential diagnosis, clinical management, and forensic utility. NeuroRehabilitation 46(2):181–194, 2020 32083596

Cummings J: The Neuropsychiatric Inventory: development and applications. J Geriatr Psychiatry Neurol 33(2):73–84, 2020 32013737

Cummings J: The role of neuropsychiatric symptoms in Research Diagnostic Criteria for neurodegenerative diseases. Am J Geriatr Psychiatry 29(4):375–383, 2021 32819825

Cummings J, Isaacson S, Mills R, et al: Pimavanserin for patients with Parkinson's disease psychosis: a randomised, placebo-controlled phase 3 trial. Lancet 383(9916):533–540, 2014 24183563

Cummings J, Mintzer J, Brodaty H, et al: Agitation in cognitive disorders: International Psychogeriatric Association provisional consensus clinical and research definition. Int Psychogeriatr 27(1):7–17, 2015 25311499

Cummings J, Ritter A, Rothenberg K: Advances in management of neuropsychiatric syndromes in neurodegenerative diseases. Curr Psychiatry Rep 21(8):79, 2019 31392434

Cummings J, Pinto LC, Cruz M, et al: Criteria for psychosis in major and mild neurocognitive disorders: International Psychogeriatric Association (IPA) consensus clinical and research definition. Am J Geriatr Psychiatry 28(12):1256–1269, 2020 32958332

Cummings J, Aisen P, Apostolova LG, et al: Aducanumab: appropriate use recommendations. J Prev Alzheimers Dis 8(4):398–410, 2021 34585212

D'Ascanio S, Alosco ML, Stern RA: Chronic traumatic encephalopathy: clinical presentation and in vivo diagnosis. Handb Clin Neurol 158:281–296, 2018 30482356

Dubois B, Burn D, Goetz C, et al: Diagnostic procedures for Parkinson's disease dementia: recommendations from the Movement Disorder Society Task Force. Mov Disord 22(16):2314–2324, 2007 18098298

Dubois B, Feldman HH, Jacova C, et al: Advancing research diagnostic criteria for Alzheimer's disease: the IWG-2 criteria. Lancet Neurol 13(6):614–629, 2014 24849862

Ducharme S, Dols A, Laforce R, et al: Recommendations to distinguish behavioural variant frontotemporal dementia from psychiatric disorders. Brain 143(6):1632–1650, 2020 32129844

Emre M, Aarsland D, Albanese A, et al: Rivastigmine for dementia associated with Parkinson's disease. N Engl J Med 351(24):2509–2518, 2004 15590953

Fischer CE, Ismail Z, Youakim JM, et al: Revisiting criteria for psychosis in Alzheimer's disease and related dementias: toward better phenotypic classification and biomarker research. J Alzheimers Dis 73(3):1143–1156, 2020 31884469

Gorno-Tempini ML, Hillis AE, Weintraub S, et al: Classification of primary progressive aphasia and its variants. Neurology 76(11):1006–1014, 2011 21325651

Herring WJ, Ceesay P, Snyder E, et al: Polysomnographic assessment of suvorexant in patients with probable Alzheimer's disease dementia and insomnia: a randomized trial. Alzheimers Dement 16(3):541–551, 2020 31944580

Höglinger GU, Respondek G, Stamelou M, et al: Clinical diagnosis of progressive supranuclear palsy: the Movement Disorder Society criteria. Mov Disord 32(6):853–864, 2017 28467028

Jack CR Jr, Bennett DA, Blennow K, et al: NIA-AA research framework: toward a biological definition of Alzheimer's disease. Alzheimers Dement 14(4):535–562, 2018 29653606

Mahalingam S, Chen MK: Neuroimaging in dementias. Semin Neurol 39(2):188–199, 2019 30925612

Manix M, Kalakoti P, Henry M, et al: Creutzfeldt-Jakob disease: updated diagnostic criteria, treatment algorithm, and the utility of brain biopsy. Neurosurg Focus 39(5):E2, 2015 26646926

Masters CL, Bateman R, Blennow K, et al: Alzheimer's disease. Nat Rev Dis Primers 1:15056, 2015 27188934

McKee AC, Cantu RC, Nowinski CJ, et al: Chronic traumatic encephalopathy in athletes: progressive tauopathy after repetitive head injury. J Neuropathol Exp Neurol 68(7):709–735, 2009 19535999

McKeith IG, Boeve BF, Dickson DW, et al: Diagnosis and management of dementia with Lewy bodies: fourth consensus report of the DLB Consortium. Neurology 89(1):88–100, 2017 28592453

McKhann GM, Knopman DS, Chertkow H, et al: The diagnosis of dementia due to Alzheimer's disease: recommendations from the National Institute on Aging-Alzheimer's Association workgroups on diagnostic guidelines for Alzheimer's disease. Alzheimers Dement 7(3):263–269, 2011 21514250

Molinuevo JL, Ayton S, Batrla R, et al: Current state of Alzheimer's fluid biomarkers. Acta Neuropathol 136(6):821–853, 2018 30488277

Norton S, Matthews FE, Barnes DE, et al: Potential for primary prevention of Alzheimer's disease: an analysis of population-based data. Lancet Neurol 13(8):788–794, 2014 25030513

Rascovsky K, Hodges JR, Knopman D, et al: Sensitivity of revised diagnostic criteria for the behavioural variant of frontotemporal dementia. Brain 134(pt 9):2456–2477, 2011 21810890

Rosenberg PB, Lanctôt KL, Drye LT, et al: Safety and efficacy of methylphenidate for apathy in Alzheimer's disease: a randomized, placebo-controlled trial. J Clin Psychiatry 74(8):810–816, 2013 24021498

Sachdev P, Kalaria R, O'Brien J, et al: Diagnostic criteria for vascular cognitive disorders: a VASCOG statement. Alzheimer Dis Assoc Disord 28(3):206–218, 2014 24632990

Tousi B, Cummings J (eds): NeuroGeriatrics: A Clinical Manual. New York, Springer, 2017

Williams MA, Malm J: Diagnosis and treatment of idiopathic normal pressure hydrocephalus. Continuum (Minneap Minn) 22(2 Dementia):579–599, 2016 27042909

12

MOVEMENT DISORDERS

Alex Eischeid, M.D.
Hokuto Morita, M.D.
Michel Medina, M.D.
Kathleen L. Poston, M.D., M.S.

Movement disorders are produced by dysfunction of the basal ganglia, and these deep gray matter structures are increasingly recognized as critically important in cognition, emotion, and motor function. There are three important corollaries with respect to the role of the basal ganglia in mental function: 1) basal ganglia disorders are frequently accompanied by abnormalities of intellectual integrity, mood, motivation, and personality; 2) many psychotropic agents affect the basal ganglia and produce movement disorders as side effects; and 3) many idiopathic psychiatric disorders have motoric manifestations. This chapter describes the neuropsychiatric disturbances that accompany movement disorders.

■ PARKINSON'S DISEASE

Demography

Parkinson's disease (PD) is a neurodegenerative condition that affects several regions of the brain, including the nuclei in the midbrain and brain stem, the olfactory tubercle, the cerebral cortex, and elements of the peripheral nervous system. The estimated prevalence of PD in industrialized countries is 0.3% in the general population, 1.0% in people older than 60 years, and 3.0% in those age 80 years and older. The lifetime risk of PD is 2% in men and 1.3% in women age 40 years and older. The median age of onset is 60 years, and the mean time between diagnosis and death is 15 years. Millions of people currently are affected worldwide, and the number of affected patients is expected to double by 2030. The cause of PD is unknown in most cases, whereas genetic risk factors can be identified in 5%–10% of patients.

Clinical Features

The four cardinal motor symptoms of PD are bradykinesia, rigidity, rest tremor, and postural instability. Together, these symptoms are referred to as "parkinsonism." *Bradykinesia* is defined as slowness of movement *and* decrement in amplitude or speed (or hesitations/halts) as movements are continued. *Rigidity* refers to "lead pipe" resistance, which is a velocity-independent resistance to passive movement. Cogwheeling is often present with rigidity, but the absence of cogwheeling does not preclude a diagnosis of PD. *Rest tremor* refers to a 4- to 6-Hz tremor in a fully resting limb. Tremor is the presenting motor symptom of PD in up to 69% of patients and affects up to 90% of patients at some point during the disease process. Tremor is typically unilateral at onset, is almost always present in the distal part of an extremity, and is classically described as "pill-rolling" (supination-pronation axis). Rest tremor can also involve the lips, chin, jaw, and legs but rarely involves the neck, head, or voice. Many PD patients (88%–92% in some studies) will also have a postural tremor; however, postural tremor in PD is differentiated from essential tremor because the appearance of the tremor in PD is usually delayed after the patient assumes an outstretched position (i.e., "re-emergent tremor"). Although postural instability is often included as a cardinal symptom of the disease, it is not included in the Movement Disorders Society's diagnostic criteria for PD and often occurs in the later stages of the illness.

Nonmotor symptoms are a common but often underappreciated feature of PD and include autonomic dysfunction, cognitive and neuropsychiatric abnormalities, and sensory and sleep disorders. Most patients with PD will experience nonmotor symptoms throughout the course of the disease, and the absence of common nonmotor features of disease despite 5 years of disease duration is a red flag for a diagnosis other than PD. Furthermore, the impact of nonmotor symptoms is often greater than that of motor symptoms. Dysautonomic features include orthostatic hypotension, constipation, urinary incontinence, gastrointestinal dysfunction, sexual dysfunction, and sweating abnormalities. Cognitive and neuropsychiatric abnormalities include depression, anxiety, apathy, impulse-control disorders, hallucinations, psychosis, executive dysfunction, memory loss, and dementia. Sensory disorders include pain (often related to rigidity) and hyposmia/anosmia. Sleep disorders include insomnia, excessive daytime sleepiness, restless legs syndrome, and rapid eye movement (REM) sleep behavior disorder. Polysomnogram-proven REM sleep behavior disorder is strongly associated with development of PD and has a likelihood ratio of +130 as a prodromal marker of a synucleinopathy disease.

Pathology

PD motor symptoms result primarily from dysfunction of the basal ganglia, which structurally includes the dorsal striatum (caudate and putamen), the external and internal globus pallidus, the subthalamic nucleus, and the substantia nigra pars reticulata and pars compacta. Dysfunction of the "motor" loop of the basal ganglia is strongly implicated in the development of the motor symptoms of PD and, more generally, parkinsonism. From a neurochemical standpoint, a number of PD symptoms are caused by the progressive loss of the dopamine neurons of the substantia nigra pars compacta, noradrenergic neurons of the locus coeruleus, and serotonergic neurons of the raphe nuclei. The hallmark pathological feature of PD is the presence of intraneuronal inclusions containing α-synuclein, which is normally a component of presynaptic terminals but, in idiopathic PD, aberrantly accumulates in neuronal cell bodies (Lewy bodies) and neuronal processes (Lewy neurites). The factors underlying α-synuclein aggregation are undetermined, and different pathogenic mechanisms causing cell death likely contribute to the complex symptomatology of the disease. Thus, PD may best be viewed as a syndrome rather than a specific disease.

Treatment

Levodopa remains the gold standard symptomatic treatment for PD (Table 12–1). It is most effective for treating bradykinesia and rigidity, with variable benefit for tremor; gait and balance show more modest improvement. It is administered along with a dopa decarboxylase inhibitor (carbidopa) to reduce its peripheral breakdown and lessen nausea. Levodopa does not hasten neurodegeneration or disease progression. There are many different formulations of levodopa—immediate- and extended-release or a combination of the two, orally disintegrating tablets, an inhalation powder, and a levodopa/carbidopa intestinal gel. Catechol-O-methyltransferase (COMT) inhibitors can be administered with carbidopa/levodopa to increase the plasma half-life of levodopa and thus improve end-of-dose wearing-off time. Dopamine agonists work by directly stimulating dopamine receptors and are utilized as both monotherapy and adjunctive therapy in the treatment of PD. Dopamine agonists are usually

TABLE 12–1. Parkinson's disease medications

Levodopa preparations
  Carbidopa/Levodopa
    (Sinemet, Sinemet CR)
  Carbidopa/Levodopa
    (Rytary); combined short
    and long-acting levodopa
    capsules
  Carbidopa/Levodopa
    (Parcopa); orally
    disintegrating tablet
  Carbidopa/Levodopa/
    Entacapone (Stalevo)
  Intestinal gel (Duopa)
  Inhalation powder (Imbrija)
Monoamine oxidase B inhibitors
  Rasagiline (Azilect)
  Selegiline (Eldepryl)
  Safinamide (Xadago)
Adenosine receptor antagonists
  Istradefylline (Nourianz)

Dopamine agonists
  Ropinirole (Requip)
  Pramipexole (Mirapex)
  Apomorphine (Apokyn)
  Rotigotine transdermal patch
    (Neupro)
NMDA antagonist
  Amantadine
Catechol-O-methyltransferase
  inhibitors
  Entacapone (Comtan)
  Opicapone (Ongentys)
Anticholinergics
  Trihexyphenidyl (Artane)
  Benztropine (Cogentin)

less efficacious than levodopa at treating PD motor symptoms, and they have a higher incidence of psychiatric side effects, including hallucinations and impulse-control disorders.

Monoamine oxidase B (MAO-B) inhibitors are used both as monotherapy in mild, early-stage disease and as adjuvant therapy in more advanced disease. MAO-B inhibition prevents catabolism of dopamine. MAO-B inhibitors were initially thought to provide neuroprotective and disease-modifying effects in patients with PD; however, their ability to alter the long-term course of PD is highly controversial. Selegiline and rasagiline are selective and irreversible MAO-B inhibitors, whereas safinamide is a reversible MAO-B inhibitor. MAO-B inhibition generates theoretical concerns about the occurrence of hypertensive crisis related to changes in tyramine metabolism; however, at recommended dosages, selective MAO-B inhibitors have limited effect on MAO-A-mediated tyramine metabolism and thus do not pose a significant risk in terms of tyramine interaction. Likewise, at therapeutic dosages, selective MAO-B inhibitors have little impact on MAO-A-mediated serotonin metabolism; therefore, serotonin syndrome occurs very rarely, and the combination of an MAO-B inhibitor and antidepressants is well tolerated provided their dosages do not exceed recommendation (see Chapter 22, "Treatments in Neuropsychiatry").

Amantadine acts as a modulator of glutamine, an excitatory neurotransmitter thought to be core in the development of dyskinesias in PD. Anticholinergics had a leading role in the treatment of PD until levodopa was introduced in the 1960s. Their side effect profile led to a decline in the use of this class of medication; their use is now generally limited to the treatment of dopamine-unresponsive tremor and PD-related dystonia, and mostly in younger patients. Deep brain stimulation (DBS) of the subthalamic nucleus or internal globus pallidus is a treatment option in some patients with PD who develop medication-associated motor complications with disease progression. These motor complications include shortened duration of medication action (i.e., "wearing off") and dyskinesias. Studies have shown that DBS can lead to improvement in overall quality of life secondary to improvement in motor and nonmotor features. Regular, consistent exercise has shown to be beneficial for patients with PD, both in vivo and in vitro. Randomized trials have indicated that several physical activities with various intensities, including treadmill training, dance, and tai-chi, improve motor symptoms of PD and health-related quality of life.

■ MILD COGNITIVE IMPAIRMENT AND PARKINSON'S DISEASE DEMENTIA

Mild cognitive impairment (MCI) is common in PD and is seen in ≤30% of patients at the time of their PD diagnosis. PD-MCI is a heterogeneous condition affecting a range of cognitive domains, with 95% of patients showing multidomain impairment. Executive dysfunction, which includes attention and working memory impairments, is common in PD and manifests as impaired verbal fluency, set shifting, and abstract thinking and planning. Progression from MCI to PD dementia (PDD) is increasingly recognized as almost an inevitable feature of the disease, and MCI is seen as a stage between normal cognition and PDD; studies have shown that ≤78% of patients with PD develop dementia over an 8-year period. PDD has a significant negative impact on quality of life for both patients and caregivers and is associated with greater risk of nursing home placement and mortality. The cognitive profile of PDD is generally similar to that of PD-MCI. No standard pharmacological treatments are available currently for cognitive deficits in patients with PD-MCI, but it is good practice to discontinue medications with cognition-decaying side effects when cognitive dysfunction becomes evident. The use of cholinesterase inhibitors can also provide modest benefit for cognition. Memantine has limited evidence of providing slight improvement in attention and episodic recognition memory, but data are conflicting.

◼ NEUROPSYCHIATRIC DISORDERS IN PARKINSON'S DISEASE

Depression

Depression is common in PD, with ≥50% of patients having it in some form. Depression is associated with a worse prognosis for both motor and cognitive function and has a greater effect on quality of life than motor dysfunction. Although depression is common in PD, data are lacking as to the efficacy of antidepressants; a 2013 meta-analysis stated that no specific antidepressant class was superior to placebo and that antidepressants *may* be efficacious in the treatment of PD-related depression. With the currently available data, there are no clear recommendations for treatment; the selective serotonin reuptake inhibitors (SSRIs) are generally preferred because they have a more benign side effect profile.

Anxiety

Anxiety is observed in >40% of patients with PD. It can be a nonmotor "off" symptom, and studies have found that patients with motor fluctuations are more likely to have generalized anxiety. No medications have been approved by the FDA for the treatment of anxiety in PD, and a few small studies have suggested that the antidepressants approved for treating anxiety and depression in the general population are not beneficial for anxiety in PD. Despite this, SSRIs and benzodiazepines are typically prescribed to treat anxiety in patients with PD. Benzodiazepines should be utilized only with great caution in elderly individuals due to the risk of confusion, falls, and development of dementia.

Apathy

Apathy is considered a disorder of motivation and therefore is closely related to both depression and fatigue. Apathy is highly prevalent in PD, seen in ≤70% of patients. Treatment of apathy in patients with PD is generally unknown and is largely anecdotal. If apathy is associated with dementia, then a trial of an acetylcholinesterase inhibitor may be warranted; if depression is a possible concomitant syndrome, a trial of an antidepressant can be entertained. Bupropion, a norepinephrine-dopamine re-uptake inhibitor, can be considered; however, no clinical trials have yet supported its use for apathy specifically. When counseling family members of patients with PD-associated apathy, it should be explained that apathy is common in this patient population and does not have clearly beneficial treatment.

Fatigue

Fatigue is particularly common in PD, seen in ≤50% of patients. It is frequently a disabling symptom of PD, and up to one-third of patients rate fatigue as their most disabling symptom. Treatment with levodopa can sometimes improve fatigue in patients with PD. Fatigue is also confounding because it is often comorbid with depression, anxiety, or apathy, making it difficult to determine whether the fatigue is a distinct symptom or part of a larger syndrome. If it is associated with depression or anxiety, these psychiatric comorbidities should be treated with the hope of improving fatigue; however, currently no data support this theory. Although data are conflicting on the use of modafinil in patients with PD, the American Academy of Neurology recommends that it be considered for PD with fatigue. Furthermore, a 2007 study showed that methylphenidate at a dosage of 10 mg three times per day was effective in reducing fatigue scores over a 6-week period in patients with idiopathic PD.

Psychosis

Psychosis can occur secondary to medication treatment for motor symptoms or as part of the underlying disease. Visual hallucinations affect about 20%–30% of medication-treated patients; auditory hallucinations are much less common and usually affect patients with visual hallucinations. Dementia appears to be the most significant risk factor for development of psychotic symptoms, and the occurrence of visual hallucinations increases the risk of developing dementia within the next few years. In evaluating a patient with PD and psychosis, if PD medications have been minimized to the lowest possible dosage and psychotic symptoms persist, addition of an antipsychotic should be considered. Quetiapine and, more recently, pimavanserin are most often used to treat PD psychosis. Pimavanserin is an atypical antipsychotic that acts as a selective serotonin 5-HT$_{2A}$ inverse agonist and is the first drug to be FDA-approved for the treatment of PD psychosis. Although often used, quetiapine has limited data on its ability to reduce visual hallucinations and, in some cases, can worsen motor symptoms. Olanzapine has been studied and shown to be ineffective at treating PD psychosis. It can also worsen motor symptoms and thus is not recommended for the treatment of PD psychosis. Clozapine was the first drug studied for the treatment of PD psychosis and has the strongest efficacy data; however, despite its proven effectiveness, it remains underused because it requires patient registry, coordination with pharmacies, and frequent lab visits due to the rare development of neutropenia. Typical antipsychotics (e.g., haloperidol) should not be used for PD psychosis because of the increased risk of worsening motor symptoms.

Treatment-Associated Neuropsychiatric Disorders

The management of PD may be complicated by unwanted behavioral side effects. Dopaminergic medications have the ability to produce neuropsychiatric problems. Such dopaminergic side effects can manifest in many forms, including psychosis, impulse-control disorders, dopamine dysregulation syndrome, and dopamine agonist withdrawal syndrome.

Psychosis may be intrinsically related to PD or be drug induced and is seen in ≤30% of medically treated patients with PD. The management of PD psychosis was discussed in the previous section, including the reduction or elimination of PD medications that have a high propensity to worsen psychosis and the addition of an antipsychotic if necessary.

Impulse-control disorders encountered in patients with PD include pathological gambling, compulsive sexual behavior, compulsive buying, and compulsive or binge eating, among others. They are seen in an estimated 13.6% of patients with PD, more commonly in men. Dopamine agonists are highly implicated in the development of impulse-control disorders.

Dopamine dysregulation syndrome is a behavioral disorder resulting from the compulsive use of dopaminergic medication and often manifesting as hoarding, deceit, impulsivity, impatience, manipulation, aggression, and poor insight. Risk factors include previous drug abuse, sensation-seeking personalities, and depression. Treatment is aimed at reduction in dopaminergic medications, and, given that many patients will lack insight into this problem, assistance from caregivers to provide supervision is essential.

Dopamine agonist withdrawal syndrome is a widely recognized constellation of symptoms related to the withdrawal

of dopamine agonists. Symptoms include anxiety, mood disturbances (e.g., irritability, dysphoria), and autonomic symptoms
(e.g., diaphoresis, flushing). The frequency of this syndrome in
PD ranges from 7.8% to 19%, and it is strongly correlated with
a prior history of impulse-control disorder. Dopamine agonist
withdrawal syndrome has been associated with higher dopamine agonist dosages and longer dopamine agonist exposure.

ATYPICAL PARKINSONISM

Parkinsonism refers to a constellation of motor symptoms consisting of bradykinesia, rigidity, and resting tremor. While PD is
the most common cause, red flag symptoms such as dopamine
unresponsiveness, early and severe autonomic failure, early
postural instability, or supranuclear gaze palsy may suggest an
alternative etiology. Atypical causes of parkinsonism include
tauopathies, such as progressive supranuclear palsy (PSP) and
corticobasal syndrome, and synucleinopathies, such as multiple system atrophy and dementia with Lewy bodies (DLB).

Progressive Supranuclear Palsy

PSP is a tauopathy with a prevalence of 5–7 cases per 100,000
people and a mean age at onset between 63 and 66 years. In recent years it has been recognized that PSP encompasses a wide
range of clinical phenotypes involving behavioral, language,
and movement abnormalities. In classic PSP, the most common
reported symptoms at onset are unexplained falls (classically
backward), gait and balance dysfunction, bradykinesia, personality changes (e.g., apathy, disinhibition), cognitive slowing
and executive dysfunction, and impaired ocular movements
(e.g., slowing of vertical saccades, difficulty reading, apraxia of
eyelid opening). Vertical supranuclear gaze palsy is the definitive clinical feature, but this might not be present until at least
3–4 years after disease onset. Most individuals with PSP syndromes eventually develop some or all of the clinical features of
classic PSP. Current PSP treatment is limited to symptom-targeted
therapies, and it is considered a fatal disease with a mean survival of 6–9 years (see Chapter 11, "Dementia").

Corticobasal Syndrome

Corticobasal syndrome is a tauopathy defined by widespread
tau deposition in various cell types in neurons and glia. Its pathology can manifest as a number of clinical phenotypes. It typ-

ically presents during the sixth decade, with a mean age at onset of 63.5 years, with men and women equally affected. Common motor features at presentation are asymmetric limb rigidity, bradykinesia, or postural instability. Limb rigidity and bradykinesia classically do not have sustained dopaminergic responsiveness. Other motor features include dystonia, tremor (often a mixture of resting, postural, and action), and myoclonus (typically stimulus- or action-induced and considered to be of cortical origin). Cortical dysfunction can manifest as limb apraxia, cortical sensory loss (e.g., agraphesthesia, astereognosis), and alien limb phenomenon as well as cognitive impairment (executive dysfunction with relative preservation of memory), or behavioral changes (e.g., apathy, antisocial behavior, personality changes, irritability, disinhibition) (see Chapter 11).

Multiple System Atrophy

Multiple system atrophy is a synucleinopathy with typical onset during the sixth decade of life. Clinical diagnosis requires autonomic dysregulation (i.e., urinary incontinence or retention, orthostatic hypotension, anhidrosis, or erectile dysfunction in males) with either parkinsonism or cerebellar abnormalities such as ataxia, dysmetria, or nystagmus. Although dementia is not typical, ≤30% of patients have MCI with frontal executive dysfunction. Moderate to severe depression affects ≤50% of patients. REM sleep behavior disorder is common. Regarding management, poor dopaminergic medication response is characteristic of the disease and is included as a diagnostic feature. For cerebellar symptoms such as gait ataxia, no efficient drug treatment is available; however, there are limited data in case reports and small series for amantadine, buspirone, riluzole, and varenicline (see Chapter 11).

Dementia With Lewy Bodies

DLB is the second most common form of neurodegenerative dementia after Alzheimer's disease. According to the 2017 Dementia with Lewy Bodies Consortium, in addition to dementia, the core clinical features of DLB are cognitive fluctuations, visual hallucinations, parkinsonism, and REM sleep behavior disorder. Fluctuations include spontaneous alterations in cognition, attention, and arousal. Psychosis with visual hallucinations develops in ≤80% of patients, and these hallucinations are typically well formed, featuring people, children, or animals, but they may also include sense of presence hallucinations and visual illusions.

REM sleep behavior disorder is included as a core clinical feature of DLB because it has been seen in ≤76% of autopsy-proven cases compared with 4% of autopsy-negative cases.

Pathologically, DLB is a synucleinopathy that largely overlaps with PD, with abnormal intraneuronal collection of the protein α-synuclein forming Lewy bodies. The distinction between DLB and PD with dementia as clinical phenotypes is based on the temporal sequence in which symptoms appear; patients who develop dementia prior to or within 1 year of clinical parkinsonism are diagnosed with DLB, whereas those who present with at minimum 1 year of parkinsonism prior to dementia are diagnosed with PD with dementia. Because patients with DLB have shown a high sensitivity to typical and atypical antipsychotics, this class of medication should be avoided whenever possible for the acute management of behavioral disturbance, delusions, or visual hallucinations (see Chapter 11).

■ SECONDARY PARKINSONISM

In addition to the neurodegenerative causes, various secondary forms of parkinsonism are most commonly attributable to certain drugs and vascular lesions (i.e., vascular parkinsonism). In contrast to neurodegenerative forms, most secondary causes aside from chronic traumatic brain injuries (TBIs) have not been linked to abnormal protein aggregation. Management of secondary forms of parkinsonism often differs from that of idiopathic PD, and therefore these should always be considered as differential diagnoses.

Drug-Induced Parkinsonism

Drug-induced parkinsonism is a parkinsonian syndrome related to the intake of distinct drugs and is thought to be the second most common cause of parkinsonism after idiopathic PD. It can be seen at any point after initiation of the offending agent. Unlike PD, nonmotor symptoms (e.g., cognitive dysfunction, constipation, olfactory dysfunction) are uncommon. Regarding management, suspected causative drugs should be reconsidered and discontinued if possible. If patients require antipsychotic treatment for psychiatric conditions, then second-generation antipsychotic medications are preferred and should be prescribed at the lowest possible dosage. In most cases, parkinsonian symptoms will resolve within 6 months of withdrawal of the offending agent, but in ≤25% of patients symptoms persist longer than 6 months.

Vascular Parkinsonism

Vascular parkinsonism, or parkinsonism due to vascular lesions, is the fourth most common cause of parkinsonism after PD, drug-induced parkinsonism, and DLB. Clinically, vascular parkinsonism is described as having primarily lower-body-predominant features with pronounced gait dysfunction and relatively minimal symptoms affecting the upper extremities. Dopamine transporter single-photon emission computed tomography can help to differentiate vascular parkinsonism from PD; one 2014 meta-analysis reported a sensitivity of 86.2% and a specificity of 82.9% for establishing a diagnosis of vascular parkinsonism.

Posttraumatic Parkinsonism

Parkinsonism has been related to repetitive mild TBI. Chronic traumatic encephalopathy presents with irritability, impulsivity, aggression, short-term memory loss, depression, and an increased risk of suicidality that typically begin about a decade after the injuries, with parkinsonism commonly seen with more advanced disease. Treatment is symptomatic, based on adopting treatment practices from other disorders that target similar symptoms.

■ HUNTINGTON'S DISEASE

Clinical Features

Huntington's disease is an autosomal-dominant neurodegenerative disease characterized by movement, personality, affect, and cognitive dysfunction. Initial motor symptoms range from mild clumsiness or dysarthria to frank choreiform movements (see Table 12–2 for differential diagnosis of chorea). Less common presenting motor features include dystonia, ataxia, and parkinsonism, which are associated with larger CAG repeat expansions and earlier age at onset.

Neuropsychiatric changes are seen in most patients with Huntington's disease and include abnormalities in behavior, affect, and cognition. Irritability is often the first noted behavioral change, with apathy, aggression, and rigid thinking commonly seen many years before motor manifestation. Cognitive dysfunction usually includes impaired executive function. Impaired verbal fluency is another early indicator of cognitive impairment.

TABLE 12–2. Differential diagnosis of chorea

Choreic disorder	Key clinical features
Acquired hepatocerebral degeneration	Liver failure
Anticonvulsant-induced chorea	Phenytoin, phenobarbital, carbamazepine, or ethosuximide history
Antiphospholipid antibody syndrome	Positive lupus anticoagulant and anticardiolipin A and B antibodies
Benign familial chorea	Early onset, nonprogressive, no dementia
Cerebral palsy	Anoxic early life episode
Chorea gravidarum	Pregnancy, history of Sydenham's chorea
Chorea with stroke	Acute onset, hemiballismus early
Chorea with systemic lupus erythematosus	Positive antinuclear antibody and anti-double-stranded DNA
Edentulous dyskinesia	Oral-buccal lingual dyskinesia in elderly
Huntington's disease	Autosomal dominant, dementia, atrophy of caudate on CT or MRI
Hyperthyroidism	Low thyroid-stimulating hormone, elevated thyroxine (T_4)
Kernicterus	Elevated bilirubin in infancy
Levodopa-induced chorea	Chorea in "on" periods of patients with Parkinson's disease treated with dopaminergic agents
Neuroacanthocytosis	Chorea and tics, peripheral neuropathy, acanthocytes
Polycythemia vera	Elevated hematocrit
Stimulant-induced chorea	Amphetamine or methylphenidate use
Sydenham's chorea	Follows streptococcal A infection, positive anti-DNase B titer
Tardive dyskinesia	Prolonged exposure to dopamine-blocking agents
Wilson's disease	Kayser-Fleischer ring; liver disease

Pathology

Huntington's disease is an autosomal dominant condition resulting from a CAG trinucleotide repeat expansion of *HTT* on chromosome 4, which encodes for the huntingtin protein. Nor-

mal huntingtin alleles have <30 repeats of the CAG trinucleotide repeat, whereas 30–35 repeats are considered premutations;
generally, individuals with ≤35 CAG repeats will not manifest
symptoms or signs of the illness. Mutant huntingtin protein is
more resistant to protein degradation, and incomplete protein
degradation products form cytoplasmic aggregates that can
translocate into the nucleus and form intranuclear aggregates.

Management

Currently, no treatment has been shown to alter disease course
in Huntington's disease, but several symptomatic therapies are
available. Tetrabenazine and deutetrabenazine have FDA approval for the treatment of chorea in Huntington's disease. Evidence from a retrospective study and a meta-analysis suggests
that deutetrabenazine is a potentially better tolerated option
than tetrabenazine because it has fewer depressive symptoms
and less somnolence. Both are contraindicated in patients with
suicidal behavior and in those with untreated or inadequately
controlled depression. Atypical antipsychotics, including olanzapine, aripiprazole, risperidone, quetiapine, and ziprasidone
can be considered for the treatment of chorea, particularly when
patients have associated personality, behavioral, or psychotic
disorders. Amantadine has mixed data regarding its efficacy in
reducing chorea. The management of Huntington's disease–
associated cognitive dysfunction is challenging, and treatment
options remain limited, with mixed evidence supporting use of
the acetylcholinesterase inhibitors. Ongoing investigations are
looking at a new treatment specifically targeting the messenger
RNA encoding the mutant huntingtin protein.

■ NON–HUNTINGTON'S DISEASE CHOREAS

Tardive Dyskinesia

Tardive dyskinesia (TD) is a late-onset movement disorder affecting the face, mouth, trunk, and limbs with rhythmic, purposeless choreoathetoid movements. Patients who have been
taking an antipsychotic for at least 3 months have a 20%–35%
risk of developing TD. The risk is approximately 32.4% for patients taking typical antipsychotics and 13.1% for those taking
atypical antipsychotics. TD is one of several tardive movement
disorders that can develop secondary to the prolonged use of
dopamine-blocking drugs; others include tardive dystonia, tar-

dive tremor, tardive akathisia, tardive tourettism, tardive tics, tardive myoclonus, tardive chorea, and tardive parkinsonism. The mechanism underlying TD remains uncertain. Risk factors for the development of TD include old age and female sex.

For management of TD, once tardive symptoms have been identified, slowly taper down the causative medication to avoid medication withdrawal symptoms. A 2018 meta-analysis demonstrated that the severity of TD was reduced by transitioning from a typical antipsychotic to clozapine. Valbenazine and deutetrabenazine are FDA-approved for treatment of TD; a 2018 meta-analysis showed that these drugs are effective for treatment without any clear increased risk of depression or suicide. Thus, they can be used long-term, if necessary, to treat ongoing tardive movements. Other medication options studied include clonazepam, baclofen, and amantadine. A 2016 study showed that internal globus pallidus DBS was both an effective and a well-tolerated treatment option for patients with medically refractory TD.

Sydenham's Chorea and Chorea Gravidarum

Sydenham's chorea follows group A streptococcal infections, although the original episode may not be recognized clinically. Chorea typically begins 1–6 months after the original infection. It is a small-amplitude chorea that affects primarily the distal muscles (the hands and fingers). The patient's sedimentation rate and antistreptolysin O titer may be normal; a test for anti-DNase B is usually positive. The condition typically resolves in 4–6 months but may occasionally persist. Sydenham's chorea is accompanied by irritability, and both the acute and the post-choreic states may be associated with obsessional and compulsive symptoms. Most of the patients who exhibit chorea during pregnancy (chorea gravidarum) or while taking oral contraceptives have a previous history of Sydenham's chorea, and these disorders represent reactivation of a latent movement disorder.

■ DYSTONIC DISORDERS

Dystonia is characterized by sustained or intermittent muscle contractions that cause abnormal, often repetitive movements, postures, or both and is often initiated or worsened by voluntary action. Its clinical manifestation varies widely depending on the severity and muscle distribution and can range from slow and twisting movements with abnormal fixed posture to more rapid and jerky movements resembling a tremor. A *geste antagoniste,* or a sensory trick, is unique to dystonia and can be a diagnostic clue; however, these are not always present. The pathophysiology underlying dystonia is not entirely understood but is thought to be due to muscle overcontraction, with proposed mechanisms including loss of inhibitory influence in the CNS. Another proposed mechanism includes altered spatial and temporal discrimination of tactile stimuli and distorted body representation in the primary sensory cortex.

Evaluation

Investigation into the underlying etiology of dystonia is almost always warranted in patients who are younger than 40 years and may include laboratory testing, a brain MRI, and genetic testing. Given the growing number of recognized dystonic syndromes, which frequently have overlapping features, and with known genetic mutations causing many clinical phenotypes, a growing trend is to use broad dystonia panels or whole-exome sequencing during the workup.

Management

The treatment of dystonia is symptomatic and is usually chosen depending on the distribution and severity of symptoms. Botulinum toxin is the gold standard treatment for focal and segmental dystonia. There are no FDA-approved oral medications for treatment of dystonia, nor have there been large-scale studies of their efficacy, so their use is off-label. Anticholinergics (trihexyphenidyl, benztropine) are often used, particularly in adolescents with dystonia. Baclofen has limited data supporting its benefit. VMAT2 inhibitors (tetrabenazine, valbenazine, deutetrabenazine) have been shown to be effective for other hyperkinetic movement disorders, including dystonia. Levodopa is highly effective, even at small dosages (300 mg/day), for the treatment of levodopa-responsive dystonia, and there are case reports of other dystonias responding to levodopa. Clonazepam can be effective for various types of dystonia, such as myoclonus dystonia. Anticonvulsants such as oxcarbazepine and carbamazepine are used in patients with paroxysmal kinesigenic dyskinesia. Surgical interventions are available for patients with medication and botulinum toxin–refractory dystonia and include pallidotomy and internal globus pallidus DBS.

TABLE 12–3. Classification of tic syndromes

Idiopathic tic disorders	Symptomatic tic disorders
Gilles de la Tourette's syndrome	Post-rheumatic tics (after rheumatic fever) with PANDAS
Transient tic disorder	Carbon monoxide exposure
Nonspecific tic disorder	Drug-induced tics
Chronic multiple motor tic or phonic tic disorder	Tardive tic disorders
Chronic single tic disorder	Levodopa
Neurodegenerative syndromes	Stimulants (amphetamines, methylphenidate)
Neuroacanthocytosis	Anticonvulsants (phenytoin, carbamazepine, phenobarbital)
Lesch-Nyhan syndrome	

PANDAS=pediatric autoimmune neuropsychiatric disorders associated with streptococcal infection.

■ TIC SYNDROMES

Tics are sudden, rapid, recurrent, nonrhythmic motor movements or vocalizations with two broad categories: motor and phonic (Table 12–3). Hallmark characteristics of tics include a waxing and waning pattern with variable severity, a mixture of new and old tics developing over time, and a premonitory urge that resolves with tic completion. Patients have described the premonitory urge as an urge, a pressure, an itch, or a tension. Although tics tend to improve in adolescence and early adulthood, one-third of them disappear, one-third improve, and one-third continue to fluctuate. Tourette's disorder is a specific diagnosis with criteria that include multiple motor tics and at least one vocal tic, a waxing and waning course, a duration of >1 year, and onset before 18 years of age. Up to 90% of patients with Tourette's disorder have at least one comorbid psychiatric condition, including ADHD, OCD, anxiety and mood disorders, disruptive behaviors, and various sleep disorders. Depression is also common. The exact etiology of tics remains to be determined, but they are likely secondary to polygenic and environmental risk factors. There is also limited and controversial evidence suggesting that tics may be an immune-mediated condition associated with a preceding group-A β-hemolytic streptococcal infection, known as pediatric autoimmune neuropsychiatric disorder associated with streptococcal infections (PANDAS).

Management

Treatment rarely leads to complete resolution of tics, and a realistic goal is a reduction in tic frequency and severity. Nondisabling, mild tics warrant patient education, counseling, and supportive care. Treatment of tics is generally indicated if they disrupt social interactions, school or job performance, or activities of daily living or cause discomfort or injury. First-line treatment includes habit reversal training with comprehensive behavioral intervention for tics. If behavioral intervention is unsuccessful, there are several medications options; currently, pimozide, haloperidol, and aripiprazole are the only agents FDA-approved for use as tic-suppressing agents. Medications are commonly chosen based on comorbid psychiatric conditions (e.g., ADHD) and can be divided into tier 1 (less efficacious, fewer side effects) and tier 2 (more efficacious, more side effects) treatment options.

Tier 1 medications include clonidine and guanfacine, both α_2-adrenergic receptor agonists; these may be particularly beneficial for patients with comorbid ADHD. Other tier 1 agents with limited data suggesting tic suppression include topiramate, clonazepam, and baclofen.

Tier 2 medications include dopamine receptor antagonists (antipsychotics) and dopamine depleters (VMAT2 inhibitors). The typical antipsychotics include haloperidol and pimozide, whereas the atypical antipsychotics commonly utilized for tic suppression include aripiprazole and risperidone. The risk of TD seems to be lower in patients with Tourette's disorder than in other psychiatric populations. Tetrabenazine, a VMAT2 inhibitor, was shown to significantly improve tics in open-label studies, and deutetrabenazine and valbenazine are currently being investigated. DBS targeting the internal globus pallidus remains a treatment option in patients with disabling tics that are refractory to optimal behavioral and medical management.

■ ATAXIA

Ataxia is a physical finding rather than a specific disease or diagnosis. It describes impaired coordination of voluntary muscle movement (Table 12–4). Ataxia is often caused by cerebellar dysfunction but can also the result of impaired vestibular function or a lack of proprioceptive input to the cerebellum. Many different clinical terms are utilized when describing ataxia, in-

TABLE 12–4. Common inherited ataxias
Autosomal dominant ataxia (spinocerebellar ataxias 1, 2, 3, 6, 7, 8, 17)
Autosomal recessive ataxia (with predominant sensory neuronopathy)
Freidrich ataxia
SANDO (sensory ataxic neuropathy, dysarthria, and ophthalmoparesis) syndrome
Autosomal recessive ataxia (with sensorimotor axonal neuropathy)
Ataxia telangiectasia
Autosomal-recessive spastic ataxia of Charlevoix-Saguenay
Ataxia with oculomotor apraxia type 1 and type 2
Ataxia with vitamin E deficiency
Cerebrotendinous xanthomatosis
Autosomal recessive ataxia (without sensory neuropathy)
Autosomal recessive cerebellar ataxia type 1 and type 2
Niemann-Pick type C
Episodic ataxia (types 1–7)
X-linked ataxia
Fragile X tremor-ataxia syndrome

cluding gait ataxia, sensory ataxia, truncal ataxia, limb ataxia, dysdiadochokinesia, intention tremor, scanning speech, dysmetria, and nystagmus. Ataxia can be categorized by age at onset, tempo of onset, clinical course, focal or generalized distribution, and acquired or inherited etiology.

Evaluation

In patients with a family history of ataxia and onset of symptoms before age 60, determining the inheritance pattern can aid in planning genetic testing (see Table 12–4). If patients have no family history and onset occurs when the patient is older than 60, the utility of genetic testing is not well established. Most patients with ataxia should have a brain MRI to identify any structural or vascular lesions. Cerebellar atrophy is a common image finding but nonspecific and not always present.

Management

Several drugs have been studied for symptomatic treatment of cerebellar ataxia, including riluzole and 4-aminopyridine. Riluzole was examined in two randomized, double-blind, placebo-controlled studies that showed small but statistically significant improvement in ataxia rating scales. 4-Aminopyridine has been shown to potentially reduce the frequency of ataxia episodes in patients with episodic ataxia type 2, based upon a randomized, double-blind, placebo-controlled crossover study. Other drugs with insignificant or conflicting results in the treatment of ataxia include L-tryptophan, L-acetylcarnitine, choline, buspirone, varenicline, and amantadine.

■ MYOCLONUS

Myoclonus is a hyperkinetic movement disorder characterized by sudden, brief, involuntary jerks of a single muscle or group of muscles caused by muscular contraction (positive myoclonus) or interruption of muscle activity (negative myoclonus). Myoclonus has a wide spectrum of clinical manifestations and numerous causes (Table 12–5). *Physiological myoclonus* is a normal phenomenon seen in almost all people, including normal startle response, hiccups and sleep myoclonus, or muscle jerks occurring during sleep or sleep transition. *Essential myoclonus* is characterized by a relatively stable course in which myoclonus is a prominent or the only neurological symptom; an example of essential myoclonus includes the autosomal dominant myoclonus-dystonia syndrome. Essential palatal myoclonus, another example of essential myoclonus, is due to disruption in the Guillain-Mollaret triangle. *Epileptic myoclonus*, caused by myoclonic epilepsy, is often paroxysmal and unpredictable. *Symptomatic myoclonus* is the largest category with a long list of potential etiologies, with myoclonus secondary to medical or neurological illnesses.

Management

Very little evidence supports specific treatment of myoclonus, but generally, the best treatment approach is tailored to the physiology of the patient's illness. In cortical myoclonus, levetiracetam is usually first-line treatment based on a few small studies. Clonazepam (1–3 mg/day) or valproic acid (500–2,000 mg/day) may be effective in combination with levetiracetam or may be tried if levetiracetam must be discontinued. DBS may be used for medication-refractory subcortical myoclonus in myoclonus-dystonia syndrome. Segmental myoclonus (e.g., palatal myoclonus, spinal segmental myoclonus) is often treatment resistant;

TABLE 12–5. Causes of symptomatic myoclonus

Category	Specific condition
Drug-induced	Psychiatric medications
	Antibiotics
	Narcotics
	Anticonvulsants
	Cardiac medications
Inflammatory	Opsoclonus-myoclonus syndrome
	Antibody-mediate
	Various infections
Metabolic	
Nervous system damage	Stroke, demyelinating lesions
Neurodegeneration	Basal ganglia disease
	Alzheimer's disease
	Creutzfeldt-Jakob disease
	Frontotemporal dementia
Progressive myoclonic epilepsy (PME) syndromes	Unverricht-Lundborg disease
	Lafora body disease
	NHLRC1 mutations
	Sialidosis type 1
	Neuronal ceroid lipofuscinoses

clonazepam is usually tried first. Peripheral myoclonus, particularly hemifacial spasm, often responds to botulinum toxin injections or, occasionally, to carbamazepine.

■ TREMOR

Tremors have no specific neuropsychiatric associations but may be induced by drugs that are commonly used in neuropsychiatry. Table 12–6 lists the features of two major types of tremor and their etiologies and treatment.

■ CATATONIA

Catatonia is a syndrome of abnormal speech, movements, and behavioral disturbances. It should be considered whenever the clinical features outlined in Table 12–7 are present. In addition, the Bush-Francis Catatonia Rating Scale can be used to confirm the diagnosis. Historically, catatonia had been classified as a subtype of schizophrenia, but it is now recognized that it may

TABLE 12–6. Characteristics of tremors

Characteristic	Rest tremor	Action tremor
Amplitude	Variable	Variable
Frequency	4–6 Hz	10–12 Hz
Present at rest	Yes	No
Increased by action	No	Yes
Increased by stress	Yes	Yes
Associated disorders	Parkinson's disease and parkinsonism	Essential tremor, exaggerated physiological tremor
Drugs that induce the tremor	Neuroleptics	Lithium, tricyclic antidepressants, stimulants, ephedrine, caffeine, valproate
Treatment	Reduce dosage of neuroleptic, dopaminergic agents	Propranolol, primidone, clonazepam

TABLE 12–7. Clinical features of catatonia

Agitation or excitement that is not influenced by external stimuli

Catalepsy/posturing, or the passive adoption of a posture, including mundane (e.g., standing for long period without reacting) or voluntarily maintaining a bizarre posture

Echolalia (senseless repetition of the words of others)

Echopraxia (mimicking the movements of others)

Grimacing (maintenance of odd facial expressions)

Immobility or stupor (minimally responsive to stimuli)

Mannerisms (odd purposeless motor activity or acts, e.g., walking tiptoe, saluting passerby)

Mutism (verbally unresponsive, refusal to speak)

Negativism (motiveless resistance to instructions or contrary behavior)

Stereotypy (repetitive, non-goal-directed movements)

Waxy flexibility (slight resistance to being moved, as in bending a candle)

manifest in a number of other psychiatric (especially mood disorders) and neurological or general medical conditions (e.g., infections, autoimmune or toxic-metabolic conditions, poisoning, CNS diseases, drugs). For example, anti-NMDA receptor encephalitis with catatonia is increasingly recognized. Overall, catatonia has been reported in more than 100 different general medical conditions; the most common of these are outlined in Table 12–7.

When catatonia is suspected, response to lorazepam challenge can help make the diagnosis because partial or transient resolution of catatonia is seen with lorazepam administration. With an intravenous bolus of lorazepam 1–2 mg, dramatic temporary relief of catatonia may be seen within 10 minutes.

The presence of catatonia reflects that a patient is severely ill and frequently requires hospitalization. Special attention is needed to prevent and manage dehydration and malnutrition, venous thromboembolisms, pressure ulcers, and catatonic excitement and impulsivity. Etiological differential diagnoses are listed in Table 12–8. The pathophysiology of catatonia is not well established, but $GABA_A$ deficiency and glutamate hyperactivity may be causative.

Treatment of catatonia involves treating the underlying etiology as soon as it is identified and pursuing an appropriate laboratory and radiological investigation if the cause is unknown. Dopamine-blocking medications and other possible culprits (e.g., metoclopramide) should be avoided because they carry an overall risk of precipitating and worsening catatonia, are a risk factor for neuroleptic malignant syndrome, and are contraindicated in malignant catatonia. After catatonia has resolved, restarting an antipsychotic drug may be indicated.

First-line treatment of catatonia includes a benzodiazepine (usually lorazepam) at dosages starting at 2–3 mg/day and increasing up to 20–30 mg/day if necessary. Electroconvulsive therapy (ECT), depending on clinical urgency, may be the treatment of choice. ECT is the most effective treatment option and should be expeditiously used if catatonia is not responding to medications or if malignant catatonia is present. Most patients receiving ECT regardless of the indication typically remit with 6–12 treatments. Patients with chronic schizophrenia may need a longer course. If benzodiazepines interfere with ECT, flumazenil may be used. Prognosis is generally favorable with early recognition and appropriate treatment.

TABLE 12–8. Etiologies of catatonia

Drug-induced
  Amphetamines
  Neuroleptic malignant syndrome
  Neuroleptic medications
  Phencyclidine (PCP)
Neurological disorders
  Encephalitis (especially herpes encephalitis)
  Epilepsy
  General paresis
  Globus pallidus lesions
  Medial frontal infarctions or hemorrhage
  Parkinson's disease
  Subacute sclerosing panencephalitis
  Thalamic infarction
Psychiatric disorders
  Depression
  Mania
  Schizophrenia
Systemic disorders
  Diabetic ketoacidosis
  Hepatic encephalopathy
  Hypercalcemia
  Mononucleosis
  Systemic lupus erythematosus
  Thrombocytopenic purpura
  Uremia

■ NEUROLEPTIC-INDUCED MOVEMENT DISORDERS

In addition to classic TD, several of the disorders discussed in this chapter can be induced by dopamine-blocking drugs. The widespread use of neuroleptic-type dopamine-blocking agents to treat psychotic and agitated patients results in a plethora of drug-induced movement abnormalities of which the clinician must be aware (summarized in Table 12–9).

TABLE 12–9. Neuroleptic-induced movement disorders

Movement disorder	Clinical features
Acute dystonia	Onset 12–36 hours after starting or increasing neuroleptic; jaw, tongue, or trunk dystonia or oculogyric crises; relieved by anticholinergics or benzodiazepine
Akathisia	Onset 1–3 days after starting or increasing neuroleptic; restlessness; relieved by anticholinergic or propranolol
Akinesia	Onset 1–3 months after starting or increasing neuroleptic; slowness in initiating movements, diminished gesturing, reduced arm swing when walking; relieved by anticholinergics or amantadine
Neuroleptic malignant syndrome	Rigidity, obtundation, fever, and autonomic abnormalities; elevated creatine phosphokinase
Parkinsonism	Onset 1–3 months after starting or increasing neuroleptic; rigidity and bradykinesia most common; relieved by anticholinergics or amantadine
Rabbit syndrome	Perioral tremor; part of parkinsonian syndrome
Rest tremor	Occasionally sole manifestation of drug-induced parkinsonism
Tardive akathisia	Uncommon variant of TD; restless movements with less subjective distress than acute akathisia
Tardive dyskinesia (TD)	Onset after a minimum of 3 months of treatment; oral-lingual dyskinesia; poorly responsive to treatment; made worse by anticholinergics
Tardive dystonia	Common variant of TD; torticollis, blepharospasm, and jaw dystonia (Meige's syndrome) are most common; sometimes relieved by high-dosage anticholinergics; best response is to local botulinum toxin injections
Tardive myoclonus	Rare variant of TD; involuntary random jerking
Tardive tics	Rare variant of TD; involuntary tics
Tardive Tourette syndrome	Rare variant of TD; involuntary tics and vocalizations

230

■ REFERENCES

Aboukarr A, Giudice M: Interaction between monoamine oxidase B inhibitors and selective serotonin reuptake inhibitors. Can J Hosp Pharm 71(3):196–207, 2018 29955193

American Psychiatric Association: Diagnostic and Statistical Manual of Mental Disorders, 5th Edition. Arlington, VA, American Psychiatric Association, 2013

Armstrong MJ, Litvan I, Lang AE, et al: Criteria for the diagnosis of corticobasal degeneration. Neurology 80(5):496–503, 2013 23359374

Azzam PN, Gopalan P: Prototypes of catatonia: diagnostic and therapeutic challenges in the general hospital. Psychosomatics 54(1):88–93, 2013 23218059

Bashir HH, Jankovic J: Treatment of tardive dyskinesia. Neurol Clin 38(2):379–396, 2020

Bush G, Fink M, Petrides G, et al: Catatonia, I: rating scale and standardized examination. Acta Psychiatr Scand 93(2):129–136, 1996 8686483

Cholerton B, Zabetian CP, Wan JY, et al: Evaluation of mild cognitive impairment subtypes in Parkinson's disease. Mov Disord 29(6):756–764, 2014 24710804

Cholerton B, Johnson CO, Fish B, et al: Sex differences in progression to mild cognitive impairment and dementia in Parkinson's disease. Parkinsonism Relat Disord 50:29–36, 2018 29478836

de Bie RMA, Clarke CE, Espay AJ, et al: Initiation of pharmacological therapy in Parkinson's disease: when, why, and how. Lancet Neurol 19(5):452–461, 2020

Deuschl G, Schade-Brittinger C, Krack P, et al: A randomized trial of deep-brain stimulation for Parkinson's disease. N Engl J Med 355(9):896–908, 2006 16943402

Factor SA, Burkhard PR, Caroff S, et al: Recent developments in drug-induced movement disorders: a mixed picture. Lancet Neurol 18(9):880–890, 2019

Fahn S, Oakes D, Shoulson I, et al: Levodopa and the progression of Parkinson's disease. N Engl J Med 351(24):2498–2508, 2004 15590952

Fink M, Taylor MA: The catatonia syndrome: forgotten but not gone. Arch Gen Psychiatry 66(11):1173–1177, 2009 19884605

Fink M, Fricchione G, Rummans T, Shorter E: Catatonia is a systemic medical syndrome. Acta Psychiatr Scand 133(3):250–251, 2016 26426740

Friedman JH: Parkinson disease psychosis: update. Behav Neurol 27(4):469–477, 2013 23242358

Heinzel S, Berg D, Gasser T, et al: Update of the MDS research criteria for prodromal Parkinson's disease. Mov Disord 34(10):1464–1470, 2019 31412427

Heo YA, Scott LJ: Deutetrabenazine: a review in chorea associated with Huntington's disease. Drugs 77(17):1857–1864, 2017 29080203

Hirschtritt ME, Lee PC, Pauls DL, et al: Lifetime prevalence, age of risk, and genetic relationships of comorbid psychiatric disorders in Tourette syndrome. JAMA Psychiatry 72(4):325–333, 2015 25671412

Höglinger GU, Respondek G, Stamelou M, et al: Clinical diagnosis of progressive supranuclear palsy: The movement disorder society criteria. Mov Disord 32(6):853–864, 2017 28467028

Jankovic J, Tan EK: Parkinson's disease: etiopathogenesis and treatment. J Neurol Neurosurg Psychiatry 91(8):795–808, 2020

Kuo SH: Ataxia. Continuum (Minneap Minn) 25(4):1036–1054, 2019 31356292

Linortner P, McDaniel C, Shahid M, et al: White matter hyperintensities related to Parkinson's disease executive function. Mov Disord Clin Pract (Hoboken) 7(6):629–638, 2020 32775508

Lundbeck Inc: Xenazine (Tetrabenazine): U.S. Prescribing Information. Deerfield, IL, Lundbeck Inc., 2017

McColgan P, Tabrizi SJ: Huntington's disease: a clinical review. Eur J Neurol 25(1):24–34, 2018 28817209

McKeith IG, Boeve BF, Dickson DW, et al: Diagnosis and management of dementia with Lewy bodies: Fourth consensus report of the DLB Consortium. Neurology 89(1):88–100, 2017 28592453

Meltzer HY, Mills R, Revell S, et al: Pimavanserin, a serotonin(2A) receptor inverse agonist, for the treatment of Parkinson's disease psychosis. Neuropsychopharmacology 35(4):881–892, 2010 19907417

Olanow CW, Rascol O, Hauser R, et al: A double-blind, delayed-start trial of rasagiline in Parkinson's disease. N Engl J Med 361(13):1268–1278, 2009 19776408

Palma JA, Norcliffe-Kaufmann L, Kaufmann H: Diagnosis of multiple system atrophy. Auton Neurosci 211:15–25, 2018 29111419

Perlman SL: Update on the treatment of ataxia: medication and emerging therapies. Neurotherapeutics 17(4):1660–1664, 2020 33021724

Pringsheim T, Holler-Managan Y, Okun MS, et al: Comprehensive systematic review summary: treatment of tics in people with Tourette syndrome and chronic tic disorders. Neurology 92(19):907–915, 2019 31061209

Rafferty MR, Schmidt PN, Luo ST, et al: Regular exercise, quality of life, and mobility in Parkinson's disease: a longitudinal analysis of National Parkinson Foundation Quality Improvement Initiative data. J Parkinsons Dis 7(1):193–202, 2017 27858719

Schrock LE, Mink JW, Woods DW, et al: Tourette syndrome deep brain stimulation: a review and updated recommendations. Mov Disord 30(4):448–471, 2015 25476818

Stahl CM, Feigin A: Medical, surgical, and genetic treatment of Huntington disease. Neurol Clin 38(2):367–378, 2020

Stamelou M, Edwards MJ, Hallett M, Bhatia KP: The non-motor syndrome of primary dystonia: clinical and pathophysiological implications. Brain 135(Pt 6):1668–1681, 2012 21933808

Testa CM, Jankovic J: Huntington disease: a quarter century of progress since the gene discovery. J Neurol Sci 396:52–68, 2019

Teva Pharmaceuticals USA, Inc.: Austedo (Deutetrabenazine): U.S. Prescribing Information. North Wales, PA, Teva Pharmaceuticals USA Inc., 2017

Ward KM, Citrome L: Antipsychotic-related movement disorders: drug-induced parkinsonism vs. tardive dyskinesia—key differences in pathophysiology and clinical management. Neurol Ther 7(2):233–248, 2018 30027457

Wilcox JA, Reid Duffy P: The syndrome of catatonia. Behav Sci (Basel) 5(4):576–588, 2015 26690229

Zesiewicz TA: Parkinson disease. Continuum (Minneap Minn) 25(4):896–918, 2019 31356286

13

CEREBROVASCULAR DISEASE—STROKE

Gregory W. Albers, M.D.
John J. Barry, M.D.

Cerebrovascular disease is one of the most common causes of acquired behavior change in adults. With the marked expansion of the cerebral cortex that occurred in human evolution, the cerebral vasculature was stretched and contorted, creating border zones and end arterial zones with little collateral circulation and a consequent vulnerability to ischemic injury. Moreover, lateralization of cognitive functions in humans reduced redundancy and further increased the chance of intellectual dysfunction with focal lesions. These two themes in human evolution converge to make the brain vulnerable to ischemic injury and create a high likelihood of disability after stroke.

Tumors are a less common but important source of neurological disability and behavior change in both adults and children. This chapter describes common stroke syndromes and their behavioral correlates, and Chapter 14 discusses brain tumors and their associated neuropsychiatric morbidity.

■ CEREBROVASCULAR DISEASE-STROKE

Types of Cerebrovascular Disease

In 2018, approximately 795,000 total strokes were reported in the United States, with 610,000 people experiencing their first stroke. One in four patients had had a prior event, and 87% of these were ischemic in origin. Stroke is an age-related disorder, becoming increasingly common among older individuals. The frequency of stroke in the general population increases from 0.9% in persons ages 20–39 years to 29.8% in those age 80 and older. Males are at greater risk for stroke than females with increasing age, but overall females have a slightly increased incidence and an increased rate of concomitant disability. Seventy percent of stroke survivors have a permanent occupational disability, and approximately 25% have vascular dementia. However, the rate of stroke is decreasing, as is that of hypertension, which is the most prominent risk factor.

There are several major types of stroke syndromes (Table 13–1). *Atherothrombotic occlusions* result from atherosclerotic (large vessels) or arteriosclerotic (arterioles) in situ obstruction of cerebral vessels. *Cerebral emboli* arise from the heart and are carried distally in the arterial circulation to the brain. Emboli occasionally arise from plaques in the carotid, vertebral, or basilar arteries. *Intracerebral hemorrhage* is typically associated with hypertension and rupture of small aneurysms on the arterioles in the deep gray nuclei of the brain. *Subarachnoid hemorrhage* results from rupture of congenital aneurysms of the circle of Willis at the base of the brain. *Transient ischemic attacks* (TIAs) are produced by temporary interruption of the blood supply to the brain, usually from disease of the carotid arteries. TIAs occasionally occur with occlusion of small vessels and mark the occurrence of a lacunar infarction in deep brain structures.

The type of stroke syndrome seen clinically depends upon the size of the cerebral vessel involved. Occlusion of the carotid arteries usually leads to a border-zone infarction at the junction of the middle cerebral artery territory and the territories of the anterior and posterior cerebral arteries or an infarction in the combined territories of the middle and anterior cerebral arteries. Occlusion of a stem or surface branch of the anterior, middle, or posterior cerebral artery produces a regional syndrome (e.g., aphasia, aprosodia, homonymous hemianopsia). Occlusion of the proximal branches of the intracerebral vessels that supply the basal ganglia, thalamus, and deep white matter produces lacunar infarctions and white matter ischemic injury. Vertebral or basilar compromise produces brain stem and posterior cerebral artery signs (e.g., nystagmus, dysarthria, diplopia). Figures 13–1 and 13–2 illustrate the locations of typical ischemic and hemorrhagic strokes, respectively.

Risk Factors for Cerebrovascular Disease

The most common risk factor for stroke is hypertension. Congestive heart failure, arrhythmias, coronary artery disease, and electrocardiographic abnormalities are also highly correlated with stroke occurrence. Elevated blood lipids, cigarette smoking, diabetes, obesity, high serum homocysteine levels, and elevated hematocrit also contribute to risk. Cerebral emboli arise

TABLE 13–1. Relative frequency of types of stroke syndromes

Syndrome	Frequency, %
Atherothrombotic vascular occlusion	60
Cerebral embolus	15
Subarachnoid hemorrhage	10
Transient ischemic attacks	7
Intracerebral hemorrhage	5
Other	3

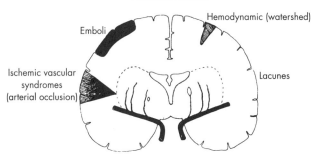

FIGURE 13–1. Locations of ischemic strokes.

Source. Reprinted from Hachinski V, Norris JW: *The Acute Stroke.* Philadelphia, PA, FA Davis, 1985, p. 98. Used with permission.

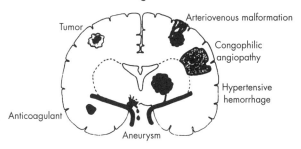

FIGURE 13–2. Locations of hemorrhagic strokes.

Source. Reprinted from Hachinski V, Norris JW: *The Acute Stroke.* Philadelphia, PA, FA Davis, 1985, p. 98. Used with permission.

from the heart as a consequence of valvular disease, myocardial infarction with mural thrombus, cardiac arrhythmia (particularly atrial fibrillation), and cardiac surgery.

Among younger patients, a history of migraine and use of oral contraceptives are risk factors for stroke. Nonatherosclerotic vascular disorders, such as collagen vascular diseases, are also more common in younger stroke victims. Table 13–2 provides a list of disorders to be considered in younger individuals who have a stroke syndrome.

■ ASSESSMENT OF PATIENTS WITH STROKE

Evaluation of patients with stroke should include a complete blood count, prothrombin time with international normalized ratio and partial thromboplastin time, erythrocyte sedimentation rate, electrolytes, blood sugar, blood urea nitrogen, serum cholesterol, electrocardiogram, and CT (often with angiography and perfusion) or MRI. Patients who sustain strokes but have no identifiable risk factors or who have a history of spontaneous abortions or migraine should be studied for the antiphospholipid antibody syndrome by obtaining anticardiolipin antibodies. Patients with TIAs or minor strokes may be candidates for carotid endarterectomy and should have CT angiography, magnetic resonance angiography, or Doppler studies of the carotid arteries. Echocardiography may be required to identify a source of emboli within the heart.

■ TREATMENT OF CEREBROVASCULAR DISEASE

Thrombolytic therapy with intravenous tissue plasminogen activator (tPA) was originally approved for treatment of stroke within 3 hours of symptom onset in 1996. Subsequent studies have reported benefits of intravenous tPA up to 4.5 hours, and current U.S. guidelines recommend tPA for eligible patients if the stroke occurred within 4.5 hours of assessment. Recent studies suggest that an extended window thrombolysis with tPA, up to 9 hours, is effective in patients with imaging evidence of salvageable tissue on neuroimaging. Mechanical thrombectomy was initially shown to be effective for treatment of patients with an internal carotid or middle cerebral artery occlusion ≤6 hours following onset in a series of studies published in 2015. In 2018, two studies showed that those with evidence of salvageable tissue can benefit for up to 16–24 hours after onset.

TABLE 13–2. Etiologies of stroke in young individuals

Arteriovenous malformation
Cardiac disorders
  Atrial fibrillation
  Atrial myxoma
  Cardiomyopathy
  Marantic endocarditis
  Mitral valve prolapse
  Patent foramen ovale
  Prosthetic mitral valve
  Rheumatic heart disease
Cerebral autosomal dominant arteriopathy with subcortical infarcts
  and leukoencephalopathy
Cerebral venous thrombosis (may occur during pregnancy)
Ehlers-Danlos syndrome
Fibromuscular dysplasia
Hematological disorders
  Dysproteinemias
  Hypercoagulation (idiopathic or with systemic cancer)
  Leukemia with leukocytosis
  Polycythemia vera
  Sickle-cell disease
  Waldenström's macroglobulinemia
Infectious arteritis
  Chronic basal meningitis
  Syphilis
Inherited metabolic defects
  Fabry's disease
  Homocystinuria
  Mitochondrial encephalopathy
Medication- and drug-induced
  Cocaine (oral or intravenous)
  Ergot derivatives
  Heroin (intravenous)
  Methylphenidate (Ritalin) (intravenous)
  Oral contraceptives
  Pentazocine (Talwin) (intravenous)
Migraine
Moya-Moya disease
Neoplastic angioendotheliosis
Pseudoxanthoma elasticum

TABLE 13–2.	Etiologies of stroke in young individuals *(continued)*

Systemic disorders
  Diabetes
  Hypertension
Trauma
  Carotid artery dissection
Vasculitis
  Antiphospholipid antibody syndrome
  Behçet's disease
  Disseminated intravascular coagulation
  Granulomatous angiitis
  Microangiopathy of retina and brain
  Polyarteritis nodosa
  Sarcoidosis
  Sneddon's syndrome (seronegative vasculitis with livido reticularis)
  Systemic lupus erythematosus
  Takayasu's disease
  Thrombotic thrombocytopenic purpura

Patients who present with a high-risk TIA or minor stroke are typically treated with a combination of aspirin and clopidogrel for the first 3 weeks and then converted to a single antiplatelet agent.

Long-term oral anticoagulation therapy should be ordered for patients with high-risk cardiac disorders, such as atrial fibrillation. Patients with atherothrombotic strokes should be treated with platelet antiaggregants, such as aspirin, clopidogrel, or combined aspirin and dipyridamole. Physical therapy, speech therapy, and occupational therapy will optimize outcome.

■ NEUROPSYCHIATRIC SYNDROMES ASSOCIATED WITH STROKE

The neuropsychiatric consequences of a stroke depend on the extent of the brain injury, the existence of other ischemic damage, and the premorbid intellectual and emotional functioning of the patient. Lesion location has been put forth as a significant factor, but contrary observations exist; this is discussed further in the sections that follow. Stroke-related frontal lobe syndromes (see Chapter 5), aphasia (Chapter 6), visuospatial disorders (Chapter 7), and memory disorders (Chapter 8) have been described. Vascular dementia is discussed in Chapter 10 ("Delir-

TABLE 13–3.	Principal behavioral alterations occurring after a stroke	
Cognitive disorders	**Neuropsychiatric disorders**
Aphasia	Anosognosia
Aprosodia	Anxiety
Constructional disturbances	Apathy
Delirium	Catastrophic reaction
Executive dysfunction	Depression
Memory impairment	Emotional lability
Pseudobulbar affect	Hallucinations
Unilateral neglect	Mania
	Psychosis

ium"). This chapter emphasizes abnormalities of mood and emotional function after a stroke. Neuropsychiatric disorders may be accompanied by motor and sensory abnormalities or may be the only manifestations of ischemic brain injury. Emotional and cognitive disorders may coexist or occur independently. Table 13–3 lists the major behavioral disorders that occur after a stroke.

Depression, mania, anxiety, and apathy are the most common neuropsychiatric disorders to occur following a stroke. Of these disorders, depression is the most common, occurring with a cumulative incidence of 39%–52% within 5 years. Valid diagnosis can be garnered with the Patient Health Questionnaire (PHQ-9) with a sensitivity of 90.6% and specificity of 88.6%. (PHQ-2 can also be used and has a similar sensitivity and specificity.) The Center for Epidemiologic Studies Depression Scale and Hamilton Depression Rating Scale are also valid. Aphasia can be assessed with the Stroke Aphasia Depression Questionnaire. Another 24% of patients develop anxiety disorders that are often comorbid with depression, sleep apnea, and fatigue. About half of patients meet the criteria for major depressive episode, and half have minor depression that is similar to dysthymic disorder. Major depression is not correlated with degree of disability, whereas minor depression is more closely related to patients' deficit syndrome.

Depression

Differences in the mechanisms of post-stroke depression may be reflected in the time interval from the event and the location associated with the lesion. Depression that occurs as a result of lesion location has been proposed, with left-hemisphere lesions associated with depression more than right-hemisphere lesions. This has been debated in recent systematic reviews of the literature. It appears that only strokes occurring in the subacute phase (i.e., 1–6 months post injury) had hemispheric localization for depression, and these were to the right hemisphere.

Mania

Mania is less common than depression after stroke, occurring at a frequency of around 2%. It occurs almost exclusively with right-hemisphere lesions, in 77%, with left-hemisphere lesions in 17%, and with lesions in both in 6%. Right-hemisphere dysfunction is responsible for ventral limbic circuit dysfunction and associated network abnormalities. Phenomenologically, secondary mania appears similar to idiopathic bipolar disorder. Lesions may affect the inferior medial frontal cortex, caudate nucleus, thalamus, or basal temporal region. Mania may be the first manifestation of cerebral autosomal dominant arteriopathy, with leukoencephalopathy and subcortical infarcts. Lithium and anticonvulsant agents provide efficacious antimanic effects (see Chapter 22, "Treatments in Neuropsychiatry").

Anxiety

Anxiety accompanies the cortical (but not subcortical) lesions that produce depression. Post-stroke anxiety is found in 21% of patients and is associated with comorbid depression, fatigue, and poor social support. Post-stroke depression and anxiety respond to conventional psychotropics (see Chapter 15, "White Matter Diseases"). Several recent MRI studies have found an increased prevalence of periventricular white matter lesions in patients with late-onset "idiopathic" depression. The changes may be vascular in origin, suggesting that the associated depression is a manifestation of subtle ischemic brain injury.

Psychosis

Psychosis may develop in 4.8% of individuals with post-acute strokes, with a 12-year incidence of 6.7%. Typical time of onset is >6 months after a stroke. The most common types of psychosis are delusions, schizophrenia-like psychosis, and mood disorder with psychotic features. Lesions are most common in the frontal (30%), temporal (26%), and parietal lobes (15.2%) and the right caudate (5.3%). "Silent strokes" are also found in about 8% of patients. In addition, concomitant lesions may occur in the left temporal region, producing Wernicke's aphasia. Patients with post-stroke depression and psychosis have a higher mortality, especially from cardiovascular disease. Seizures appear in 3.1% of patients who manifest post-stroke psychosis and are associated with a higher mortality. Psychosis is more common in patients with bilateral cerebrovascular lesions. Post-stroke delusions should be treated with traditional antipsychotic agents (see Chapter 22). Complete resolution of the psychosis usually occurs about 3.5 months after treatment.

Hallucinations

Visual hallucinations occur with retinal ischemia in amaurosis fugax, midbrain lesions in the syndrome of peduncular hallucinosis, optic nerve lesions in ischemic optic neuritis, and lesions of the geniculocalcarine radiations that produce homonymous visual-field defects (i.e., "release" hallucinations). Stroke-related seizures of the temporal, parietal, or occipital cortex may produce visual hallucinations. *Auditory hallucinations* may occur with pontine or temporal lobe ischemic injuries and may accompany post-stroke delusions.

Apathy and Pseudobulbar Affect

Post-stroke depression and fatigue are comorbid, and apathy (see Chapter 22) occurs in one-third of patients after a stroke, often without concomitant depression. This has a significant effect on patients' quality of life and must be distinguished from depression, in particular because each may be treated differently. *Apathy* is defined as a disorder of diminished motivation and can be diagnosed using the Apathy Evaluation Scale. Its pathophysiology includes orbitofrontal and anterior cingulate abnormalities. Treatment includes positive randomized controlled trials of acetylcholinesterase inhibitors and stimulants, such as methylphenidate, especially when prompt response is necessary, but safety concerns warrant continued evaluation (see Chapter 22).

As in other CNS diseases, patients who experience strokes frequently are affected by pseudobulbar affect. This is discussed further in Chapter 3, "Neuropsychiatric Symptoms and Syndromes."

■ RISKS OF TREATMENT

Atypical Antipsychotic Agents in Elderly Patients With Dementia

Typical and atypical neuroleptic drugs have been used for the treatment of psychological and behavioral dysfunction in elderly patients with dementia. At present, there is an FDA black box warning regarding use of these drugs for this purpose. Several studies have demonstrated an increased odds ratio for the occurrence of cardiovascular events with atypical agents, with a mortality rate of 4.5% in patients treated with secondary atypical antipsychotics versus 2.6% in patients given placebo. Current recommendations emphasize the use of alternative interventions. Patients with dementia may still benefit from the use of atypical antipsychotics, but they must be monitored closely and their continued necessity for these medications reviewed.

Selective Serotonin Reuptake Inhibitors in Patients With Post-Stroke Depression

Use of selective serotonin reuptake inhibitors in patients with post-stroke depression carries the possible risk of bleeding, especially for patients with acute intracerebral hemorrhage and those who are concurrently taking anticoagulant medication. The mechanism for this effect appears to be the depletion of platelet serotonin, which limits platelet adhesion and results in impaired hemostasis. The frequency of this event appears to be extremely low, with only one episode of increased intracerebral bleeding reported in 10,000 patients treated for 1 year. In another study of ischemic stroke, no increased risk of death or of intracranial bleeding was recorded during a 180-day observation period. Although the literature is controversial, the risk appears to be low. However, this risk may be increased with the concurrent use of anticoagulants.

Electroconvulsive Therapy and Transcranial Magnetic Stimulation in Patients With Post-Stroke Depression

Patients with post-stroke depression that is refractory to treatment may be candidates for electroconvulsive therapy (ECT; see Chapter 23, "Interventional Psychiatry"). ECT may also be effective in patients with treatment-refractory behavioral disturbance following stroke. Issues of optimal long-term maintenance treatment remain.

Patients with treatment-refractory depression following stroke may also be candidates for transcranial magnetic stimulation (TMS; see Chapter 23). TMS has been demonstrated to be safe and effective for post-stroke depression and results in improved quality of life, possibly by repairing damaged neural networks and increasing brain-derived neurotrophic factor. In addition, TMS may be a helpful intervention for treatment of aphasia after stroke.

■ REFERENCES

Ayerbe L, Ayis S, Wolfe CDA, Rudd AG: Natural history, predictors and outcomes of depression after stroke: systematic review and meta-analysis. Br J Psychiatry 202(1):14–21, 2013 23284148

Ayerbe L, Ayis S, Crichton CDA, et al: The long-term outcome of depression up to 10 years after stroke; the South London Stroke Register. J Neurol Neuropsychiatry 85:514–521, 2014

Beckson M, Cummings JL: Neuropsychiatric aspects of stroke. Int J Psychiatry Med 21(1):1–15, 1991 2066251

Bornstein RA, Brown G (eds): Neurobehavioral Aspects of Cerebrovascular Disease. New York, Oxford University Press, 1991

Centers for Disease Control and Prevention: Stroke Facts (online). Atlanta, GA, Centers for Disease Control and Prevention, 2018. Available at: https://www.cdc.gov/stroke/facts.htm. Accessed February 8, 2022.

Fridriksson J, Rordon C, Elm J, et al: Transcranial direct current stimulation vs stimulation to treat aphasia after stroke: a randomized clinical trial. JAMA Neurol 75(12):1470–1476, 2018 30128538

Gorman DG, Cummings JL: Neurobehavioral presentations of the antiphospholipid antibody syndrome. J Neuropsychiatry Clin Neurosci 5(1):37–42, 1993 8094019

Grotta J, Albers GW, Broderick J, et al: Stroke: Pathophysiology, Diagnosis, and Management, 7th Edition. Amsterdam, Elsevier, 2021

Guzik A, Bushnell C: Stroke epidemiology and risk factor management. Continuum (Minneap Minn) 23(1):15–39, 2017 28157742

Jones M, Corcoran A, Jorge RE: The psychopharmacology of brain vascular disease/poststroke depression. Handb Clin Neurol 165:229–241 2019 31727214

Kaufman DM, Geyey HL, Milstein MJ: Kaufman's Clinical Neurology for Psychiatrists, 8th Edition. Amsterdam, Elsevier, 2017

Kölmel HW: Complex visual hallucinations in the hemianopic field. J Neurol Neurosurg Psychiatry 48(1):29–38, 1985 3973619

Kuehn BM: FDA warns antipsychotic drugs may be risky for elderly. JAMA 293(20):2462, 2005 15914734

Lepore FE: Spontaneous visual phenomena with visual loss: 104 patients with lesions of retinal and neural afferent pathways. Neurology 40(3 Pt 1):444–447, 1990 2314586

Lim HK, Millar ZA, Zaman R: Cadasil and bipolar affective disorder. Psychiatr Danub 31(suppl 3):591–594, 2019

McKee AC, Levine DN, Kowall NW, et al: Peduncular hallucinosis associated with isolated infarction of the substantia nigra pars reticulata. Ann Neurol 27:500–504, 1990

Powers WJ, Rabinstein AA, Ackerson T, et al: Guidelines for the early management of patients with acute ischemic stroke: 2019 update to the 2018 guidelines for the early management of acute ischemic stroke: a guideline for healthcare professionals from the American Heart Association/American Stroke Association. Stroke 50:e344–e418, 2019

Robinson RG, Starkstein SE: Current research in affective disorders following stroke. J Neuropsychiatry Clin Neurosci 2(1):1–14, 1990 2136055

Rodenbach KE, Varon D, Denko T, et al: Use of ECT in major vascular neurocognitive disorder with treatment-resistant behavioral disturbance following an acute stroke in a young patient. Case Rep Psychiatry 2019:9694765, 2019 31139486

Sanner Beauchamp JE, Casameni Montiel T, Cai C, et al: A retrospective study to identify novel factors associated with post-stroke anxiety. J Stroke Cerebrovasc Dis 29(2):104582, 2020 31859033

Santos CO, Caero L, Ferro JM, et al: Mania and stroke: a systematic review. Cerebrovasc Dis 32(1):11–21, 2011 21576938

Satzer D, Bond DJ: Mania secondary to focal brain lesions: implications for understanding the functional neuroanatomy of bipolar disorder. Bipolar Disord 18(3):205–220, 2016 27112231

Shen X, Liu M, Cheng Y, et al: Repetitive transcranial magnetic stimulation for the treatment of post-stroke depression: a systematic review and meta-analysis of randomized controlled clinical trials. J Affect Disord 211:65–74, 2017 28092847

Spiegel DR, Warren A, Takakura W, et al: Disorders of diminished motivation: what they are, and how to treat them. Curr Psychiatry 17:11–20, 2018

Stangeland H, Orgeta V, Bell V: Poststroke psychosis: a systematic review. J Neurol Neurosurg Psychiatry 89(8):879–885, 2018 29332009

Starkstein SE, Robinson RG: Depression in cerebrovascular disease, in Depression in Neurologic Disease. Edited by Starkstein SE, Robinson RG. Baltimore, MD, Johns Hopkins University Press, 1993, pp 28–49

Starkstein SE, Robinson RG: Stroke, in Textbook of Geriatric Neuropsychiatry, 2nd Edition. Edited by Coffey CE, Cummings JL. Washington, DC, American Psychiatric Publishing, 2000, pp 601–620

Starkstein SE, Pearlson GD, Boston J, Robinson RG: Mania after brain injury: a controlled study of causative factors. Arch Neurol 44(10):1069–1073, 1987 3632381

Syed MJ, Farooq S, Siddiqui S, et al: Depression and the use of selective serotonin reuptake inhibitors in patients with acute intracerebral hemorrhage. Cureus 11(10):e5975, 2019 31803557

Szaflarski JP, Rackley AY, Kleindorfer DO, et al: Incidence of seizures in the acute phase of stroke: a population-based study. Epilepsia 49(6):974–981, 2008 18248443

Wei N, Yong W, Li X, et al: Post-stroke depression and lesion location: a systematic review. J Neurol 262(1):81–90, 2015 25308633

Williams LS, Brizendine EJ, Plue L, et al: Performance of the PHQ-9 as a screening tool for depression after stroke. Stroke 36(3):635–638, 2005 15677576

14

BRAIN TUMORS

Reena P. Thomas, M.D., Ph.D
John J. Barry, M.D.

Intracranial neoplasms can present with neuropsychiatric disturbances or behavioral alterations that may evolve as the tumor enlarges. Detection of an underlying tumor is important because increased intracranial pressure can be life threatening, and treatment of the tumor must be implemented. Some tumors are benign and curative following complete resection, whereas others are malignant and necessitate adjuvant therapy, including radiation and chemotherapy, in order to extend patients' survival.

■ TYPES OF BRAIN TUMORS

Table 14–1 presents the major types of brain tumors and relative frequencies of their occurrence. Primary brain tumors represent the seventh most common neoplasm. The 2016 *World Health Organization Classification of Tumors of the Central Nervous System* uses molecular parameters in addition to histology in the diagnostic process. This classification facilitates clinical decision making and prognostication and has significance for therapeutic discovery as well.

Gliomas arise from the nonneural CNS cell lines, including astrocytes (gliomas, astrocytomas), arachnoid cells (meningiomas), ependymal cells (ependymomas), oligodendrocytes (oligodendrogliomas), and embryonic cerebellar cells (medulloblastomas). Gliomas and meningiomas usually occur around age 55 years and make up two-thirds of primary brain tumors. Glioblastomas are most frequently seen in the frontal lobes and are usually diagnosed at a median age of 64 years. When symmetric corpus callosal invasion occurs, the term *butterfly glioma*

TABLE 14–1. Relative frequency of major types of primary brain and CNS tumors

Tumor type	Frequency, %
Tumors of meninges	36.6
Tumors of neuroepithelial tissue	29.9
Glioblastoma	14.9
Glioma and others	14.9
Astrocytomas	5.6
Ependymal tumors	1.9
Oligodendroglioma	1.5
Tumors of sella region—pituitary and craniopharyngioma	17
Tumors of cranial and spinal nerves	8.1
Lymphomas and hematopoietic tumors	2
Unclassified	5.6

Source. Adapted from Ostrom QT, Gittleman H, Fulop J, et al: "CBTRUS Statistical Report: Primary Brain and Central Nervous System Tumors Diagnosed in the U.S. in 2008–2012." *Neuro-Oncology* 17(suppl 4):iv1–iv62, 2015

is often used. Medulloblastoma occurs before age 20 years. Gliomas are the most malignant and most common intracranial tumors. Gliomas, including ependymomas, astrocytomas, and oligodendrogliomas, comprise 81% of malignant brain tumors and have a 5-year survival rate of 21.3%.

Meningiomas are generally benign tumors, although they may recur after surgical resection if removal is incomplete or if tumor fragments are left in place because of their proximity to critical structures. Calcification is found in 25%. Medulloblastomas usually occur in the first decade of a patient's life and are radiosensitive.

Metastases to the CNS arise from lung tumors, breast malignancies, melanomas, gastrointestinal tract neoplasms, and kidney tumors (in decreasing order of frequency). Breast and prostate tumors and multiple myeloma often metastasize to the skull and dura. The discovery that a patient has intracranial tumors at more than one site favors a diagnosis of metastatic disease.

Oligodendroglias are usually found in the frontal lobes. Meningiomas are often located on the brain convexities and parasagittal or sphenoid ridges and are often seen in females and in older adults with ionizing radiation as risk factor; patients are often asymptomatic. The differential of a brain mass is described in Table 14–2.

TABLE 14–2.	Differential diagnosis of brain mass

Bacterial or fungus abscesses, including progressive multifocal leukoencephalopathy

Inflammatory and demyelinating lesions, including multiple sclerosis and vasculitis

Metastatic brain tumors

Primary brain tumor—glioma, meningioma, pituitary adenoma, and others

Vascular disease

■ CLINICAL FEATURES OF BRAIN TUMORS

The presence of a brain tumor is often insidious. Headaches are prominent and are the initial complaint in one-half of patients with CNS tumors. Headaches are typically nonpulsatile and often bifrontal; they are often constant, positional, and nocturnal, with nausea and vomiting. Only 1 patient in 1,000 who present with headache will have an associated CNS tumor. Seizures are very common in conjunction with intracranial tumors, occurring in 50%–80% of primary and 10%–20% of metastatic tumors. Increased intracranial pressure from tumor mass and impairment of cerebrospinal fluid outflow produces papilledema that is characterized by obscuration of the optic disk margins, disk hyperemia, retinal hemorrhages, cotton-wool spots, and venous engorgement. Vision is not affected by papilledema. Unilateral weakness, parasthesias, and sensory loss, ataxia, or homonymous visual-field defects may be present, depending on the location of the tumor. Thus, a patient presenting with new onset of seizures, headache, nausea or vomiting, sensory or cognitive changes, and focal neurological findings should alert the clinician to have a high index of suspicion for the presence of a brain tumor and investigate accordingly.

■ NEUROPSYCHIATRIC SYNDROMES ASSOCIATED WITH BRAIN TUMORS

Neurocognitive dysfunction is the most common feature of tumor presentation, including personality changes, apathy, and intellectual abnormalities. Any unusual presentation of a psychiatric syndrome should be viewed with suspicion and provide an impetus to look for unusual medical etiologies and the presence of a brain tumor. CNS tumors may produce behavioral disturbances similar to those that occur with stroke (see Chapter 13, "Cerebrovascular Disease—Stroke," Table 13–3), but the syndromes are usually less discrete because neoplasms and their associated edema and increased intracranial pressure tend to produce more extensive dysfunction. Mental status changes characteristic of mild delirium, with slowness of thought, reduced attention, and impaired comprehension, are typical of patients with intracranial tumors (see Chapter 10, "Delirium"). Irritability is also common. These symptoms may be combined with more focal symptoms such as aphasia.

Meningiomas sometimes rise from the floor of the anterior cranial fossa, producing orbitofrontal compression and a progressive frontal lobe syndrome. Frontal lobe tumors are particularly likely to cause depression. Specific clinical syndromes depend on tumor location, growth rate, and the production of increased intracranial pressure. Symptoms overlap, but three primary syndromes appear. The first is the orbitofrontal syndrome, which includes prominent lability of affect and poor judgment. The second relates to dysfunction in the dorsolateral prefrontal cortex, which presents with apathy, perseveration, and executive dysfunction. The third involves damage to the anterior cingulate cortex, which may result in akinetic mutism. Symptom overlap often takes place because of diaschisis, in which a damaged CNS site may affect the function of another neuronally connected undamaged location.

Major depressive disorder may occur in 15%–20% of patients, especially in the first 8 months after diagnosis, and may be maintained for 1 year after surgery. Subclinical depression may occur in 27% of patients and may result in depressed quality of life. Suicidal ideation occurs in 12% of patients, especially those with seizures and steroid use. Suicide completion in patients with brain tumor is eight times that seen in control subjects. Psychotic symptoms may occur with pituitary and frontal lobe tumors. Symptoms may resolve with surgical tumor removal. Right frontal or right hemispheric tumors may produce mania, and temporal lobe tumors may produce psychosis or atypical mood disturbances with euphoria, hypomania, and lability. Diencephalic tumors may also cause hypomania.

■ TREATMENT

Steroids are utilized to reduce the edema associated with intracranial tumors. The role of surgery, radiation therapy, and chemotherapy is dictated by the tumor type. Tumors may produce hydrocephalus that requires ventriculoperitoneal shunting for management. Seizures are treated with anticonvulsants, and behavioral disturbances are treated with psychotropic agents (see Chapter 22, "Treatments in Neuropsychiatry"). Use of antidepressants has not been supported by randomized controlled trials. The question of seizure induction with antidepressants is reviewed in Chapter 9. Brain tumors are also frequently associated with seizures. Decreasing seizure threshold is a concern, but most antidepressants can be used safely (refer to Chapter 9). Finally, increased intracranial pressure is a contraindication to the use of electroconvulsive therapy.

■ REFERENCES

Boele FW, Rooney AG, Grant R, et al: Psychiatric symptoms in glioma patients: from diagnosis to management. Neuropsychiatr Dis Treat 11:1413–1420, 2015 26089669

Caudill JS, Brown PD, Cerhan JH, et al: Selective serotonin reuptake inhibitors, glioblastoma multiform, and the impact on toxicities and overall survival. Am J Clin Oncol 34:4, 2011

Dalmau JO, Posner JB: Paraneoplastic syndromes. Arch Neurol 56(4):405–408, 1999 10199327

Fleminger S, Greenwood RRJ, Olover DL: Pharmacological management for agitation and aggression people with acquired brain injury (review). Cochrane Database Syst Rev 4:1–60, 2006

Irle E, Peper M, Wowra B, Kunze S: Mood changes after surgery for tumors of the cerebral cortex. Arch Neurol 51(2):164–174, 1994 8304842

Kaufman DM, Geyey HL, Milstein MJ: Kaufman's Clinical Neurology for Psychiatrists, 8th Edition. Amsterdam, Elsevier, 2017

Louis DN, Perry A, Reifenberger G, et al: The 2016 World Health Organization Classification of Tumors of the Central Nervous System: a summary. Acta Neuropathol 131(6):803–820, 2016 27157931

Madhusoodanan S, Ting MB, Wilson SY: The psychopharmacology of primary and metastatic brain tumor and paraneoplastic syndromes. Handb Clin Neurol 165:269–283, 2019 31727214

McNeill KA: Epidemiology of brain tumors. Neurol Clin 34(4):981–998, 2016 27720005

Ostrom QT, Gittleman H, Xu J, et al: CBTRUS statistical report: primary brain and other central nervous system tumors diagnosed in the United States in 2009–2013. Neuro Oncol 18(suppl 5):v1–v75, 2016 28475809

Rooney AG: Brain tumors, in Textbook of Neuropsychiatry and Clinical Neurosciences, 6th Edition. Edited by Arciniegas DB, Yudofsky SC, Hales RE. Washington, DC, American Psychiatric Association Publishing, 2018, pp 333–351

Rooney AG, Grant R: Pharmacological treatment of depression in patients with a primary brain tumor (review). Cochrane Database Syst Rev (5):CD006932, 2013

Rooney AG, McNamara S, Mackinnon M, et al: Screening for a major depressive disorder in adults with glioma using the PHQ-9: a comparison of patient versus proxy reports. J Neurooncol 113:49–55, 2013

Satzer D, Bond DJ: Mania secondary to focal brain lesions: implications for understanding the functional neuroanatomy of bipolar disorder. Bipolar Disord 18(3):205–220, 2016 27112231

Wang KY, Chen MM, Malayil Lincoln CM: Adult primary brain neoplasm, including 2016 World Health Organization classification. Radiol Clin North Am 57(6):1147–1162, 2019 31582041

15

WHITE MATTER DISEASES

Les Dorfman, M.D.
John J. Barry, M.D.

The white matter of the brain and spinal cord consists mainly of myelinated neuronal axons, together with the oligodendrocytes that make and support the myelin and some structural elements such as astrocytes, microglia, and blood vessels. The high lipid content of myelin gives this tissue its white color. The electrical insulation provided by myelin increases the velocity of impulse propagation along the axon; damage to myelin slows or blocks impulse transmission. Diseases may selectively destroy myelin (*acquired demyelination*) or cause production of abnormal myelin (*dysmyelination*) or insufficient myelin (*hypomyelination*); these latter two categories are mainly genetic disorders of childhood. The salient clinical features of CNS white-matter disorders (Table 15–1) are spasticity and blindness, in contrast to gray-matter disorders, which tend to cause seizures and dementia. Note that the myelin on the peripheral nerves is structurally similar to that in the CNS but is chemically and immunologically distinct, so that disorders of CNS myelin infrequently involve the peripheral nerves, and vice versa.

■ MULTIPLE SCLEROSIS

Multiple sclerosis (MS) is the most common white-matter disease, with a prevalence on the order of 1 in 1,000 persons in North America. It tends to affect adults in the third and fourth decades of life, with a 3:1 female preponderance. MS is an autoimmune-inflammatory disorder of unknown cause, with predisposing factors that include female sex, genetic predisposition (especially human leukocyte antigen–DR subtype), exposure to Epstein-Barr virus, tobacco smoking, vitamin D deficiency, and perhaps the so-called hygiene hypothesis. MS is most prevalent

TABLE 15–1. Major categories of CNS white-matter diseases and representative examples

Autoimmune/Inflammatory
    Multiple sclerosis
    Neuromyelitis optica
    Acute disseminated encephalomyelitis
    Acute transverse myelitis
    Optic neuritis
Infectious
    Progressive multifocal leukoencephalopathy
    Human T lymphotropic virus type 1–associated myelopathy
    Subacute sclerosing panencephalitis
Toxic/Metabolic
    Vitamin B_{12}/Folate deficiency
    Central pontine myelinolysis
    Copper deficiency
Genetic leukoencephalopathies
    Adrenoleukodystrophy
    Metachromatic leukodystrophy
    Globoid cell leukodystrophy (Krabbe disease)

in temperate regions of the world and rare in equatorial regions, possibly related to sun exposure and vitamin D.

There is currently no reliable biomarker for MS, so diagnosis continues to rest on characteristic symptoms, abnormal neurological examination findings, and demonstration of multiple CNS white-matter lesions disseminated in both space and time; coupled with the elimination of alternative diagnostic considerations. Symptoms at onset are highly variable and can include weakness, numbness, imbalance, incoordination, incontinence, and diplopia or vision loss. Suggestive findings on examination include disturbances of eye movements (especially internuclear ophthalmoplegia), Lhermitte's phenomenon (electric shock–like sensation elicited by neck flexion), and optic atrophy. An MRI of the brain and spinal cord is central to diagnosis in most cases, often supplemented by cerebrospinal fluid analysis for evidence of immune activation (the presence of mononuclear cells, excessive intrathecal immunoglobulin G, and oligoclonal bands on protein electrophoresis). Sensory-evoked potential testing is sometimes a helpful adjunct. Consensus algorithms have evolved over time to allow earlier and more specific diagnosis (and treatment). Tables 15–2 and 15–3 cover the diagnostic criteria for making the diagnosis.

TABLE 15–2. Laboratory tests used in the diagnosis of multiple sclerosis

Test	Patients with abnormal early test results, %[a,b]
Cerebrospinal fluid	
Increased immunoglobulin level	90
Oligoclonal bands	90
Raised lymphocyte count	33
Evoked potentials	
Somatosensory	40–50
Visual	30
Auditory	10–20
Magnetic resonance imaging	
High-signal lesions	90–95

[a]Percentages are approximate.
[b]All values higher late in the disease course.

TABLE 15–3. McDonald criteria in multiple sclerosis*

Attacks	Lesions with objective clinical evidence, N	Additional criteria for diagnosis
Two or more	≥2	None
Two or more	1	Dissemination in space: further attack or MRI
One	≥2	Dissemination in time: further attack, MRI, oligoclonal bands
One	1	Dissemination in space and in time
Zero		1 year of disease progression and two of the following:
		One or more cranial lesions: periventricular, cortical/juxtacortical, or infratentorial
		Two or more cord lesions
		Positive cerebrospinal fluid

*2017 revision.

MS can take one of three courses. In the *relapsing-remitting* form (~80% at onset), patients experience episodes of neurological dysfunction that usually evolve over several days, last for weeks to months, and spontaneously resolve either completely or partially. Treating these episodes (attacks, relapses) with corticosteroids early in the course can hasten their resolution. In the *primary-progressive* form (15%–20% at onset), the symptoms come on insidiously and do not remit but slowly and progressively worsen over time (years). Approximately half of relapsing-remitting cases later transition to a more slowly progressive phase, referred to as *secondarily progressive*. The most frequent long-term consequences of either repeated relapses or slow progression are difficulties with ambulation, continence, and cognition.

Prophylactic immunotherapy is the principal long-term management of MS. Currently, more than 15 immunomodulatory and immunosuppressive agents have been proven to reduce the frequency of relapses in the relapsing-remitting form. Whether any slow the progression of the primary-progressive or secondarily progressive forms is unclear. These agents come with different degrees of potency and various side effect and safety profiles; thus, the selection of therapy must be matched to disease factors, including the type and apparent severity, the presence of comorbidities, and the risk tolerance of the patient (and physician), among others.

The management of specific symptoms is another important aspect of long-term care. Table 15–4 lists some of the common problems and the type(s) of treatment available. Note the inclusion of some neuropsychiatric issues.

Neuropsychiatric Aspects

Psychiatric comorbidities are common in individuals with MS, with up to 95% presenting with neuropsychiatric symptoms. Depressive symptoms are the most common (79%), followed by anxiety complaints (37%), apathy (20%), and psychosis (10%). Unselected patients admitted to a psychiatric ward who were evaluated by MRI were noted to have radiological findings consistent with MS in 0.83%. This is 15 times the frequency of the condition in the general population.

Mood Disorders

The incidence of major depressive disorder (MDD) in patients with MS has been evaluated with structured psychometric tools and variously estimated to be about 25%. Depression is the major factor in the assessment of quality of life. The occurrence of MDD is somewhat lower when fatigue and cognitive difficulties, which may be symptoms of the condition, are removed

TABLE 15–4. Common long-term problems in patients with multiple sclerosis, and some management strategies

Problem	Management strategy
Walking	Physical therapy, exercise, orthotics, canes/walkers, wheeled devices
Continence	Bladder relaxants, botulinum toxin, catheters
Fatigue	Sleep evaluation, amantadine, 4-aminopyridine, sympathomimetics
Neuropathic pain	Specific medications, pain consultation and interventions
Paresthesias	Specific medications (mainly anticonvulsants)
Weakness	Exercise
Spasticity	Tizanidine, baclofen, botulinum toxin, benzodiazepines, physical therapy
Depression	Psychiatric assessment, antidepressants, counseling
Sensation loss	None
Cognitive impairment	Neuropsychological assessment and counseling
Anxiety	Antidepressants, counseling
Emotional lability	Antidepressants, dextromethorphan/quinidine

from the sample. MDD frequency may be lower still depending on the patient's age, with a lower frequency found with increasing age. The lifetime prevalence in tertiary-care clinics is three times that seen in the general population.

Lifetime incidence of suicidal ideation and intent in patients with MS may be as high as 30%. Six percent to 12% of patients attempt suicide, especially within the first year after their diagnosis; this is 2–7.5 times higher than in the general population. Factors include lesion location (especially the left inferior medial frontal and left anterior temporal areas), hippocampal neuroinflammation, proinflammatory cytokines, hypothalamic-pituitary-adrenal (HPA) axis functioning, and brain-derived neurotrophic factor depletion. Concerns about the depressive effects of interferon β1b appear to have been disproven.

Several psychometric tools are available to aid in the diagnosis of a probable depressive disorder in people with MS, including the self-administered Beck Depressive Inventory and

Patient Health Questionnaire–9 or the clinician-administered Hamilton Depression Rating Scale.

Treatment has been poorly investigated. Only three randomized controlled trials have evaluated the utility of paroxetine, sertraline, or desipramine, with mixed results. Open trials point to the utility of duloxetine, fluvoxamine, moclobemide, and sertraline. Selection of an antidepressant should be made according to most salient physical manifestation of the disease. For example, in patients with nausea, insomnia, sexual dysfunction, or severe anxiety, mirtazapine is a reasonable first choice. In patients with pain, duloxetine or venlafaxine is reasonable. For those with prominent fatigue, bupropion is recommended unless seizures are a complaint (see Chapter 9, "Epilepsy and Limbic System Disorders"). Evaluation of the effectiveness of antidepressants in MS has been hampered by the exclusion of patients with more severe depressive illness and the decreased efficacy of antidepressants in some subgroups, such as those with primary-progressive and secondarily progressive types. Antidepressants with prominent anticholinergic properties would be reasonably avoided, such as paroxetine or the tricyclic antidepressants.

Electroconvulsive therapy (ECT) may be effective as an intervention for treatment-resistant depression in a patient with MS. However, a recent MRI with contrast enhancing lesions may be associated with disease exacerbation (see Chapter 23, "Interventional Psychiatry").

Cognitive-behavioral therapy can be utilized as a singular intervention or as an augmentation to antidepressant treatment. Supportive therapy may also be useful.

Bipolar Affective Disorder

The incidence of bipolar affective disorder in people with MS is unclear. It appears that bipolar subtypes are more prevalent in patients with MS, especially bipolar II disorder. Difficulty in the recognition of bipolar depression and mixed states may be the reason for controversy (see Chapter 22, "Treatments in Neuropsychiatry"). MS lesion location may be important. For example, lesions in the dorsolateral prefrontal cortex may result in depression, whereas lesions in the orbitofrontal cortex may result in impulsivity and cognitive dysfunction due to anterior cingulate impairment.

Treatment is anecdotal and similar to that for idiopathic bipolar affective disorder, but response may be more unpredictable. Of great importance is the recognition of depression as part of the clinical picture because antidepressants are often ineffective and some may induce manic mood states (see Chapter 22 on recognition of depression in bipolar affective disorder). Mood stabilizers are generally the treatments of choice. In addition, suicide may be more prominent with a bipolar affective disorder type II depression.

Anxiety Disorders

Anxiety disorders occur with a frequency of 15.4% and are generally treated with antidepressants. Benzodiazepines should be avoided when possible to prevent exacerbating cognition, fatigue, and balance dysfunction.

Psychotic Disorders

The presence of psychosis associated with MS has not yet been fully established. Alternative diagnoses must be investigated, such as anti-NMDA receptor encephalitis (see Chapter 20, "Limbic Encephalitis"). Periventricular white matter and temporal demyelination have been implicated. Treatment is the same as in idiopathic presentations, but first-generation and some secondary atypical antipsychotics, such as olanzapine with its high anticholinergic and sedative effects, may be problematic.

Cognitive Dysfunction

Nearly 50% of people with MS experience cognitive dysfunction, with ≤20% developing mild or more severe forms of dementia. Deficits are most often seen with declines in attention, episodic memory, speed of processing, and executive function. Patients with early evidence of gray matter atrophy are particularly susceptible. Although MS does not selectively impair cholinergic activity, some decrease may occur, and acetylcholinesterase inhibitors (e.g., donepezil) have been evaluated to improve this condition. Generally, the results have been disappointing. Other medications, such as amphetamines, may have some positive effects, but pemoline, amantadine, and ginkgo biloba have been generally ineffective.

Fatigue

Fatigue is the single most frequent complaint of patients with MS. Psychometric scales can be utilized to quantify and qualify fatigue, including the Fatigue Severity Scale, Fatigue Impact Scale, and Fatigue Descriptive Scale. When present, a search for secondary causes includes the presence of comorbid depression and medications used to treat the side effects of the disease. These include gabapentin and pregabalin for neurogenic pain and baclofen for muscle spasms. Sleep dysfunction is also often a problem with MS, along with heat exposure (Uhthoff phenomenon) and infections. Primary causes include brain atrophy progression, lesion load, functional cortical reorganization, immune activation, elevated cytokines, and HPA axis and dopamine dysregulation. Treatment is controversial. Modafinil is a stimulant that is not an amphetamine and has the most positive literature advocating its use in MS; clinicians should start patients at 100 mg/day and gradually increase to 400 mg/day. Amantadine may also be effective at dosages ≤200 mg/day, as well as methylphenidate ≤40 mg/day. Transcranial magnetic stimulation may be useful and is discussed in Chapter 23. Nonpharmacological interventions such as self-management techniques are particularly effective and preferable.

Pseudobulbar Affect

Pseudobulbar affect is discussed in Chapter 3 ("Neuropsychiatric Symptoms and Syndromes"). Its prevalence ranges from 7% to 29% in MS depending on disease duration and the criteria, psychometric tools, and cutoff scores used (i.e., Pathological Laughing and Crying Scale vs. Center for Neurologic Study–Lability Scale). Treatment consists of either selective serotonin reuptake inhibitors or tricyclic antidepressants, with one FDA intervention approved: NMDA receptor antagonist and sigma-1 receptor agonist dextromethorphan/quinidine (Nuedexta).

Steroids

Corticosteroids are often used for acute exacerbations of MS. Psychiatric side effects seem to be dosage dependent, with patients taking ≤40 mg of prednisone having 1.3% incidence of side effects compared with 4.6% of those taking 41–80 mg and 18.4% of those taking dosages >80 mg. Steroid-induced dementia may occur with dosages >60 mg and resolves slowly with drug discontinuation. Hypomania and mania are the most common presentations, and depression is more prominent as the intervention becomes chronic. Treatment should include dosage reduction below 40 mg/day, with eventual discontinuation. If drug reduction is not possible, then antipsychotics and mood stabilizers, including lithium, seem effective. If drug re-institution is considered, lithium pretreatment may be effective.

■ NEUROMYELITIS OPTICA

Long referred to as Devic's disease and generally considered to be a variant of MS (opticospinal MS), *neuromyelitis optica* (NMO) is now understood to be a separate autoimmune disorder with a known pathogenesis, distinct clinical and radiological features, and different treatment. NMO is particularly prevalent in Asia, where MS is less common, but it does occur worldwide. The principal manifestations are relapsing attacks of optic neuritis—often severe, recurrent, or bilateral—and of myelitis, either together or separately. MRI findings are distinctive, with long segments of inflammation in the spinal cord or optic nerve and sometimes elsewhere in the CNS.

NMO in most cases (80%) is caused by a circulating autoantibody to the aquaporin-4 water channel found in various parts of the CNS, including the optic nerve, the spinal cord, and, notably, the astroglia. NMO is therefore an autoimmune astrocytopathy that gives rise to myelinopathy. About 10% of NMO-like cases are caused by a circulating autoantibody to the myelin-oligodendrocyte glycoprotein (MOG), and these tend to have a more benign course, whereas true NMO can cause severe long-term disability.

Diagnosis of NMO (or MOG) is made from the characteristic clinical and radiological features, together with the presence of the circulating autoantibody. Otherwise-typical cases that lack one or the other antibody are referred to as NMO-spectrum disorder. As in MS, acute attacks are treated with corticosteroids (or sometimes with plasma exchange), and long-term management is usually immunoprophylaxis with azathioprine, rituximab, or eculizumab. The distinction between MS and NMO is important because a number of MS therapies have been found to worsen NMO.

■ PROGRESSIVE MULTIFOCAL LEUKOENCEPHALOPATHY

Progressive multifocal leukoencephalopathy (PML) is an uncommon but severe and sometimes fatal disease that usually occurs in the setting of immunosuppression or immunodeficiency. Its incidence rose during the pretreatment phase of the AIDS epidemic but has declined since the introduction of therapies for HIV. PML is caused by the John Cunningham (JC) virus, which resides dormant and inactive in about half of the North American population but can mutate and invade the CNS, where it infects oligodendroglia, leading to destruction of myelin. Common symptoms include hemiplegia, aphasia, hemianopia, seizures, and cognitive impairment. MRI shows large areas of myelin destruction in the brain. Diagnosis is based on clinical and MRI features and detection of JC virus DNA in the cerebrospinal fluid. There is no specific therapy for this condition, but some patients have survived when immunosuppression could be reversed.

PML is a dreaded complication of some contemporary therapies for MS, notably natalizumab. Risk-assessment paradigms have been developed based on the duration of exposure to the potential sensitizing immunosuppressant and the titer of circulating antibody to JC virus.

◼ VITAMIN B$_{12}$ DEFICIENCY

Vitamin B$_{12}$ (cobalamin) deficiency is an uncommon (but not rare) disorder that can be fully reversed if it is diagnosed and treated early. It serves as a model for other types of nutritional and toxic leukoencephalopathies, such as folate deficiency, copper deficiency (which is often related to zinc overload), and glue-sniffing encephalopathy. Vitamin B$_{12}$ is required for the formation and maintenance of CNS myelin. Deficiency can cause degeneration of myelin, most prominently in the posterior and lateral columns of the spinal cord but in the brain as well and occasionally also in peripheral nerves. Dietary deficiency of vitamin B$_{12}$ is rare; most cases are caused by intestinal malabsorption due to a lack of intrinsic factor produced by the parietal cells of the stomach. Parietal cells may be lost following gastric surgery or as a result of autoimmune attack (pernicious anemia). Diagnosis can be confirmed by measuring methylmalonic acid and homocysteine in the blood and by the coexistence of megaloblastic anemia. Treatment consists of replenishment, preferably parenterally.

◼ LEUKOARAIOSIS

Many people manifest small subcortical white-matter hyperintensities on brain MRI. These tend to increase in number and volume with age and are more prominent in persons with migraine. They are often referred to as "microangiopathic," suggesting a vascular origin, but it is usually unclear whether these truly represent small infarcts or merely prominent Virchow-Robin perivascular spaces due to normal brain shrinkage. They are often considered to be benign and incidental findings, but there is some evidence that the number, volume, and location of these hyperintensities may be related to declining cognition with aging. In extreme cases there may be overt vascular dementia, sometimes referred to as Binswanger disease.

■ LEUKODYSTROPHIES

The leukodystrophies are genetic disorders of myelin formation or maintenance that tend to affect children but, in some cases, may occasionally present in adulthood, usually as dementia. Metachromatic leukodystrophy, due to deficiency of arylsulfatase A, and globoid cell leukodystrophy (Krabbe disease), due to deficiency of galactocerebrosidase, are examples. These two can involve peripheral and central myelin, making diagnosis easier from study of the peripheral nerves, although contemporary diagnosis more often involves going directly to the genome when the condition is suspected. Enzyme replacement therapy or gene therapy for these disorders is still in its infancy.

■ REFERENCES

Ahmed A, Simmons Z: Pseudobulbar affect: prevalence and management. Ther Clin Risk Manag 9:483–489, 2013 24348042

Asghar-Ali AA, Taber KH, Hurley RA, Hayman LA: Pure neuropsychiatric presentation of multiple sclerosis. Am J Psychiatry 161(2):226–231, 2004 14754769

Brochet B (ed): Neuropsychiatric Symptoms of Inflammatory Demyelinating Diseases (Neuropsychiatric Symptoms of Neurological Disease), 1st Edition. Berlin, Springer, 2016

Carta MG, Moro MF, Lorefice L, et al: The risk of bipolar disorders in multiple sclerosis. J Affect Disord 155:255–260, 2014 24295600

Chalah MA, Ayache SS: Cognitive behavioral therapies and multiple sclerosis fatigue: a review of literature. J Clin Neurosci 52:1–4, 2018 29609859

Chan KH: Diagnosis and Treatments of Neuromyelitis Optica Spectrum Disorders. Republic of Moldova, Lambert Academic Publishing, 2016

Cheema J, Huynh AC, Prat SS: Multiple sclerosis and psychosis: a case report. Mult Scler Relat Disord 34:158–161, 2019 31302591

Confavreux C, Lassmann H, McDonald I, et al (eds): McAlpine's Multiple Sclerosis, 4th Edition. London, Churchill Livingstone, 2005

Cummings JL, Lyketsos CG, Peskind ER, et al: Effects of dextromethorphan-quinidine on agitation in patients with Alzheimer disease dementia: a randomized clinical trial. JAMA 314 (12):1242–1254, 2015

Feinstein A: Multiple sclerosis and depression. Mult Scler 17(11):1276–1281, 2011 22058085

Grech LB, Butler E, Stuckey S, Hester R: Neuroprotective benefits of antidepressants in multiple sclerosis: are we missing the mark?. J Neuropsychiatry Clin Neurosci 31(4):289–297, 2019 30945589

Greeke EE, Chua AS, Healy BC, et al: Depression and fatigue in patients with multiple sclerosis. J Neurol Sci 380(15):236–241, 2017

Harel Y, Appleboim N, Lavie M, Achiron A: Single dose of methylphenidate improves cognitive performance in multiple sclerosis patients with impaired attention process. J Neurol Sci 276(1–2):38–40, 2009 18817930

Kalb R, Feinstein A, Rohrig A, et al: Depression and suicidality in multiple sclerosis: red flags, management strategies, and ethical considerations. Curr Neurol Neurosci Rep 19(10):77, 2019 31463644

Kenna HA, Poon AW, de los Angeles CP, Koran LM: Psychiatric complications of treatment with corticosteroids: review with case report. Psychiatry Clin Neurosci 65(6):549–560, 2011 22003987

Kos D, Kerckhofs E, Nagels G, et al: Origin of fatigue in multiple sclerosis: review of the literature. Neurorehabil Neural Repair 22(1):91–100, 2008 17409388

Krupp LB, Christodoulou C, Melville P, et al: Multicenter randomized clinical trial of donepezil for memory impairment in multiple sclerosis. Neurology 76(17):1500–1507, 2011 21519001

Manning KJ: Hippocampal neuroinflammation and depression: relevance to multiple sclerosis and other neuropsychiatric illnesses. Biol Psychiatry 80:e1–e2, 2016

Marrie RA: What is the risk of suicide in multiple sclerosis? Mult Scler 23(6):755–756, 2017 28299962

Marrie RA, Fisk JD, Tremlett H, et al: Differences in the burden of psychiatric comorbidity in MS vs the general population. Neurology 85(22):1972–1979, 2015 26519542

Murray ME, Senjem ML, Petersen RC, et al: Functional impact of white matter hyperintensities in cognitively normal elderly subjects. Arch Neurol 67(11):1379–1385, 2010 21060015

Nannucci S, Donnini I, Pantoni L: Inherited leukoencephalopathies with clinical onset in middle and old age. J Neurol Sci 347(1–2):1–13, 2014 25307983

Nathoo N, Mackie A: Treating depression in multiple sclerosis with antidepressants: a brief review of clinical trials and exploration of clinical symptoms to guide treatment decisions. Mult Scler Relat Disord 18:177–180, 2017 29141805

O'Brien JT, Thomas A: Vascular dementia. Lancet 386(10004):1698–1706, 2015 26595643

Patten SB: Antidepressant treatment for major depression in multiple sclerosis: the evolving efficacy literature. Int J MS Care 11:174–179, 2009

Patten SB: Psychopharmacology of multiple sclerosis. Handb Clin Neurol 165:309–314, 2019

Patten SB, Beck CA, Williams JVA, et al: Major depression in multiple sclerosis: a population-based perspective. Neurology 61(11):1524–1527, 2003 14663036

Pietropaolo V, Prezioso C, Bagnato F, Antonelli G: John Cunningham virus: an overview on biology and disease of the etiological agent of the progressive multifocal leukoencephalopathy. New Microbiol 41(3):179–186, 2018 29620790

Pucak ML, Carroll KAL, Kerr DA, Kaplin AI: Neuropsychiatric manifestations of depression in multiple sclerosis: neuroinflammatory, neuroendocrine, and neurotrophic mechanisms in the pathogenesis of immune-mediated depression. Dialogues Clin Neurosci 9(2):125–139, 2007 17726912

Shangyan H, Kuiqing L, Yumin X, et al: Meta-analysis of the efficacy of modafinil versus placebo in the treatment of multiple sclerosis fatigue. Mult Scler Relat Disord 19:85–89, 2018 29175676

Stabler SP: Clinical practice: vitamin B12 deficiency. N Engl J Med 368(2):149–160, 2013 23301732

Thompson AJ, Banwell BL, Barkhof F, et al: Diagnosis of multiple sclerosis: 2017 revisions of the McDonald criteria. Lancet Neurol 17(2):162–173, 2018 29275977

Whitehouse CE, Fisk JD, Bernstein CN, et al: Comorbid anxiety, depression, and cognition in MS and other immune-mediated disorders. Neurology 92(5):e406–e417, 2019 30635487

Work SS, Colamonico JA, Bradley WG, Kaye RE: Pseudobulbar affect: an under-recognized and under-treated neurological disorder. Adv Ther 28(7):586–601, 2011 21660634

Zabad RK, Patten SB, Metz LM: The association of depression with disease course in multiple sclerosis. Neurology 64(2):359–360, 2005 15668442

Zifko UA: Management of fatigue in patients with multiple sclerosis. Drugs 64(12):1295–1304, 2004 15200345

16

HEAD INJURY AND ITS SEQUELAE

Aryandokht Fotros, M.D.
Sepideh N. Bajestan, M.D., Ph.D.

Sixty-nine million individuals worldwide are estimated to sustain a traumatic brain injury (TBI) from all causes each year. North America has the greatest incidence of TBI per 100,000 in the world (1,299 cases). Almost 8% of these injuries may be considered severe. Falls, being struck by or against an object, and motor vehicle crashes are the most common mechanisms of injury contributing to a TBI diagnosis in the emergency department. TBI contributes to 2.2% of all injury-related deaths in the United States. Morbidity depends on several factors, including the severity of the injury, the patient's sociodemographic and medical background, and the availability and speed of medical care after the injury.

The measure used most often to assess injury severity is the Glasgow Coma Scale (GCS), which evaluates three areas of neurological function: eye opening, verbal responses, and motor responses (Table 16–1). Other clinically relevant factors not included in the GCS include duration of altered mental status or loss of consciousness, duration of posttraumatic amnesia, and imaging finding (Table 16–2). Of note, the terms *mild TBI* and *concussion* have been used by clinicians interchangeably.

The pathophysiology of TBI is divided into two categories: primary and secondary brain injury. *Primary brain injury* occurs at the time of the trauma and leads to focal injuries, such as epidural hematoma, subdural hematoma, and subarachnoid hemorrhage. Common mechanisms of primary brain injury include direct impact; indirect impact, which is often secondary to rapid acceleration/deceleration force (*coup contrecoup*); penetrating injury; and blast waves. The areas most commonly affected are the frontal and temporal lobes. In *secondary brain injury*, damage occurs at a neuron's cellular level, with a cascade of molecular in-

TABLE 16–1. Scales used to assess head injury

Length of posttraumatic amnesia

    <5 minutes = very mild

    ≥5 minutes to <1 hour = mild

    ≥1 hour to <24 hours = moderate

    ≥24 hours to <1 week = severe

    ≥1 week = very severe

Glasgow Coma Scale*

Eye opening	Motor response	Verbal response
1. Nil	1. Nil	1. Nil
2. To pain	2. Extensor	2. Groans
3. To speech	3. Flexor	3. Inappropriate
4. Spontaneously	4. Withdrawal	4. Confused
	5. Localizing	5. Oriented
	6. Voluntary	

*1–4=very severe; 5–8=severe; 9–12=moderate; 13 or higher=mild.

TABLE 16–2. Classification of traumatic brain injury severity

Severity	LOC, *hours*	PTA, *days*	AOC, *days*	GCS score*
Mild	≤0.5	≤1	≤1	13–15
Complicated mild	≤0.5	≤1	≤1	13–15
Moderate	>0.5 to <24	>1 to <7	>1	9–12
Severe	≥24	≥7	>1	3–8

Note. AOC=alteration of consciousness (e.g., confusion, disorientation); GCS =Glasgow Coma Scale; LOC=loss of consciousness; PTA= posttraumatic amnesia.

*1–4=very severe; 5–8=severe; 9–12=moderate; ≥13=mild.

Source. Adapted from Arciniegas DB: "Medical Evaluation," in *Clinical Manual for the Management of Adults With Traumatic Brain Injury.* Edited by Arciniegas DB, Zasler ND, Vanderploeg RD, et al. Washington, DC, American Psychiatric Publishing, 2013.

jury mechanisms that begins at the time of initial trauma and continues for hours or days, including inflammatory response, electrolyte imbalance, edema, ischemia, and apoptosis. Diffuse axonal injury can be detected on diffusion weighted imaging studies. It is associated with disorders of consciousness and poorer prognosis for recovery.

■ GENERAL ASSESSMENT AND TREATMENT RECOMMENDATIONS

The first step is to assess the severity and acuity of the brain injury and to determine necessary and appropriate neurosurgical and neurocritical care management. In acute settings, CT is the most appropriate neuroimaging test. In nonurgent chronic and mild cases, a comprehensive assessment of risk factors (i.e., predisposing, injury-related, and perpetuating factors) is important for understanding the vulnerabilities and development of neuropsychiatric symptoms. Treatment should then follow from this assessment.

- *Predisposing factors* include the person's age, sex, developmental factors, preinjury cognitive/intellectual function, medical history, psychiatric history (especially substance use), personality traits, and socioeconomic status.
- *Injury factors* include the type and location of the injury.
- *Perpetuating and postinjury factors* include the presence of subsequent and repetitive brain injuries; medical treatments, especially pain management and prolonged treatments for other injured parts of the body; the extent of cognitive deficits and physical limitations; comorbid psychiatric symptoms; rehabilitation treatments; coping style; the person's ability to adjust to changes (in identity, role, and function); support; cultural expectations; disability; and legal litigations.

Rapid improvement is usually seen within 3 months of injury. Neuropsychological testing can be helpful to assess the extent of cognitive deficits. Educating patients and their families about the symptoms and course of recovery early on is important and can reduce the likelihood of persistent symptoms.

Behavioral techniques, cognitive retraining, and psychotherapy form important parts of remedial therapy. With more severely disabled patients, relatives and caregivers usually need help and support to cope with the changed personality and behavior of the injured person. For medication treatments, the general rule is to start low and go slow for dosing, try one medication at a time, and be mindful of the sedative and cognitive impacts of medications. Patients with TBI may have an unusual response or develop side effects when using medications, and clinicians must remain open-minded.

■ NEUROPSYCHIATRIC ASPECTS AND TREATMENT RECOMMENDATIONS

Cognition

Cognitive changes are common early post-injury, especially in moderate and severe TBI. These include deficits in all areas of cognition, including arousal and awareness, attention, memory, processing speed, and executive function. In mild TBI, most of the symptoms resolve within days to weeks following the injury, with complete resolution usually happening in <3 months. In severe TBI, significant improvement is seen within 24 months after the injury. Cognitive rehabilitation is the primary treatment approach. Some studies have recommended the use of pharmacotherapy, such as stimulants or acetylcholinesterase inhibitors as adjunctive treatments.

Emotion

Depression, anxiety, and PTSD are among the most common sequelae of TBI. Another manifestation of emotional changes in TBI is emotional dyscontrol. Pathological laughing and crying (also known as pseudobulbar affect or emotional incontinence), affective lability, and irritability are examples of emotional dyscontrol. Psychotherapy may be helpful for these symptoms. For pharmacological treatment, selective serotonin reuptake inhibitors (SSRIs) are first-line treatment. When choosing the second line of treatment, comorbid conditions should be considered. For example, a patient with irritability and apathy may benefit more from starting a stimulant than a mood stabilizer.

For treatment of pathological laughing and crying or affective lability, if SSRIs are not effective, then methylphenidate, levodopa, amantadine, and mood stabilizers (e.g, lamotrigine, valproate, or carbamazepine) may be helpful. Dextromethorphan-quinidine can be used as an adjunctive treatment.

For the pharmacological treatment of irritability, second-line options include the mood stabilizers (e.g., valproate or carbamazepine), methylphenidate, amantadine, propranolol, buspirone, and antipsychotics (e.g., quetiapine or aripiprazole).

Behavior

The behavior category includes disorders of diminished motivation (apathy), behavioral dyscontrol, psychosis, and suicide.

Apathy

Apathy is manifested with deficits in motivation for emotional responses, cognition, and emotional concomitants of behaviors. The first step in assessment of apathy is differentiating it from comorbid neuropsychiatric conditions, such as depression. If pure apathy is diagnosed and psychotherapy proves to be insufficient, pharmacological intervention can be considered, such as prescription of a stimulant.

Behavioral Dyscontrol

The category of behavioral dyscontrol includes verbal and physical aggression (i.e., verbal outbursts or physical violence) and disinhibited behavior (i.e., inappropriate nonaggressive verbal, physical, or sexual responses due to lack of voluntary control). The aggression may be acute or chronic. For treatment of acute aggression, the antipsychotics and benzodiazepines have been suggested, after considering the risks and benefits, in order to maintain the safety of the patient and others around the patient. When treating chronic aggression, any comorbid and contributing conditions should be taken into consideration, such as pain, seizures, depression, anxiety, psychosis, and family dynamics. SSRIs and mood stabilizers are recommended treatments for chronic aggression and behavioral dyscontrol. Buspirone has been found to be helpful in the treatment of comorbid anxiety and aggression. Few studies to date have shown β-blockers to be safe medications in the treatment of chronic aggression.

Posttraumatic Psychosis

Posttraumatic psychosis tends to present primarily with positive psychotic symptoms in the absence of a formal thought disorder, negative symptoms, and catatonia. It has two common phenotypes: delusional disorder and schizophrenia-like psychosis. The atypical antipsychotic agents are considered to be first-line treatment for this condition.

Suicide

Suicide is one of the most devastating behavioral risks associated with TBI. Military personnel are particularly at higher risk of suicide following a brain injury.

Somatic Symptoms

Sleep Disturbances

Data show that sleep disturbances can be as high as 50% post-TBI. Circadian rhythm disturbances and obstructive sleep apnea are most commonly reported. Neuronal injury and inflammation affecting orexin metabolism are likely associated with these disturbances. The gold standard of diagnosis is polysomnography, and first-line management should remain treatment of comorbid conditions, sleep hygiene, and psychotherapy.

Posttraumatic Headache

Posttraumatic headache onset usually occurs within a week of the traumatic injury. Acute headache typically resolves within 3 months, whereas persistent headache lasts longer. Overall, headaches tend to improve in the months following the trauma. A longer duration of headache is associated with a greater likelihood of secondary adverse events (e.g., problems with sleep, cognition, irritability, and libido and mood changes). Brain injuries, even mild TBIs, can affect visuospatial function and eye movements, which may impact the patient's ability to read and thus result in headaches. If posttraumatic headache is suspected, it is crucial to refer the patient for an oculomotor examination and provide appropriate treatment. General recommendations for the assessment and treatment of posttraumatic headache are similar to those for nontraumatic headache disorders.

Balance Difficulties

Balance difficulties, including dizziness and vertigo, can be the result of damage to the vestibular system in TBI. In most cases, symptoms resolve spontaneously within a short time. If symptoms are prolonged, vestibular rehabilitation and balance exercises can be considered.

Posttraumatic Pituitary Dysfunction

Posttraumatic pituitary dysfunction is a largely underappreciated TBI sequelae. Pituitary damage can affect the hormones associated with pituitary function. Screening for these hormones can be considered 3–6 months post-TBI in symptomatic patients, and the decision for hormone replacement therapy should be made based on clinical judgment.

Posttraumatic Epilepsy

Posttraumatic epilepsy is another concerning complication. The risk of posttraumatic epilepsy is associated with the severity of trauma and other comorbid conditions (e.g., alcohol use). For higher-risk patients, prophylactic anticonvulsant medications can be considered for a duration of 1 week. Once epilepsy is established, treatment with antiepileptic medications is usually considered for a minimum of 2 years. Prognosis is known to be good overall, with 70% of patients achieving remission.

Psychogenic Nonepileptic Seizures

Psychogenic nonepileptic seizures are not uncommon in TBI, with higher risk in patients with comorbid PTSD. Treatment approach is mainly seizure-focused psychotherapy.

■ IS THERE A POST-CONCUSSIVE SYNDROME?

The term *post-concussive syndrome* has created much confusion and discrepancy in the TBI literature. Clinicians use it loosely to describe short-term or persistent symptoms that patients experience after a brain injury. One recommended approach is to assess and treat each sequela of TBI independently and not as a syndrome. That is, even though the symptoms have the same initiating event, which might justify use of this terminology, no single treatment ameliorates the "syndrome," and recovery from various sequelae is often noted to be independent of each symptom, which is further evidence that these symptoms are not always linked together as they usually should be in a syndrome. Thus, post-concussive *symptoms* might be a more accurate term.

■ REFERENCES

Capizzi A, Woo J, Verduzco-Gutierrez M: Traumatic brain injury: an overview of epidemiology, pathophysiology, and medical management. Med Clin North Am 104(2):213–238, 2020 32035565

Dewan MC, Rattani A, Gupta S, et al: Estimating the global incidence of traumatic brain injury. J Neurosurg 130(4):1–18, 2018 29701556

Groswasser Z, Peled I: Survival and mortality following TBI. Brain Inj 32(2):149–157, 2018 29200309

Headache Classification Committee of the International Headache Society: The International Classification of Headache Disorders, 3rd edition (beta version). Cephalalgia 33(9):629–808, 2013 23771276

Mathias JL, Alvaro PK: Prevalence of sleep disturbances, disorders, and problems following traumatic brain injury: a meta-analysis. Sleep Med 13(7):898–905, 2012 22705246

Peterson AB, Xu L, Daugherty J, Breiding MJ: Surveillance Report of Traumatic Brain Injury-Related Emergency Department Visits, Hospitalizations, and Deaths: United States, 2014. Atlanta, GA, Centers for Disease Control and Prevention, 2019

Silver JM, McAllister TW, Arciniegas DB (eds): Textbook of Traumatic Brain Injury. Washington, DC, American Psychiatric Association Publishing, 2018

Taylor CA, Bell JM, Breiding MJ, Xu L: Traumatic brain injury–related emergency department visits, hospitalizations, and deaths— United States, 2007 and 2013. MMWR Surveill Summ 66(9):1–16, 2017 28301451

Venkatakrishna R: Management of acute moderate and severe traumatic brain injury, in UpToDate (online). Edited by Aminoff MJ, Moreira ME, Rabinstein AA. Alphen aan den Rijn, Netherlands, Wolters Kluwer, 2020. Available at: https://www.uptodate.com/contents/management-of-acute-moderate-and-severe-traumatic-brain-injury. Accessed March 20, 2020.

Wilkins TE, Beers SR, Borrasso AJ, et al: Favorable functional recovery in severe traumatic brain injury survivors beyond six months. J Neurotrauma 36(22):3158–3163, 2019 31210093

17

ALCOHOL AND OTHER
SUBSTANCE USE DISORDERS

Amer Raheemullah, M.D.
Ori-Michael Benhamou, M.D.

Substance use disorder (SUD) treatment has not been previously included in medical training. As a result, it is poorly understood and undertreated by physicians. In a nationally representative sample, 94% of physicians failed to diagnose substance abuse. When it is diagnosed, treatment is rarely offered. Despite this, patients are more willing to enter treatment via primary care than specialty drug treatment centers, and physicians remain an important part of the front-line treatment of addiction.

This chapter offers a practical primer on SUD for integrating its diagnosis and treatment into routine medical care. There are close to a dozen categories of substances discussed in addiction medicine, including alcohol, opioids, cannabis, benzodiazepines, sedatives, stimulants, nicotine, hallucinogens, inhalants, dissociatives, and anabolic-androgenic steroids. However, the diagnostic criteria for SUD remains the same regardless of substance used. All SUDs are characterized by changes in the brain and behavior and respond to similar psychosocial treatments. Physicians play an indispensable role in being able to prescribe medications that are effective in treating SUD, and medications approved by the FDA for SUD are the focus of this review.

■ EPIDEMIOLOGY

According to the 2018 National Survey on Drug Use and Health, 14.4 million adults (5.8% of adults) have an alcohol use disorder (AUD). Between 2006 and 2010, the annual number of alcohol-associated deaths in the United States was approximately 88,000 (9.8% of all deaths), and that number has been increasing in recent years largely because of alcoholic liver disease. Alcohol is the third leading preventable cause of death in the United States. Despite the severity of this problem, only about 7.9% of adults with AUD receive treatment.

Drug overdose deaths have also been increasing overall in recent decades, and total annual U.S. drug overdose deaths have surpassed the peak death rates from HIV/AIDS, guns, and motor vehicle accidents.

■ NEUROBIOLOGY OF ADDICTION

Historically, addiction was viewed by society as a moral failing and a deficiency in willpower rather than as a medical problem with a neurobiological basis. As such, addiction has been treated in criminal justice, social work, religious, and mental health settings that were geographically, financially, and culturally segregated from medical settings such as the hospital or primary care clinic.

Technological breakthroughs in brain imaging allow neuroscientists to study the effects of addiction on the brain in greater detail, from the basic structure and function of areas to the neurotransmitters and receptors affected by addiction. For example, functional MRI allows researchers to see craving states and their associated areas in the brain. PET allows researchers to locate what brain areas are changed by chronic substance use and to monitor the effects of a treatment regimen. A practical example of how addiction is driven by changes in the brain can be seen in subjects who smoked tobacco daily and had acquired damage to the insula. They were able to stop smoking easily and without experiencing cravings or relapse compared with subjects who smoked tobacco and did not have insular lesions.

Addiction can be conceptualized as involving a recurring cycle of binge (intoxication), withdrawal (negative affect), and craving (preoccupation and anticipation). As this cycle progressively worsens, it causes neuroplastic changes in the brain's reward, stress, and executive functions. Specifically, it affects three major areas: the basal ganglia, extended amygdala, and prefrontal cortex.

The basal ganglia play an important role in motivation and the pleasurable effects of engaging in activities such as eating, socializing, and sex. These areas form the brain's "reward circuit" and are involved in the formation of habits and routines. Addictive substances excessively stimulate this circuit and produce intense rewards that are far beyond what natural rewards can produce. With repeated exposure, this circuit adapts to the presence of the addictive substance and diminishes its sensitivity and ability to reward. This makes it hard to feel pleasure from naturally rewarding activities.

The extended amygdala plays a role in stressful feelings such as anxiety, irritability, and unease. These are the cardinal features of withdrawal and act as an additional motivating factor driving a person to seek out the substance again to relieve these feelings. Over time, individuals with SUD shift their focus toward relieving dysphoria rather than achieving euphoria.

The prefrontal cortex is responsible for problem solving, planning, and exerting impulse control. This part of the brain is the last to mature; thus, the adolescent brain is especially vulnerable to the effects of substance use.

The cycle of addiction perpetuates changes in the prefrontal cortex, basal ganglia, and extended amygdala, resulting in deficits in reward, stress, and self-control. These deficits drive the behavior to seek the addictive substance compulsively, with reduced impulse control. *Compulsivity* is characterized by perseverative, repetitive actions that are excessive and inappropriate. *Impulsivity* is characterized by a predisposition to rapid, unplanned responses to internal and external stimuli without regard to negative consequences.

■ DIAGNOSIS OF SUBSTANCE USE DISORDER

Similar to other brain diseases, such as Parkinson's disease, imaging is not required to make a diagnosis of SUD. While there are deficits seen on imaging that characterize the disease, the diagnosis can be made clinically based on behavior changes.

Exploring substance use is most constructive when it is approached nonjudgmentally, with empathy, and after building rapport. Utilizing screening tools and referencing national practice guidelines can help normalize the process as a part of routine medical care.

To screen for alcohol use, the U.S. Preventive Services Task Force recommends using the Alcohol Use Disorders Identification Test (AUDIT), the concise version (AUDIT-C), or a single question, such as "How many times in the past year have you had five [for men] or four [for women] or more drinks in a day?" The AUDIT is a 10-item self-report questionnaire that asks about alcohol use and its consequences over the preceding year. Scores range from 0 to 40, and higher scores indicate harmful drinking.

The AUDIT C comprises just the first three AUDIT questions, which measure the frequency and quantity of alcohol use and has scores ranging from 0 to 12. All of these screening methods can identify binge drinking or heavy alcohol use, but the single-question and three-item AUDIT-C approaches are briefer and can be easier to use.

Other screening tests exist, and tests used should be chosen based on what is practical for each setting. For example, the Michigan Alcohol Screening Test is one of the oldest screening tools; it consists of 24 questions and also has a geriatric version. Screening for drug use can be more challenging than screening for alcohol use due to the wide range of drugs targeted and their different health consequences and risks. Patients may use prescription drugs for nonmedical reasons, such as achieving a certain experience or feeling. A single question such as "How many times in the past year have you used an illegal drug or used a prescription medication for nonmedical reasons?" is just as well validated as longer questionnaires (e.g., the 10-item Drug Abuse Screening Test).

Patients who screen positive should have a more detailed evaluation to determine whether they meet criteria for SUD. A semistructured interview using open-ended questions and the principles of motivational interviewing can help elicit the details needed to make the diagnosis and assess its severity. According to DSM-5, the diagnosis of SUD is based on 11 criteria (Table 17–1), and its severity is based on how many points are met in the criteria: mild (2–3), moderate (4–5), and severe (6 or more).

It is important to distinguish between physiological dependence and SUD because they require very different treatments. Patients taking chronic opioid or benzodiazepine therapy will become physiologically dependent but will not necessarily have SUD. This is why tolerance and withdrawal (i.e., signs of physiological dependence) are not considered part of the DSM-5 SUD criteria for patients taking prescribed medications under appropriate medical supervision (see Table 17–1). If opioids or benzodiazepines are stopped or reduced abruptly in physiologically dependent patients, they will develop withdrawal and will often seek out more of the medication to relieve their withdrawal. Because these behaviors may be misinterpreted as signs of an SUD, it is important to use the DSM-5 criteria (see Table 17–1) to guide but not replace clinical decision making.

In patients who are physiologically dependent on opioids and benzodiazepines and are not in active withdrawal after a

TABLE 17–1. DSM-5 criteria for substance use disorder[a]

A problematic pattern of use leading to clinically significant impairment or distress, as manifested by at least two of the following, occurring within a 12-month period:

1. Often taking more of the substance for a longer period than intended
2. Ongoing desire or unsuccessful efforts to reduce use
3. Great deal of time spent to obtain, use, or recover from substance
4. Craving the substance
5. Failing to fulfill obligations at work, home, or school as a result of continued use
6. Continued use despite ongoing social or relationship problems caused or worsened by use
7. Giving up or reducing social, occupational, or recreational activities because of use
8. Repeated use in physically dangerous situations (e.g., drinking or using other drugs while driving, smoking in bed)
9. Continued use despite ongoing physical or mental health problems caused or worsened by use
10. Developing tolerance (feeling less effect from the substance with continued use)
11. Experiencing withdrawal symptoms after reducing use[b] (symptoms vary by substance)

[a]This criteria is not considered to be met by patients on opioids who are under medical supervision.
[b]Withdrawal does not happen with all substances; examples include inhalants and hallucinogens.
Source. Adapted from American Psychiatric Association: *Diagnostic and Statistical Manual of Mental Disorders*, 5th Edition. Arlington, VA, American Psychiatric Association, 2013. Used with permission.

dosage decrease, certain patterns of behavior can help in making the diagnosis of SUD, such as deterioration at home and work, nonadherence with recommended nonpharmacological strategies, illegal activities, and repeated lost prescriptions. Making a definitive diagnosis of SUD in these patients is not as important as making a treatment change because long-term use of opioids and benzodiazepines is rarely indicated. The tapering of opioids and benzodiazepines should be carried out slowly in collaboration with patients and guided by their capacity to tolerate symptoms. For opioids, national guidelines such as the *Health and Human Services Guide for Clinicians on the Appropriate Dosage Reduction or Discontinuation of Long-Term Opioid Analgesics* show prescribers how to broach the conversation of tapering, provide behavioral support and alternative pain strategies to reduce reliance on opioids, and begin the process of tapering opioids. For benzodiazepines, recognized guidelines for tapering such as the *Ashton Manual* provide rationale for slow tapers and suggested tapering schedules, typically about 5%–10% every 2–4 weeks, with tapering breaks guided by the patients' capacity to tolerate symptoms.

■ PSYCHOSOCIAL TREATMENT

Once patients have been diagnosed with SUD, clinicians should assess the patients' motivation and readiness to change before developing a treatment plan. Patients' motivation to change will ultimately determine whether they will engage with and follow through with the plan. The principles that underlie motivational counseling approaches such as motivational interviewing, motivational enhancement therapy, and brief interventions have been utilized for alcohol, drugs, and tobacco. They have been applied across various settings, including primary care clinics and emergency departments, and are associated with successful outcomes, including adherence to SUD treatment, reduced substance use, and decreased consequences. Because effective motivational counseling approaches can be brief, they integrate well into medical settings.

Motivational counseling is patient-centered and is based on the understanding that patients have intimate knowledge of their own lives. This is a response to the ineffective, authority-centered approaches that use confrontation to pressure people into change. Providers empathize with patients and respect their autonomy in order to create a collaborative partnership and to bring about change. Ambivalence toward change is an expected part of the process and is approached nonjudgmentally and with compassion.

The spirit of motivational interviewing is partnership, acceptance, compassion, and evocation. The core skills are **O**pen-ended questions, **A**ffirmations, **R**eflective listening, and **S**ummarization (OARS). Motivational counseling strategies should be customized to each patient's level of motivation and stage of change (Table 17–2).

For patients who have milder SUDs or those who are not ready to commit to higher levels of care, less intensive treatments, such as cognitive-behavioral therapy with a therapist trained in addiction treatment, are a reasonable starting point.

TABLE 17–2. Stages of change

1. Precontemplation—Patient is not yet considering change
2. Contemplation—Patient is considering change but is unsure how to change
3. Preparation—Patient identifies goals for change and formulates a plan to change
4. Action—Patient takes practical steps to change
5. Maintenance—Patient meets goals of change and changes in behavior are stable

For patients who need more structure, support, and accountability or have more severe SUDs, an intensive outpatient or residential addiction treatment program may be needed to break the cycle of addiction. Before arranging entrance into a treatment program, patients should have their risk of withdrawal assessed and managed. If patients are at a high risk of severe withdrawal or have significant medical or psychiatric comorbidities, they may need their withdrawal managed at an inpatient level of care.

■ MEDICATIONS FOR SUBSTANCE USE DISORDER

The FDA has approved medications for the treatment of alcohol and opioid use disorder. These medications improve several important outcomes, such as cravings and days of abstinence, and are discussed in the sections that follow. Smaller studies have suggested medications that may be helpful for other SUDs, but these are not FDA approved and cannot be recommended for stand-alone treatment until larger studies are conducted. Examples of non-approved medications worth mentioning are gabapentin and N-acetylcysteine for cannabis use disorder and the combination of bupropion and naltrexone for methamphetamine use disorder.

Medications for Alcohol Use Disorder

Four medications (Table 17–3) are FDA-approved to treat AUD. Despite being a standard of care and recommended as a first-line treatment in practice guidelines, medications for AUD are prescribed to <9% of patients who would likely benefit from them.

Naltrexone and acamprosate are most strongly supported by placebo-controlled clinical trials in AUD. Clinical trials of

TABLE 17–3. FDA-approved alcohol use disorder medications

	Oral naltrexone	Long-acting injectable naltrexone	Acamprosate	Disulfiram
Dosing	50 mg/day (FDA-approved dosage); dosages in clinical trials were ≤100 mg/day	380 mg monthly IM gluteal injection	666 mg tid po (FDA-approved dosage 1,998 mg/day); dosages in clinical trials were 1,000–3,000 mg/day	250–500 mg/day po (FDA-approved dosage)
Considerations	May avoid side effects by starting at 25 mg/day for a few days before titrating to 50 mg/day dosage. This is an opioid blocker and should not be used in patients requiring opioids.	If there is time, start oral naltrexone to ensure patient tolerates the drug. Can increase frequency of injections or supplement with oral naltrexone if cravings return prior to next dose.	Most positive trials included a period of abstinence before starting the medication (naltrexone can be initiated while patients are still drinking).	Clinical trials suggest efficacy only when ingestion is observed. Disulfiram-ethanol reaction may not occur in some patients.
Contraindications	Decompensated cirrhosis; avoid if liver function tests are >3–5 times upper limit of normal	Same as oral naltrexone	Acute kidney injury; renally adjust dosage for chronic kidney disease	Heart disease, psychosis, liver failure
Common side effects	Somnolence, nausea, vomiting, abdominal pain, insomnia, dizziness	Injection site reactions; same side effects as oral naltrexone	Diarrhea	Drowsiness; hepatitis, confusion, neuropathy, optic neuritis, and psychosis occur rarely

acamprosate showing efficacy were mostly conducted in European countries, and trials in the United States have shown a lack of efficacy. Disulfiram is a second-line option after naltrexone and acamprosate. Multiple clinical trials have found topiramate to reduce drinking in patients with AUD. Topiramate can be associated with multiple side effects (e.g., cognitive impairment, paresthesia, dizziness; see Chapter 22, "Treatments in Neuropsychiatry") and should be started at a low dosage and gradually increased. The therapeutic range is up to 300 mg/day and requires tapering over weeks before discontinuation. Baclofen and gabapentin can be used for treatment of AUD if other options are not effective because data from clinical trials supporting their efficacy are more limited. Baclofen has been shown to be safe in patients with liver cirrhosis.

Medications for Opioid Use Disorder

For opioid use disorder (OUD), medications are usually given in conjunction with psychosocial interventions. Numerous clinical trials in patients with OUD have shown medications to reduce substance use compared with placebo; buprenorphine, methadone, and naltrexone are safe and effective and a standard of care. Fewer trials have found psychosocial treatment alone to be effective compared with control conditions. Most clinical trials of patients with OUD have found medications to result in reduced substance use and greater rates of abstinence compared with psychosocial treatment alone. Some organizations, such as the World Health Organization, use the term *psychosocially assisted pharmacological treatment* instead of *medication-assisted treatment*, emphasizing that medications have more than just an adjunctive role.

Selecting the right medication is based on shared decision-making after patients have been informed about the pros and cons of each drug and taking into consideration the patients' preference, family input, addiction severity, and risk of relapse. Withdrawal is an important initial consideration and should be completed prior to starting the opioid antagonist naltrexone. Because a significant number of patients drop out of treatment before fully withdrawing from opioids as required before starting naltrexone, treatment with buprenorphine or methadone is the first treatment of choice for most patients. For buprenorphine (partial agonist), national guidelines recommend a period of withdrawal of ≥12 hours to avoid precipitated withdrawal. However, newer induction methods starting with microdoses of buprenorphine do not require a patient to enter withdrawal before starting the drug. Methadone (full-agonist) can also be started before the patient enters withdrawal.

The first-line medication for moderate to severe OUD is usually with buprenorphine or methadone. Both of these medications are comparable in their efficacy, but both are regulated, with different requirements and settings governing their use. The choice between the two agents is often driven by the setting and previous patient experiences. Federal regulations require methadone to be administered at methadone clinics (in opioid treatment programs), and patients must travel daily to obtain the medication during the initial phase of treatment. Buprenorphine, on the other hand, can be prescribed like other prescription drugs in outpatient clinics and thus is more convenient because it does not require daily travel. Physicians must take a brief training course before they can obtain a waiver allowing them to prescribe buprenorphine. Many U.S. counties do not have a buprenorphine provider; however, telehealth options are increasing access to this medication. Methadone is a reasonable option for patients who have a poor response or who have no access to buprenorphine. For patients who decline buprenorphine or methadone treatment, long-acting injectable naltrexone is a good option. For patients who are able to complete withdrawal without relapsing, injectable naltrexone has outcomes similar to those achieved with buprenorphine. Oral naltrexone is also available and can be taken daily for highly motivated individuals who prefer naltrexone.

■ REFERENCES

Ashton CH: Benzodiazepines: How They Work and How to Withdraw (aka The Ashton Manual). Newcastle Upon Tyne, UK, Institute of Neuroscience, Newcastle University, 2002. Available at: https://www.benzo.org.uk/manual. Accessed January 31, 2022.

Barry CL, Epstein AJ, Fiellin DA, et al: Estimating demand for primary care–based treatment for substance and alcohol use disorders. Addiction 111(8):1376–1384, 2016

Koob GF, Volkow ND: Neurobiology of addiction: a neurocircuitry analysis. Lancet Psychiatry 3(8):760–773, 2016 27475769

Kranzler HR, Soyka M: Diagnosis and pharmacotherapy of alcohol use disorder: a review. JAMA 320(8):815–824, 2018 30167705

Miller WR: TIP 35: Enhancing Motivation for Change in Substance Abuse Treatment. Rockville, MD, Substance Abuse and Mental Health Services Administration, 2019

National Institute on Drug Abuse: Overdose death rates, in Trends and Statistics (online). Bethesda, MD, National Institute on Drug Abuse, 2020. Available at: https://www.drugabuse.gov/related-topics/trends-statistics/overdose-death-rates. Accessed May 11, 2020.

Substance Abuse and Mental Health Services Administration: Table 2.1B: Tobacco product and alcohol use in lifetime, past year, and past month among persons aged 12 or older, by age group: percentages, 2017 and 2018, in Results From the 2018 National Survey on Drug Use and Health (NSDUH). Rockville, MD, Substance Abuse and Mental Health Services Administration, 2018. Available at: https://www.samhsa.gov/data/sites/default/files/cbhsq-reports/NSDUHDetailedTabs2018R2/NSDUHDetTabsSect2pe2018.htm#tab2-1b. Accessed January 31, 2022.

University of Illinois at Chicago Survey Research Laboratory, Columbia University National Center on Addiction and Substance Abuse: Missed Opportunity: National Survey of Primary Care Physicians and Patients on Substance Abuse. New York, Columbia University, National Center on Addiction and Substance Abuse, 2000

U.S. Department of Health and Human Services: HHS Guide for Clinicians on the Appropriate Dosage Reduction or Discontinuation of Long-Term Opioid Analgesics. Washington, DC, U.S. Department of Health and Human Services, 2019

18

AUTISM SPECTRUM DISORDER

Jesse Adams, M.D.
Manal Khan, M.D.

Autism spectrum disorder (ASD) is a neurodevelopmental condition that comprises a constellation of symptoms associated with deficits in social communication and repetitive sensory-motor behaviors. Although often referred to as a single disorder, *autism*, ASD is a heterogeneous condition that describes a broad phenotype, with impairment ranging from mild to severe.

In DSM-5, ASD has been consolidated into one diagnosis with a spectrum of impairment, subsuming Asperger's disorder (now *autism spectrum disorder without intellectual or language impairment*) and pervasive developmental disorder not otherwise specified. Criteria have shifted to focus on two symptom categories: social communication and restrictive/repetitive behaviors (Table 18–1).

Symptoms must be present in the early developmental period even if not fully realized until later in life when demands exceed capacities. Intellectual disability and ASD frequently co-occur, in which case, social communication should be below general developmental level in order to diagnose ASD.

■ EPIDEMIOLOGY

The prevalence of ASD in developed countries is reported to be 1.5%. The international prevalence of ASD was estimated to be 0.76% by the World Health Organization in 2010. After increasing over time due to recognition of milder cases, this prevalence has plateaued. The male-to-female ratio is approximately 4:1; however, this imbalance diminishes with increasing severity of ASD. Girls with ASD show, on average, more significant impairment. Differences in symptom presentation and sex biases in diagnosis may contribute to the observed imbalance. That

TABLE 18–1.	DSM-5 diagnostic criteria for autism spectrum disorder

A. Persistent deficits in social communication and social interaction, as manifested by the following:

    1. Deficits in social-emotional reciprocity (e.g., social approach or sharing of interests or affect).

    2. Deficits in nonverbal communication (e.g., eye contact/body language or deficits in understanding gestures).

    3. Deficits in developing, maintaining, and understanding relationships (e.g., sharing imaginative play or making friends).

B. Restricted, repetitive patterns of behavior, interests, or activities, as manifested by at least two of the following:

    1. Stereotyped/repetitive movements, use of objects, or speech (e.g., stereotypies, echolalia).

    2. Insistence on sameness, inflexible adherence to routines, or ritualized patterns of behavior (e.g., extreme distress at small changes or difficulties with transitions).

    3. Highly restricted, fixated interests that are abnormal in intensity or focus (e.g., fixation with unusual objects or excessively circumscribed/perseverative interests).

    4. Hyper- or hyporeactivity to sensory input or unusual interest in sensory aspects of the environment (e.g., adverse response to specific sounds/textures or visual fascination with lights or movement).

Source. Adapted from American Psychiatric Association: *Diagnostic and Statistical Manual of Mental Disorders*, 5th Edition. Arlington, VA, American Psychiatric Association, 2013. Used with permission.

said, these findings are consistent across other populations. ASD is seen in all racial and ethnic groups.

■ ETIOLOGY

ASD encompasses a diverse spectrum of disorders with varying degrees of impairment in social/emotional processing, language, intellect, adaptive functioning, executive functioning, and more. As such, there are likely a variety of contributing factors. Although genetic and neurodevelopmental changes are thought to underlie much of the phenotypic presentation, there is no single accepted "cause" of ASD. Most frequently, the cause is not known; *<5% of patients with ASD have an identifiable etiology.* Of this 5%, most patients have tuberous sclerosis or fragile X syndrome. Other genetic comorbidities include neurofibromatosis type 1 or velocardiofacial syndrome. Encephalitis or fetal infections may also contribute.

Although widely debunked, fears of a link between vaccines and autism remain, originating from a retracted 1998 *Lancet* study that implicated the measles, mumps, and rubella vaccine as a cause. The study's credibility was suspect due to its small sample size, its selection/recall bias, and the author's conflicts of interest. Since then, several high-quality studies have refuted any such link. Thimerosal, a mercury-containing agent in vaccines, has also been the target of such concerns. Again, several studies refuted these concerns, and thimerosal has largely been removed from vaccines in the United States. Unfortunately, this myth and others persist.

■ GENETICS

ASD seems to be highly genetically based and heritable (heritability approximately 90%, with ≤90% concordance in monozygotic and 0%–24% in dizygotic twins). The likelihood of an ASD proband having ASD ranges from 2% to 6%. Relatives often demonstrate isolated behavioral or social challenges without manifesting the full disorder, termed *autistic-like traits*. Few major candidate genes have been validated. Many candidates affect neuronal migration or synaptogenesis. Findings of increased whole-blood serotonin and alterations in frontal cortical serotonin uptake have led to investigation of the serotonin transporter. Due to the 4:1 sex ratio, X-linked inheritance or imprinting has been suggested but not clearly validated. Nearly all chromosomes have shown some potential linkage. Thus, the genetics of ASD are complex, polygenic, and still not well understood.

■ NEUROANATOMY

Because it is a heterogeneous spectrum of disorders, no single, well-validated neuroanatomical model of ASD has been developed. Alterations are noted in various brain regions throughout development. Studies are frequently contradictory, further complicating attempts to create such a model. ASD also appears to be related, at least in part, to altered brain development, disordered neuronal migration, and cortical disorganization, thus rendering it difficult to identify any one discrete region or circuit responsible.

The *frontal cortex* has been an area of focus. The overgrowth of frontal cortical regions, both white and gray matter, has been observed in young children with ASD, although this may attenuate later in life. Variations in cortical thickness have also been noted.

The *cerebellum*, which is thought to modulate activity of other regions and functions, has been shown to play a significant role in cognition. Consistent findings in ASD include hypoplasia of the cerebellar vermis and reduction in the size and number of Purkinje cells. Because Purkinje cells are the cerebellum's output neurons, this deficit may impair cerebellar modulation of other functions.

The *amygdala*, which is key in emotional salience, would seem likely to be involved in social/emotional deficits. Amygdalar hypoactivity has been seen during theory-of-mind tasks and when processing faces. Amygdalae in those with ASD may have fewer neurons and may precociously enlarge, analogous to the frontal cortex.

Other abnormal findings in ASD include abnormal cortical minicolumns in the prefrontal cortex; abnormal gene expression, epigenetic alterations, abnormal gyri in the parietal lobe regions; and enlargement or hypoactivity in the fusiform gyrus with hypocellularity. *Functional connectivity* via white-matter tracts also appears to be altered. Extensive further study is needed in order to delineate the most salient underlying abnormalities.

■ DIAGNOSTIC ASSESSMENT

The presentation of ASD is very broad, expanding well beyond the clichéd description of an awkward child who has poor eye contact and stereotypies. In higher-functioning individuals, subtle manifestations including difficulty initiating conversations, the use of context-inappropriate language, or challenges understanding social constructs may be the only obvious sources of distress.

Evaluation of a child with ASD should be multidisciplinary, including assessments by a developmental pediatrician, a child psychiatrist, a child psychologist, a neuropsychologist, and a speech-language pathologist. Key data include interviews, observations, caregiver/teacher reports, screening tools, and medical assessments (Table 18–2). Due to limited access, however, most diagnoses are made by pediatricians or psychiatrists.

TABLE 18–2. Diagnostic tools for assessment of autism spectrum disorder

Screening tools

Parent report measures	Modified Checklist for Autism in Toddlers
	Social-Communication Questionnaire
	Social Responsiveness Scale
Teacher report measure	Autism Behavior Checklist
Parent interview	Autism Diagnostic Interview-Revised
	Diagnostic Instrument for Social Communication Disorders
Observational rating scales	Screening Tool for Autism in Toddlers and Young Children
	Autism Diagnostic Observation Schedule
	Childhood Autism Rating Scale

Medical assessment

Targeted at detecting genetic syndromes or comorbidities

Physical examination

Hearing/Vision examination

Genetic screening (e.g., *FMR1*)

Screening for heavy metals

Electroencephalogram

Other blood work

Neuropsychological testing

Most helpful for

Identifying areas of strength/weakness

Optimizing supports to address challenges

Assessing intelligence, attention, executive function, social cognition, and praxis

Autism Diagnostic Observation Schedule

Standardized diagnostic test; takes 40 minutes with trained proctor. Used in those older than 1 year. Series of semistructured tasks designed to expose challenges with social cognition, abstract reasoning, restrictive/repetitive behaviors, and other aspects of the broader ASD phenotype. Sensitivity between 86% and 100%; specificity between 68% and 100%.

■ NEUROPSYCHIATRIC COMORBIDITIES

Depression

An atypical presentation, alexithymia, and a blunted affect can complicate diagnosis. Depression may present with aggression, mood lability, hyperactivity, decreased adaptive functioning or self-care, regression, or increased compulsiveness. Depression may exacerbate stereotypies and lead to apathy toward previously intense/restricted interests. Self-injurious behavior, catatonia, and other changes in behavior from baseline may occur.

Anxiety

Anxiety disorders occur in about 50% of individuals with ASD. Patients may not recognize their experiences or symptoms as being anxiety, fear, or worry driven, complicating detection. Anxiety can worsen ASD symptoms such as repetitiveness or insistence on sameness. Behavioral outbursts in response to a particular stimulus (e.g., transition, social interaction) may be a key clue. The interview may need to focus on physical manifestations of anxiety (e.g., chest pain, shakiness, palpitations, or breathing changes).

Obsessive-Compulsive Disorder

OCD and ASD overlap in presentation. In OCD, individuals struggle with intrusive, unwanted, and distressing thoughts, images, and urges. This distress may be mitigated by compulsive behaviors. In ASD, individuals may have repetitive behaviors such as hand flapping and rocking. These individuals can also insist on sameness and routine. The content of and approach to these thoughts and behaviors varies between the two disorders. In OCD, obsessions are often related to contamination, aggression, religion, and sex. In ASD, obsessions are often related to a specific restricted or repetitive interest (e.g., Legos, trains) or sameness, and these thoughts do not inherently cause distress. Individuals with OCD are distressed by their obsessions, and this distress may then be relieved by engaging in compulsive behaviors. Individuals with ASD may find their compulsive/repetitive behaviors comforting "for their own sake" and engage in them regardless of whether they are have an intrusive thought. Exposure and response prevention, applied behavioral analysis, and selective serotonin reuptake inhibitors may help.

Tourette's Syndrome

Tourette's syndrome and ASD both include the presence of repetitive movements or vocalizations. Impaired socialization, impaired communication, impaired attention, hyperactivity, sleep disturbances, and sensory processing issues may occur in both disorders. Tics related to Tourette's syndrome are often unilateral and are usually associated with a premonitory build-up or "urge" to tic, followed by relief when the tic occurs. Tics are frequently simple, brief movements (e.g., blinking, grimacing, shoulder shrugging). Stereotypies in ASD more often are bilateral and complex, serve a self-stimulatory function (e.g., flapping, repetitive sounds or syllables), and lack an "urge." Patients with ASD may be soothed by stereotypies that mimic the "urge-relief" cycle in tics. Attention should be paid to the history and time-course of the symptoms; tics wax and wane, often receding with age.

Catatonia

Catatonia affects both behavior and motor function, leading to mutism, slowness/immobility/freezing, rigidity, and unusual mannerisms. This tends to develop alongside neuropsychiatric/neurodevelopmental conditions, including autism. The risk of catatonia may be associated with the severity of ASD. Onset is often in early adolescence. Self-harming or aggressive behaviors may represent agitated catatonia. High-dosage benzodiazepines (even as high as 30 mg/day in divided doses) are first-line treatment, with electroconvulsive therapy a highly effective backup.

Psychosis

Psychosis, including schizophrenia, occurs more frequently in individuals with ASD. Negative symptoms may resemble the symptoms of catatonia or autism, confusing diagnosis if positive symptoms are not also present. Careful examination of early developmental history will generally assist in identifying the underlying deficits attributable to ASD as opposed to psychosis or catatonia.

■ MANAGEMENT

Management of ASD involves improving adaptive, self-care, and prosocial behaviors while reducing disruptive or harmful behaviors in order to maximize functioning and quality of life. Outcomes vary, with high-functioning individuals able to live essentially unimpaired lives, and low-functioning individuals requiring lifelong care and assistance with basic activities of daily living. Medications may improve comorbidities, but patients benefit most from intensive behavioral therapies.

Applied Behavior Analysis

B.F. Skinner introduced the concept of behavioral shaping through consequences: if a behavior results in a favorable outcome, then that behavior is reinforced and more likely to happen again. If the behavior results in an unfavorable outcome, it is less likely to happen again. Applied behavior analysis (ABA) is a field of study as opposed to a single treatment and encompasses many different approaches. Like any other area of scientific study, ABA has undergone continual evolution with an expansion in the breadth of the approaches used and problems addressed. Interventions are implemented systematically based on the principles of ABA, early in a child's life—preferably before 3 years of age—and target a large number of skills based on typical development. Crucially, ABA interventions are supported by parent education services. ABA programs have been noted to be moderately to highly effective for improving intellectual abilities and communication skills. In addition, ABA seems to be moderately effective for improving nonverbal IQ, adaptive behavior, and socialization. ABA can also reduce the intensity of ASD-related core symptoms and behaviors and improve daily living skills. Depending on the severity of behavioral problems and skills deficits associated with ASD, ABA treatment can be administered on a spectrum from more immersive to time-limited and focused interventions.

A popular ABA-based intervention is functional behavioral assessment, which evaluates behaviors as they relate to the environments in which they occur. Through observation and informal interviewing, the evaluator can understand the antecedents and consequences of a given target behavior, which helps to identify reinforcing factors that may be maintaining it. This then allows for removal or adjustment of these reinforcers to help reduce the frequency of challenging behaviors and increase desired behaviors.

Social Skills Training

Deficits in social communication and social interaction are a core symptom of ASD and range from a patient who is completely nonverbal to one who is highly functional with more mild difficulties in understanding the nuances of nonverbal communication such as humor, sarcasm, or flirting. The social skills deficits typically associated with ASD include lack of motivation to initiate social interactions, inability to initiate and sustain interactions despite motivation, difficulties with reading facial expressions, lack of engagement in joint attention, and others. As a result of these challenges, individuals with ASD are at a significant disadvantage when it comes to peer relationships, which then can negatively impact their psychological wellness, academic functioning, and quality of life. This can contribute to depression or anxiety, which creates a vicious circle leading to further decline in social functioning.

Social skills training aims to remediate these skills deficits and prevent their many negative downstream effects. Social skills interventions can be offered in a variety of formats, such as group settings in schools and community, peer training or mentoring, social stories, and video modeling. For youth with ASD, group-based social skills interventions result in a moderate overall improvement in social competence.

Psychopharmacology

There are currently no well-validated psychopharmacological interventions for the core features of ASD; psychosocial and therapeutic options remain the mainstay for improving patients' functioning. However, medications may be useful in managing the behavioral manifestations of ASD or associated psychiatric comorbidities. The axiom "start low and go slow" holds true because children and adolescents with ASD (particularly those with more severe impairment) are often quite sensitive to the adverse effects of medications and may require much lower dosages and a much slower titration schedule than neurotypical peers. However, this hypersensitivity is not universal, and many patients will tolerate typical dosages and titration schedules. In general, psychiatric medications maintain their typical uses and indications in this population, with a few additional points of interest noted below.

Atypical Antipsychotics

Risperidone (in those age 5 years and older) and aripiprazole (age 6 years and older) are the only medications specifically FDA-approved for use in ASD and are generally used for related irritability and aggression. Some patients may see benefits in hyperactivity, restricted/repetitive behaviors, adaptive behaviors, or nonverbal communication, although these are not the primary indications. Other atypical antipsychotics, such as olanzapine, may yield some benefit but are not as well studied.

Typical Antipsychotics

Haloperidol may be helpful in reducing hyperactivity, re-stricted/repetitive behaviors, and irritability, although side ef-fects may limit its use. Dosages generally range from 0.25 mg to 4 mg daily. Notably, 34% of children in one study of haloper-idol use in children ages 2–8 years for 708 days showed with-drawal or tardive dyskinesias.

Antidepressants

Antidepressants have generally not been clearly shown to be effective (beyond their typical indications for depression, anx-iety, or OCD) in managing behaviors related to ASD.

Mood Stabilizers

Valproate has been demonstrated in small, double-blind, pla-cebo-controlled studies to improve irritability in children with autism. Lamotrigine, however, did not outperform placebo in a small double-blind study.

Stimulants

Although the magnitude of effect and the tolerability of stimu-lants may be somewhat worse in children with ASD than those without, they remain the mainstay treatment for ADHD and related symptoms in this population. Atomoxetine and α_2 ag-onists remain reasonable second-line options, although they may cause significant irritability in some patients.

Other Medications

Various other medications, including but not limited to naltrex-one, oxytocin, donepezil, L-carnitine, amantadine, cyprohepta-dine, and N-acetylcysteine have been studied, but data have generally shown mixed or poor results. Naltrexone may im-prove hyperactivity and irritability, and N-acetylcysteine may have some use for improving irritability but is not well-studied. Oxytocin has generally not shown clear efficacy for improving core symptoms. Melatonin has been well-studied for sleep dis-turbances and appears to be safe and effective. Omega-3 fatty acids may be helpful for hyperactivity and are safe but not clearly efficacious. No dietary or digestive interventions have been shown to be helpful. Chelation therapies may be harmful and are not recommended.

Brain Stimulation Therapies

Transcranial Magnetic Stimulation

Transcranial magnetic stimulation has been studied as a possible intervention for behavioral, cognitive, and core features of ASD, with some positive findings, although studies are quite limited, and this is not a widely recommended treatment at this time.

Electroconvulsive Therapy

Electroconvulsive therapy may occasionally be a lifesaving intervention for extreme, uncontrollable, repetitive self-harm or violence, possibly due to an overlap with an agitated catatonia syndrome.

■ REFERENCES

American Psychiatric Association: Diagnostic and Statistical Manual of Mental Disorders, 5th Edition. Arlington, VA, American Psychiatric Association, 2013

Bachevalier J, Loveland KA: The orbitofrontal-amygdala circuit and self-regulation of social-emotional behavior in autism. Neurosci Biobehav Rev 30(1):97–117, 2006 16157377

Bailey A, Le Couteur A, Gottesman I, et al: Autism as a strongly genetic disorder: evidence from a British twin study. Psychol Med 25(1):63–77, 1995 7792363

Baron-Cohen S, Ring HA, Wheelwright S, et al: Social intelligence in the normal and autistic brain: an fMRI study. Eur J Neurosci 11(6):1891–1898, 1999 10336657

Belsito KM, Law PA, Kirk KS, et al: Lamotrigine therapy for autistic disorder: a randomized, double-blind, placebo-controlled trial. J Autism Dev Disord 31(2):175–181, 2001 11450816

Billstedt E, Gillberg IC, Gillberg C: Autism after adolescence: population-based 13- to 22-year follow-up study of 120 individuals with autism diagnosed in childhood. J Autism Dev Disord 35(3):351–360, 2005 16119476

Bolton P, Rutter M: Genetic influences in autism. Int Rev Psychiatry 2(1):67–80, 1990

Breen J, Hare DJ: The nature and prevalence of catatonic symptoms in young people with autism. J Intellect Disabil Res 61(6):580–593, 2017 28150394

Buxhoeveden DP, Semendeferi K, Buckwalter J, et al: Reduced minicolumns in the frontal cortex of patients with autism. Neuropathol Appl Neurobiol 32(5):483–491, 2006 16972882

Campbell M, Armenteros JL, Malone RP, et al: Neuroleptic-related dyskinesias in autistic children: a prospective, longitudinal study. J Am Acad Child Adolesc Psychiatry 36(6):835–843, 1997

Campbell M, Anderson LT, Small AM, et al: The effects of haloperidol on learning and behavior in autistic children. J Autism Dev Disord 12(2):167–175, 1982 7174605

Capuano A, Valeri G: Tics and Tourette syndrome in autism spectrum disorder, in Psychiatric Symptoms and Comorbidities in Autism Spectrum Disorder. Edited by Mazzone L, Vitiello B. Cham, Springer International Publishing, 2016, pp 93–109

Chen JA, Peñagarikano O, Belgard TG, et al: The emerging picture of autism spectrum disorder: genetics and pathology. Annu Rev Pathol 10:111–144, 2015 25621659

Chisholm K, Pelton M, Duncan N, et al: A cross-sectional examination of the clinical significance of autistic traits in individuals experiencing a first episode of psychosis. Psychiatry Res 282:112623, 2019 31685288

Chow ML, Pramparo T, Winn ME, et al: Age-dependent brain gene expression and copy number anomalies in autism suggest distinct pathological processes at young versus mature ages. PLoS Genet 8(3):e1002592, 2012 22457638

Chugani DC, Muzik O, Rothermel R, et al: Altered serotonin synthesis in the dentatothalamocortical pathway in autistic boys. Ann Neurol 42(4):666–669, 1997 9382481

Chugani DC, Muzik O, Behen M, et al: Developmental changes in brain serotonin synthesis capacity in autistic and nonautistic children. Ann Neurol 45(3):287–295, 1999 10072042

Critchley HD, Daly EM, Bullmore ET, et al: The functional neuroanatomy of social behaviour: changes in cerebral blood flow when people with autistic disorder process facial expressions. Brain 123(pt 11):2203–2212, 2000 11050021

D'Agati D, Chang AD, Wachtel LE, Reti IM: Treatment of severe self-injurious behavior in autism spectrum disorder by neuromodulation. J ECT 33(1):7–11, 2017 27428475

DeFilippis M, Wagner KD: Treatment of autism spectrum disorder in children and adolescents. Psychopharmacol Bull 46(2):18–41, 2016 27738378

Ecker C, Marquand A, Mourão-Miranda J, et al: Describing the brain in autism in five dimensions—magnetic resonance imaging-assisted diagnosis of autism spectrum disorder using a multiparameter classification approach. J Neurosci 30(32):10612–10623, 2010 20702694

Fatemi SH, Aldinger KA, Ashwood P, et al: Consensus paper: pathological role of the cerebellum in autism. Cerebellum 11(3):777–807, 2012 22370873

Gates JA, Kang E, Lerner MD: Efficacy of group social skills interventions for youth with autism spectrum disorder: a systematic review and meta-analysis. Clin Psychol Rev 52:164–181, 2017 28130983

Gerber JS, Offit PA: Vaccines and autism: a tale of shifting hypotheses. Clin Infect Dis 48(4):456–461, 2009 19128068

Geschwind DH: Genetics of autism spectrum disorders. Trends Cogn Sci 15(9):409–416, 2011 21855394

Giannitelli M, Levinson DF, Cohen D, et al: Developmental and symptom profiles in early onset psychosis. Schizophr Res 216:470–478, 2020 31874744

Gotham K, Risi S, Pickles A, Lord C: The Autism Diagnostic Observation Schedule (ADOS). J Autism Dev Disord 2006

Hare DJ, Malone C: Catatonia and autistic spectrum disorders. Autism 8(2):183–195, 2004 15165434

Harris G: Journal retracts 1998 paper linking autism to vaccines. The New York Times, February 2, 2010

Harrison JE, Bolton PF: Annotation: tuberous sclerosis. J Child Psychol Psychiatry 38(6):603–614, 1997 9315970

Hollander E, Chaplin W, Soorya L, et al: Divalproex sodium vs placebo for the treatment of irritability in children and adolescents with autism spectrum disorders. Neuropsychopharmacology 35(4):990–998, 2010 20010551

Kern JK, Geier DA, King PG, et al: Shared brain connectivity issues, symptoms, and comorbidities in autism spectrum disorder, attention deficit/hyperactivity disorder, and Tourette syndrome. Brain Connect 5(6):321–335, 2015 25602622

Kincaid DL, Doris M, Shannon C, Mulholland C: What is the prevalence of autism spectrum disorder and ASD traits in psychosis? A systematic review. Psychiatry Res 250:99–105, 2017 28152400

Krumm N, O'Roak BJ, Shendure J, Eichler EE: A de novo convergence of autism genetics and molecular neuroscience. Trends Neurosci 37(2):95–105, 2014 24387789

Lord C, Rutter M, DiLavore PC, et al: Autism Diagnostic Observation Schedule, 2nd Edition. Torrence, CA, Western Psychological Services, 2012

Lyall K, Croen L, Daniels J, et al: The changing epidemiology of autism spectrum disorders. Annu Rev Public Health 38:81–102, 2017 28068486

Magnuson KM, Constantino JN: Characterization of depression in children with autism spectrum disorders. J Dev Behav Pediatr 32(4):332–340, 2011 21502871

Makrygianni MK, Gena A, Katoudi S, Galanis P: The effectiveness of applied behavior analytic interventions for children with autism spectrum disorder: a meta-analytic study. Research in Autism Spectrum Disorders 51:18–31, 2018

McDougle CJ, Scahill L, Aman MG, et al: Risperidone for the core symptom domains of autism: results from the study by the autism network of the research units on pediatric psychopharmacology. Am J Psychiatry 162(6):1142–1148, 2005 15930063

Medda JE, Cholemkery H, Freitag CM: Sensitivity and specificity of the ADOS-2 algorithm in a large German sample. J Autism Dev Disord 49(2):750–761, 2019 30238180

Nagaraj R, Singhi P, Malhi P: Risperidone in children with autism: randomized, placebo-controlled, double-blind study. J Child Neurol 21(6):450–455, 2006 16948927

Ohta M, Kano Y, Nagai Y: Catatonia in individuals with autism spectrum disorders in adolescence and early adulthood: a long-term prospective study. Int Rev Neurobiol 72:41–54, 2006 16697290

Postorino V, Kerns CM, Vivanti G, et al: Anxiety disorders and obsessive-compulsive disorder in individuals with autism spectrum disorder. Curr Psychiatry Rep 19(12):92, 2017 29082426

Ritvo ER, Yuwiler A, Geller E, et al: Increased blood serotonin and platelets in early infantile autism. Arch Gen Psychiatry 23(6):566–572, 1970 5482649

Roane HS, Fisher WW, Carr JE: Applied behavior analysis as treatment for autism spectrum disorder. J Pediatr 175:27–32, 2016 27179552

Rodgers J, Ofield A: Understanding, recognising and treating co-occurring anxiety in autism. Curr Dev Disord Rep 5(1):58–64, 2018 29497597

Schultz RT, Gauthier I, Klin A, et al: Abnormal ventral temporal cortical activity during face discrimination among individuals with autism and Asperger syndrome. Arch Gen Psychiatry 57(4):331–340, 2000 10768694

Schumann CM, Hamstra J, Goodlin-Jones BL, et al: The amygdala is enlarged in children but not adolescents with autism; the hippocampus is enlarged at all ages. J Neurosci 24(28):6392–6401, 2004 15254095

Schumann CM, Bloss CS, Barnes CC, et al: Longitudinal magnetic resonance imaging study of cortical development through early childhood in autism. J Neurosci 30(12):4419–4427, 2010 20335478

Siu MT, Weksberg R: Epigenetics of autism spectrum disorder. Adv Exp Med Biol 978:63–90, 2017 28523541

Skuse DH: Imprinting, the X-chromosome, and the male brain: explaining sex differences in the liability to autism. Pediatr Res 47(1):9–16, 2000 10625077

van Kooten IAJ, Palmen SJMC, von Cappeln P, et al: Neurons in the fusiform gyrus are fewer and smaller in autism. Brain 131(Pt 4):987–999, 2008 18332073

Vissers MEX, Cohen MX, Geurts HM: Brain connectivity and high functioning autism: a promising path of research that needs refined models, methodological convergence, and stronger behavioral links. Neurosci Biobehav Rev 36(1):604–625, 2012 21963441

Volkmar FR, Szatmari P, Sparrow SS: Sex differences in pervasive developmental disorders. J Autism Dev Disord 23(4):579–591, 1993 8106301

Waiter GD, Williams JHG, Murray AD, et al: A voxel-based investigation of brain structure in male adolescents with autistic spectrum disorder. Neuroimage 22(2):619–625, 2004 15193590

Wassink TH, Brzustowicz LM, Bartlett CW, Szatmari P: The search for autism disease genes. Ment Retard Dev Disabil Res Rev 10(4):272–283, 2004 15666342

Williams SK, Scahill L, Vitiello B, et al: Risperidone and adaptive behavior in children with autism. J Am Acad Child Adolesc Psychiatry 45(4):431–439, 2006 16601648

Wing L, Shah A: Catatonia in autistic spectrum disorders. Br J Psychiatry 176(4):357–362, 2000 10827884

WPS Publishing: Autism Diagnostic Observation Schedule, 2nd Edition. Torrance, CA, WPS Publishing, 2012

Zheng Z, Zheng P, Zou X: Association between schizophrenia and autism spectrum disorder: a systematic review and meta-analysis. Autism Res 11(8):1110–1119, 2018 30284394

Zwick GP: Neuropsychological assessment in autism spectrum disorder and related conditions. Dialogues Clin Neurosci 19(4):373–379, 2017 29398932

19

EVALUATION AND TREATMENT OF ENDOCRINE DISORDERS WITH NEUROPSYCHIATRIC SYMPTOMS (THYROID AND ADRENAL)

Katherine E. Williams, M.D.

Multiple common endocrine disorders present with a variety of neuropsychiatric symptoms that range in presentation and severity. The purpose of this chapter is to review the neuropsychiatric presentations, evaluation, and treatment of two of the most common neuroendocrine disorders, thyroid and adrenal disease.

■ HYPOTHYROIDISM

Overt hypothyroidism is defined as an elevated serum thyrotropin (thyroid-stimulating hormone, TSH) level and decreased free thyroxine levels (T_4). In subclinical hypothyroidism, the TSH is only slightly elevated, while free T_4 is normal.

Prevalence rates for overt hypothyroidism range from 0.3% to 5% and for subclinical hypothyroidism are ≤10% of the general population worldwide. High rates of subclinical hypothyroidism are found in the elderly (~10%–14%).

Both overt and subclinical hypothyroidism conditions are more common in women, especially during the perinatal period and menopausal transition. Although overt hypothyroidism is relatively rare in pregnancy (estimated to occur in 0.3%–0.5% of pregnancies), subclinical hypothyroidism is more common, occurring in 3%–5% of pregnant women. Postpartum thyroiditis occurs in 7.5% of postpartum women, and 5%–8% of these women per year progress to permanent hypothyroidism.

TABLE 19–1. Causes and risk factors for hypothyroidism
Age 60 years or older
Female sex
High anti-thyroid peroxidase antibody and anti-thyroglobulin antibody titers
Low-iodine diet
Medications such as lithium, amiiodarone, dopamine agonists
Personal or family history of thyroid disease or autoimmune disorder
Postpartum thyroiditis
Surgical or medical hyperthyroidism treatment

Hypothyroidism is common in patients of either sex with bipolar disorder. The use of lithium further elevates this higher prevalence because ≤20% of patients taking lithium develop hypothyroidism. Other risk factors for hypothyroidism include surgical or medical treatment of hyperthyroidism with insufficient thyroid replacement therapy and a personal family history of thyroid disease or autoimmune disorders. Risk factors are outlined in Table 19–1.

Pathophysiology of Neuropsychiatric Symptoms

Chronic autoimmune thyroiditis (Hashimoto's thyroiditis) is the most common cause of hypothyroidism in populations with sufficient iodine intake. The condition is associated with high serum concentrations of autoantibodies to the enzymes thyroglobulin (TgAb) and thyroid peroxidase (TPOAb).

Neuroimaging and biopsy studies correlate the neuropsychiatric symptoms of Hashimoto's encephalopathy with vasculitis, in which blood vessels throughout the brain, including the cerebellum and brain stem, are infiltrated by lymphocytes and immune complexes. High autoantibodies against TPO and thyroglobulin and a variety of other autoantibodies against neuronal antigens and enzymes also appear to play a role in Hashimoto's encephalopathy vasculitis through cytotoxic effects on vascular endothelium and neurons. High levels of TPOAb are found in the blood and cerebrospinal fluid.

Neuropsychiatric symptoms in patients with hypothyroidism without vasculitic encephalopathy may be related to changes in cerebral blood flow and glucose metabolism because single-photon emission computed tomography studies have shown changes in regional cerebral blood flow. Thyroid hormones also have a complex role in regulation of neuroplasticity.

TABLE 19–2.	Physical and neuropsychiatric symptoms of hypothyroidism
Cardiovascular	Bradycardia
	Diastolic or systolic hypertension
Cognitive	Decreased attention
	Decreased verbal and motor memory
	Impaired working memory
Constitutional	Cold intolerance
	Fatigue
	Weight gain
Dermatological	Coarse hair and hair loss, especially lateral third of eyebrow
	Dry skin
Genitourinary/ Gastrointestinal	Amenorrhea and recurrent miscarriage
	Sexual dysfunction (libido/arousal/premature ejaculation)
Musculoskeletal	Arthralgias
	Myalgias
	Constipation
Psychiatric	Anxiety (especially thyroiditis)
	Depressed mood, including suicidal ideation
	Rare: delirium, hallucinations, catatonia

Physical and Neuropsychiatric Symptoms

Common physical and neuropsychiatric signs and symptoms of hypothyroidism vary in type and intensity (Table 19–2). Hypothyroidism is classically associated with depression symptoms; however, hypothyroidism is also often associated with anxiety symptoms. Many studies have reported that even patients with thyroid antibodies who are euthyroid are at a higher risk for mood disorders.

Neuropsychiatric testing studies confirm patients' frequent subjective cognitive complaints that occur even when the patients are taking thyroid replacement therapy. Common findings include impairment in complex attention tasks, verbal memory tests, verbal divergent thinking (phonemic fluency), and categorical fluency. Impairment in working memory, implicit learning, and motor learning have also been reported. Meta-analyses report that subclinical hypothyroidism is also associated with cognitive impairment, but this occurs primarily in patients who are younger than 75 years.

Autoimmune encephalitis or vasculitis can occur in patients with chronic autoimmune thyroiditis, leading to severely altered mental status, often labeled Hashimoto's encephalopathy. In this rare condition, patients may present with delusions, auditory hallucinations, and catatonia, as well as cognitive dysfunction and altered sensorium. Coma may also develop. Patients may present with acute episodes of focal neurological deficits, suggesting a stroke. Generalized tonic clonic seizures and even status epilepticus have been reported.

Diagnostic Workup

Hypothyroidism should be high in the differential diagnosis of all patients with affective or cognitive symptoms, especially patients who have a family history or other risk factors for thyroid disorders. Screening for hypothyroidism begins with a serum TSH; normal values range from 0.3 to 7.5 mIU/L in most labs. Upper limit of normal increases with age and obesity. See Figure 19–1 for workup.

When the patient's free T_4 level is low but the TSH level is normal, this suggests the rarer diagnosis of central hypothyroidism, which is caused by hypothalamic or pituitary dysfunction. In patients who are not perinatal, the rates of conversion from subclinical hypothyroidism to overt hypothyroidism vary from 4.3% to 17.7%. The risk increases with higher baseline TSH levels and the presence of TPOAb. Measurement of TPO and Tg antibodies is useful to confirm the immunological cause and to evaluate the risk of conversion to overt hypothyroidism.

Treatment

Overt and central hypothyroidism are both treated with oral synthetic T_4 replacement therapy. Starting dosages are adjusted to the patient's age, comorbid medical conditions, body weight, and severity and duration of hypothyroidism. Serum TSH and free T_4 are checked every 4–6 weeks, and dosages are adjusted until T_4 concentrations have increased and TSH serum levels have decreased to normal values.

Treatment of subclinical hypothyroidism with thyroxine is recommended when the TSH level is ≥10 mIU/L; however, the treatment of patients with values of 4.5–10 mIU/L is controversial. Most studies have not found improvement in depression or hypothyroid physical symptoms in patients with subclinical hypothyroidism treated with thyroid hormone when their TSH is

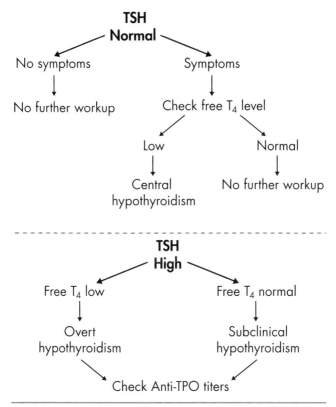

FIGURE 19–1. Proposed evaluation of thyroid-stimulating hormone (TSH) levels.

<10 mIU/L. Nevertheless, in nonelderly patients, those with goiters, and those with infertility issues, treatment with thyroid hormone despite a TSH level below 10 mIU/L may be indicated.

   Treatment of primary subclinical and overt hypothyroidism may not lead to full remission of neuropsychiatric symptoms, despite normalization of the patient's TSH and free T_4 levels. Treatment-resistant depression is often associated with subclinical hypothyroidism, and treatment with triiodothyronine (T_3) has been shown to be beneficial for treatment response and remission when added to either serotonin reuptake inhibitors or tricyclic antidepressants. Hashimoto's encephalopathy is treated with corticosteroids, and 90%–98% of patients respond to this treatment.

TABLE 19–3. Common causes and risk factors for hyperthyroidism

Cause	Risk factors
Graves' disease	Family/personal history autoimmune disorder
	Female ages 30–40
	Smoking
	Stress
Iatrogenic	Excessive thyroid hormone intake
	Increased iodine intake
Thyroiditis	
Toxic multinodular goiter	

■ HYPERTHYROIDISM

The prevalence of hyperthyroidism in the general population is approximately 1%. The most common cause is Graves' disease (80% of cases), which is caused by thyroid-stimulating antibody–induced inflammation of the thyroid gland and the excessive production of thyroid hormones. Graves' disease is more common among females, and the risk increases in individuals ages 30–40 years; a number of other risk factors have been identified (Table 19–3).

Elevated estrogen levels, as with pregnancy or estrogen replacement therapy, can increase thyroid-binding globulin, leading to decreased free T_4. Consequently, when estrogen levels fall, thyroid dosages need to be adjusted downward to avoid iatrogenic hyperthyroidism.

Pathophysiology of Neuropsychiatric Symptoms

In Graves' disease, autoantibodies activate the thyrotropin receptor, leading to increased thyroid hormone synthesis and secretion and thyroid follicular cell hyperplasia, causing a diffuse goiter. Increased thyroid hormone upregulates α-adrenergic receptors, resulting in symptoms of anxiety, agitation, and mood lability.

Clinical Presentation

Signs and symptoms of hyperthyroidism are numerous and diverse, affecting many body systems and functions (Table 19–4).

TABLE 19–4. Physical and neuropsychiatric signs/symptoms of hyperthyroidism

Cardiovascular	Atrial fibrillation
	Systolic hypertension
	Tachycardia
Cognitive	Decreased attention
	Impaired working memory
Constitutional	Frequent sweating
	Heat intolerance
	Weight loss
Eyes	Exophthalmos
	Frequent blinking
	Lid lag
Gastrointestinal/Genitourinary	Frequent bowel movements
Neurological	Exaggerated startle response
	High frequency action tremor
	Hyperactive deep tendon reflexes
	Muscle weakness
Psychiatric	Agitation
	Anxiety (60%)
	Depressed mood (30%–50%)
	Insomnia
	Irritability
	Delirium, seizures, coma (rare)
Thyroid gland	Enlarged (Graves' disease)
	Single painful nodule (adenoma)

Diagnostic Workup

In overt hyperthyroidism, serum TSH level is low, and total and free serum T_4 and free T_3 are elevated. In subclinical hyperthyroidism, the TSH is below normal, but the serum free T_4 and T_3 and free T_3 are all normal. Elevated thyrotropin receptor antibodies confirm Graves' disease. Toxic multinodular goiter and adenomas are diagnosed via radioactive iodine uptake scans.

Treatments

β-Blockers, such as propranolol, can improve tremor, systolic hypertension, and other signs of sympathetic overdrive, including anxiety. Definitive treatments for Graves' disease include medications that inhibit synthesis of thyroid hormone, such as propylthiouracil and methimazole (Tapazole). Radioactive iodine and total or subtotal thyroidectomy may be needed, especially when patients have a large goiter, are pregnant, or have ophthalmopathy or potentially malignant nodules. Total thyroidectomy rather than subtotal bilateral thyroidectomy recently has been recommended because total thyroid removal decreases the risk of Graves' disease recurrence. Thyroid hormone levels should be closely monitored post surgery and throughout the patient's life, as many will need long-term thyroid hormone replacement medication.

■ HYPOCORTISOLEMIA

Common Causes and Risk Factors

Adrenocortical insufficiency results from the inadequate production of glucocorticoids, mineralocorticoids, and sex steroids from the adrenal gland. The prevalence of primary adrenocortical insufficiency, or Addison's disease, is estimated as 35–144 cases per 1 million population, and the condition affects women and men equally. Approximately 70%–90% of cases of primary adrenocortical deficiency are the result of autoimmune destruction of the adrenal cortex. Approximately 10%–20% of cases are due to tuberculosis; other causes include other infections and cancer metastasis.

Secondary adrenal insufficiency caused by suppression of the hypothalamic-pituitary-adrenal axis as a result of chronic use of glucocorticoids for medical conditions is now one of the most common causes of adrenal insufficiency. Another cause is deficient ACTH secretion because of pituitary tumors, trauma, infectious diseases, infarction, or surgical ablation. It has been estimated that this occurs in 1 in 8,000 people. *Tertiary adrenal insufficiency* refers to deficient hypothalamic secretion of cortisol-releasing hormone.

Pathophysiology of Neuropsychiatric Symptoms

There are likely multiple causes of neuropsychiatric symptoms in adrenal insufficiency, including the frequent complications of hypoglycemia and hyponatremia. Several studies have demonstrated electroencephalographic abnormalities in patients with adrenal insufficiency, most commonly diffuse slowing.

Acute adrenocortical insufficiency, or "adrenal crisis," is a medical emergency that is associated with hypotension, hypovolemia, and shock. It requires immediate glucocorticoid treat-

TABLE 19–5. Physical and neuropsychiatric signs/symptoms of adrenal insufficiency

Decreased appetite

Excessive fatigue

Loss of body hair

Orthostatic hypotension

Psychiatric

  Anxiety

  Depressed mood

  Mania (rare)

  Memory problems

  Psychosis (rare)

Salt craving

Skin hyperpigmentation

ment. Patients abruptly withdrawn from chronic glucocorticoid use are at risk. The physical signs and symptoms include weakness, fever, and gastrointestinal symptoms such as diarrhea and nausea. Delirium can be the presenting symptom (Table 19–5). Chronic adrenal insufficiency is more common, and symptom onset is usually insidious. Symptoms are frequently nonspecific, leading to frequent lack of diagnosis or misdiagnosis.

Diagnosis

A diagnosis of adrenal insufficiency is likely if plasma cortisol levels drawn in the early morning (when cortisol levels should be peaking) are low (<3 µg/dL). In cases of primary adrenal insufficiency, ACTH levels are elevated, and cortisol levels do not rise after ACTH stimulation test. Cosyntropin, 250 µg, is administered intravenously, and cortisol levels normally peak within 30–90 minutes. A "normal" test is defined as a baseline cortisol level of ≥ 5 µg/dL, a rise between baseline and stimulated cortisol levels of >7 µg/dL, and a stimulated cortisol level >18 µg/dL. Low cortisol responses indicate adrenal insufficiency. If the insufficiency results from hypothalamic disease, the ACTH response to administration of cortisol-releasing hormone is adequate, but cortisol levels may fail to rise because of adrenal atrophy after prolonged ACTH deficiency.

    Common laboratory results include low serum levels of sodium, elevated levels of potassium, and low or normal plasma cortisol levels.

Treatment

Acute adrenal insufficiency requires immediate treatment with intravenous hydrocortisone (Hydrocortone) and fluid replacement with saline solution and potassium supplementation. In primary insufficiency, a mineralocorticoid (e.g., fludrocortisone [Florinef]) is also needed. In chronic insufficiency, prednisone or hydrocortisone is given orally as maintenance treatment.

Because abrupt withdrawal of glucocorticoids is a common cause of adrenal insufficiency, discontinuation should be slow and tapered.

Supplemental dehydroepiandrosterone (DHEA) in women with adrenal insufficiency improves their quality of life, with some improvement in depressive symptoms but not in anxiety or sexual interest. Use of DHEA in these patients for this reason remains controversial.

■ HYPERCORTISOLEMIA

The most common cause of hypercortisolemia is iatrogenic, resulting from corticosteroid use. Other causes include adrenal adenomas and neuroendocrine tumors. Endogenous hypercortisolemia, also known as Cushing's syndrome, is rare; the incidence is estimated as 0.7–2.4 per 1 million population per year. It is most commonly caused by pituitary adenomas (60%–70%).

Pathophysiology of Neuropsychiatric Symptoms

Affective and cognitive impairments in patients with hypercortisolemia are thought to result from hippocampal neuron damage. Neuroimaging studies have reported smaller hippocampal, anterior cingulate cortex, and medial frontal gyrus volumes in patients exposed to prolonged elevated steroid levels. In animal models, glucocorticoids also downregulate brain-derived neurotrophic factor, which is involved in neuronal growth and synaptic plasticity and facilitates memory and mood. Both autopsy studies and CT and MRI scans demonstrate global loss of cerebral cortex and cerebellar volume in patients who are endogenously or exogenously exposed to corticosteroids.

Clinical Presentation

Cognitive deficits do not correlate with depression severity and appear to be related to the deleterious effects of high glucocorti-

TABLE 19–6. Physical and neuropsychiatric signs/symptoms of hypercortisolemia

Cognitive	Declarative memory impairment
	Decreased attention and concentration
	Spatial memory impairment
	Verbal memory impairment
	Working memory impairment
Constitutional	Excessive sweating
	Systolic hypertension
	Weight gain (face, trunk, back)
Genitourinary	Amenorrhea
Metabolic/Inflammatory	Osteoarthritis
	Osteoporosis
Neurological signs/ symptoms	Exaggerated startle response
	Excessive sweating
	Heat intolerance
	High frequency action tremor
	Hyperactive deep tendon reflexes
	Muscle wasting and muscle weakness
Psychiatric	Anxiety (12%–79%), including panic attacks
	Depressed mood (50%–80%), including suicidal ideation
	Hypomania (30%)
	Sleep: decreased total time/early morning awakening
Skin	Hirsutism/Acne
	Hyperpigmentation
	Thinning, easy bruising, stria

coid levels on hippocampal neurons. Approximately 20%–25% of patients continue to have residual mood and cognitive complaints after treatment, and brain volume often does not completely return to normal. The rapid withdrawal of exogenous steroids can also produce psychiatric disturbances, particularly depression, emotional lability, memory impairment, and even delirium and adrenal crisis. The physical signs and symptoms are diverse (Table 19–6).

Diagnostic Workup

Initial screening includes at least two 24-hour urinary free cortisol levels or late-night salivary cortisol levels. If the levels are elevated, the dexamethasone suppression test is used to distinguish adrenal from pituitary causes of hypercortisolemia. One milligram of the synthetic steroid dexamethasone (Decadron) is administered at night, and the serum cortisol level is collected the following morning, 8–9 hours later. If dexamethasone does not lead to cortisol suppression through the expected negative feedback, then further workup of the cause of hypercortisolemia is required, and serum adrenocorticotropic hormone (ACTH) levels should be measured. Low ACTH levels in hypercortisolemia confirm a disease process that is independent from the adrenal gland. High ACTH levels confirm a likely pituitary or exogenous source, such as lung cancer. High-dose dexamethasone further clarifies the high-ACTH etiology because complete nonsuppression of cortisol is consistent with an extrapituitary source, such as lung cancer, whereas pituitary adenomas have some negative feedback responsivity. Once the source of cortisol is identified, further workup includes imaging studies of the organs of interest for adenomas or tumors.

Treatment and Course

The treatment of choice for pituitary ACTH-producing tumors is surgical resection and then, if unsuccessful, pituitary irradiation. Adrenal adenomas and carcinoma are also removed surgically. Medications that inhibit cortisol production are utilized when patients are awaiting surgery or radiation or if these first-line treatments have been unsuccessful. Mifepristone (RU486), a progesterone and glucocorticoid receptor antagonist, is associated with early (within the first week), high rates of improvement in depressive symptoms (80%).

The treatment of iatrogenic steroid-induced psychosis and mood disorders involves tapering off the medication, if possible, and the use of antipsychotics and mood stabilizers such as lithium. Prednisone should be tapered rather than discontinued abruptly to allow for the pituitary gland, which has been suppressed, to resume its production of ACTH.

■ REFERENCES

Anglin RE, Rosebush PI, Mazurek MF: The neuropsychiatric profile of Addison's disease: revisiting a forgotten phenomenon. J Neuropsychiatry Clin Neurosci 18(4):450–459, 2006 17135373

Bartalena L, Piantanida E, Gallo D, et al: Epidemiology, natural history, risk factors, and prevention of Graves' orbitopathy. Front Endocrinol (Lausanne) 11:615993, 2020 33329408

Bauduin SEEC, van der Wee NJA, van der Werff SJA: Structural brain abnormalities in Cushing's syndrome. Curr Opin Endocrinol Diabetes Obes 25(4):285–289, 2018 29746308

Biondi B, Cappola AR, Cooper DS: Subclinical hypothyroidism: a review. JAMA 322(2):153–160, 2019 31287527

Burmeister LA, Ganguli M, Dodge HH, et al: Hypothyroidism and cognition: preliminary evidence for a specific defect in memory. Thyroid 11(12):1177–1185, 2001 12186506

Chen H, Lombès M, Le Menuet D: Glucocorticoid receptor represses brain-derived neurotrophic factor expression in neuron-like cells. Mol Brain 10(1):12, 2017 28403881

Churilov LP, Sobolevskaia PA, Stroev YI: Thyroid gland and brain: enigma of Hashimoto's encephalopathy. Best Pract Res Clin Endocrinol Metab 33(6):101364, 2019 31801687

Feldman AZ, Shrestha RT, Hennessey JV: Neuropsychiatric manifestations of thyroid disease. Endocrinol Metab Clin North Am 42(3):453–476, 2013 24011860

Feller M, Snel M, Moutzouri E, et al: Association of thyroid hormone therapy with quality of life and thyroid-related symptoms in patients with subclinical hypothyroidism: a systematic review and meta-analysis. JAMA 320(13):1349, 2018

George KM, Lutsey PL, Selvin E, et al: Association between thyroid dysfunction and incident dementia in the atherosclerosis risk in communities neurocognitive study. J Endocrinol Metab 9(4):82–89, 2019 32411312

Giannouli V, Toulis KA, Syrmos N: Cognitive function in Hashimoto's thyroiditis under levothyroxine treatment. Hormones (Athens) 13(3):430–433, 2014 25079471

Göbel A, Heldmann M, Göttlich M, et al: Effect of mild thyrotoxicosis on performance and brain activations in a working memory task. PLoS One 11(8):e0161552, 2016 27536945

Grozinsky-Glasberg S, Fraser A, Nahshoni E, et al: Thyroxine-triiodothyronine combination therapy versus thyroxine monotherapy for clinical hypothyroidism: meta-analysis of randomized controlled trials. J Clin Endocrinol Metab 91(7):2592–2599, 2006 16670166

Guo Z, Yu P, Liu Z, et al: Total thyroidectomy vs bilateral subtotal thyroidectomy in patients with Graves' diseases: a meta-analysis of randomized clinical trials. Clin Endocrinol (Oxf) 79(5):739–746, 2013

Kothbauer-Margreiter I, Sturzenegger M, Komor J, et al: Encephalopathy associated with Hashimoto thyroiditis: diagnosis and treatment. J Neurol 243(8):585–593, 1996 8865025

Leyhe T, Mussig K: Cognitive and affective dysfunctions in autoimmune thyroiditis. Brain Behav Immun 41:261–266, 2014 24685840

Lin TY, Hanna J, Ishak WW: Psychiatric symptoms in Cushing's syndrome: a systematic review. Innov Clin Neurosci 17(1–3):30–35, 2020 32547845

Loh HH, Lim LL, Yee A, Loh HS: Association between subclinical hypothyroidism and depression: an updated systematic review and meta-analysis. BMC Psychiatry 19(1):12, 2019

Miller KJ, Parsons TD, Whybrow PC, et al: Verbal memory retrieval deficits associated with untreated hypothyroidism. J Neuropsychiatry Clin Neurosci 19(2):132–136, 2007 17431058

Munawar M, Iftikhar PM, Hasan CA, et al: Neuropsychiatric manifestation of Addison's disease: a rare case report. Cureus 11(4):e4356, 2019

Nieman LK, Biller BM, Findling JW, et al: The diagnosis of Cushing's syndrome: an Endocrine Society Clinical Practice Guideline. J Clin Endocrinol Metab 93(5):1526–1540, 2008 18334580

Pasqualetti G, Pagano G, Rengo G, et al: Subclinical hypothyroidism and cognitive impairment: systematic review and meta-analysis. J Clin Endocrinol Metab 100(11):4240–4248, 2015 26305618

Pazderska A, Pearce SH: Adrenal insufficiency: recognition and management. Clin Med (Lond) 17(3):258–262, 2017 28572228

Pivonello R, Simeoli C, De Martino MC, et al: Neuropsychiatric disorders in Cushing's syndrome. Front Neurosci 9:129, 2015 25941467

Samuels MH: Psychiatric and cognitive manifestations of hypothyroidism. Curr Opin Endocrinol Diabetes Obes 21(5):377–383, 2014 25122491

Samuels MH, Schuff KG, Carlson NE, et al: Health status, psychological symptoms, mood, and cognition in L-thyroxine-treated hypothyroid subjects. Thyroid 17(3):249–258, 2007 17381359

Sapolsky RM: Glucocorticoids and hippocampal atrophy in neuropsychiatric disorders. Arch Gen Psychiatry 57(10):925–935, 2000 11015810

Tang A, O'Sullivan AJ, Diamond T, et al: Psychiatric symptoms as a clinical presentation of Cushing's syndrome. Ann Gen Psychiatry 12(1):23, 2013 23866099

Udovcic M, Pena RH, Patham B, et al: Hypothyroidism and the heart. Methodist DeBakey Cardiovasc J 13(2):55–59, 2017 28740582

Wekking EM, Appelhof BC, Fliers E, et al: Cognitive functioning and well-being in euthyroid patients on thyroxine replacement therapy for primary hypothyroidism. Eur J Endocrinol 153(6):747–753, 2005 16322379

LIMBIC ENCEPHALITIS

Scheherazade Le, M.D.

Limbic encephalitis (LE) is an inflammatory brain disorder. LE should be considered when patients present with subacute on-set (<12 weeks) of altered mental status, short-term memory deficits, seizures, or psychiatric symptoms suggestive of limbic dysfunction, such as psychosis. This chapter reviews the epidemiology, etiology, and diagnostic workup of LE and treatment options for patients (focusing on autoimmune LE). LE is most common type of encephalitis to mimic primary psychiatric disease. Patients often have florid psychiatric symptoms such as audiovisual hallucinations, bizarre personality changes, agitation, aggressiveness, and emotional lability. LE affects patients of all ages, preferentially affects women and children, and may be either infectious or noninfectious. Noninfectious etiologies discovered increasingly since 2006 have been mostly autoimmune. The estimated incidence of acute encephalitis is approximately 5–10 per 100,000 per year. In 2007, the California Encephalitis Project was established to study the epidemiology of encephalitis. It found that autoimmune NMDA receptor (NMDAR) encephalitis was the leading etiology in the cohort, identified more than four times as often as herpes simplex virus (HSV-1), West Nile virus, or varicella zoster virus. Early recognition of the syndrome of autoimmune LE is critical because earlier diagnosis and treatment are correlated with better outcomes.

■ PATHOGENESIS

Limbic encephalitis may be associated with pathogenic antibodies against neuronal (i) cell-surface or (ii) intracellular antigens. Well-defined antibody syndromes, such as a cell-surface antibodies against the NMDAR or targeting leucine-rich glioma inactivated 1 (LGI1), are generally more responsive to immunotherapy than intracellular syndromes such as glutamic acid decarboxylase encephalitis. However, patients with autoimmune LE may initially have an unrevealing serum, cerebrospinal fluid (CSF), and neuroimaging workup that does not exclude the disorder. Many forms of LE are actually paraneoplastic; therefore, depending on the clinical scenario and the suspected antibody, searching for an underlying malignancy may be warranted.

■ CLINICAL PRESENTATION

Guidelines for a clinical approach to diagnosing autoimmune encephalitis have been published by Dr. Josep Dalmau's group. A subacute time course (<12 weeks) of new-onset neuropsychiatric symptoms and signs is characteristic of the clinical presentation of autoimmune LE. Many patients have the prodromal symptoms of headache, fever, nuchal rigidity, or a viral process. The key features of autoimmune LE are altered cognition and fluctuating or decreasing levels of consciousness, which may progress to coma (Table 20–1). Psychiatric manifestations may occur early and range from personality or behavioral changes, disinhibition, and agitation to frank psychosis. Movement disorders can occur and range from dyskinesias (involuntary jerky writhing), to dystonia (an abnormal fixed, sustained posture), to choreoathetosis (twisting, sinuous, dance-like movements), to myoclonus (transient, shock-like upward increases in tone), to stiffness or rigidity (increased tone). The limbic system is preferentially involved; therefore, seizures are common and may be refractory to antiseizure medications. Patients often present with high numbers of seizures or status epilepticus. "Immune epilepsy" is now recognized by the International League Against Epilepsy classification, defined as a condition in which seizures are a core symptom and are the direct result of an immune disorder. Patients often exhibit autonomic dysfunction, such as tachycardia, bradycardia, asystole, orthostatic hypotension, labile blood pressure, or hyperhidrosis. Psychiatrists may need to investigate the possibility of LE if patients present with unusual features of psychiatric symptoms, such as atypical age of onset, viral prodrome, subacute florid psychosis with neurological deficits, and autonomic lability.

Case Example

A 36-year-old previously healthy woman developed a low-grade fever, sore throat, and rhinorrhea, followed a week later by outbursts of profane language, disorganized thinking, and

TABLE 20–1. Key features of autoimmune limbic encephalitis
Limbic encephalitis presents with a characteristic subacute time course (<12 weeks)
Prodromal symptoms include headache, fever, viral illness
Core symptoms include altered mental status, memory deficits, seizures, and/or neuropsychiatric symptoms suggestive of limbic dysfunction

memory loss. She started singing in inappropriate situations and developed involuntary writhing, dance-like choreoathetoid movements. Two weeks later, she had a generalized tonic-clonic seizure and was brought to the emergency department.

This patient's new, subacute onset (<12 weeks) of florid psychosis with associated neurological symptoms after viral prodrome were a clue to possible LE. Psychosis at this age is also unusual because patients with schizophrenia are usually much younger. This patient was found to have anti-NMDA antibodies in the serum and an inflammatory CSF. She received early immunotherapy with high-dose steroids, plasmapheresis, intravenous immunoglobulin (IVIg), and rituximab. She spent several months in the intensive care unit due to decreased responsiveness and autonomic dysfunction. Two years after presentation, her physician discovered that she had an ovarian teratoma, which was surgically removed. The patient eventually made a full recovery.

■ DIAGNOSTIC WORKUP

Patients with new subacute mental status changes accompanied by seizures or new CNS findings should undergo a workup for infectious and noninfectious causes of LE (Table 20–2). The diagnostic workup should specifically include both serum and CSF autoimmune/paraneoplastic antibody panels, lumbar puncture to assess for inflammatory pleocytosis (>5 white blood cells/dL or protein >50 mg/dL, elevated immunoglobulin G (IgG) index or oligoclonal bands, bacterial gram stain and cultures, HSV-1 polymerase chain reaction), electroencephalography, and neuro-imaging with a brain MRI with and without contrast for features suggestive of LE. A classic MRI finding of LE on T2-weighted fluid-attenuated inversion recovery MRI consists of bilateral hyperintensities of the medial temporal lobes; contrast enhancement is rare. Electroencephalography should be performed to exclude nonconvulsive seizures or nonconvulsive status epilepticus. Common but nonspecific electroencephalographic abnor-

---
TABLE 20–2. Clinical approach to limbic encephalitis (LE)

In a patient with a compelling presentation for LE:

1. Assess for evidence of brain inflammation: MRI brain ± contrast: abnormalities such as unilateral/bilateral hippocampal T2 FLAIR hyperintensities; lumbar puncture CSF pleocytosis >5 cells/dL or CSF protein >50 mg/dL

2. Perform infectious workup, including CSF HSV-1 PCR, bacterial gram stain, and cultures

3. Send autoimmune/paraneoplastic antibody panels in both serum and CSF

4. Obtain EEG to rule out ongoing nonconvulsive seizures, status epilepticus

5. Consider causes on the differential diagnosis for LE including infectious, autoimmune, neoplastic/paraneoplastic etiologies.

Patients may be responsive to early treatment with immunotherapy, especially if the LE is autoimmune in etiology and an underlying cell-surface antibody is discovered. Empirical treatment should not be delayed if there is a high index of clinical suspicion for autoimmune LE because test results may not return for weeks.

CSF=cerebrospinal fluid; EEG=electroencephalogram; FLAIR=fluid attenuated inversion recovery; HSV-1=herpes simplex virus-1; PCR= polymerase chain reaction.

malities include focal or diffuse slowing, epileptiform activity, or lateralized periodic discharges. About one-third to one-half of patients with anti-NMDAR encephalitis may have a typical electroencephalographic pattern called "extreme delta brush"; however, this finding has also been described in other encephalopathies, such as hypoxic-ischemic injury.

■ DIFFERENTIAL DIAGNOSIS

Exclusion of other etiologies, such as infectious and noninfectious causes (i.e., other autoimmune disorders, malignancy, medical issues), is necessary (Table 20–3). A triad of subacute fever or rigors, headache with or without nuchal rigidity, and altered mental status should raise suspicion for a CNS infection such as viral or bacterial encephalitis. HSV-1 encephalitis is the most important infectious viral encephalitis for which to evaluate and exclude because it is the most often fatal but the most treatable encephalitis worldwide. HSV-1 has a predilection for the orbitofrontal and temporal lobes; therefore, patients may also present with prominent behavioral syndromes including

TABLE 20–3. Differential diagnosis for limbic encephalitis

Infectious	Bacterial
	Creutzfeldt-Jakob disease
	Viral (herpes simplex virus-1, varicella zoster virus)
Inflammatory/ Demyelinating	Acute disseminated encephalomyelitis
	Autoimmune
	CNS lupus
	CNS vasculitis or primary CNS angiitis
	Hashimoto's encephalopathy
	Neurosarcoidosis
Neoplastic	Carcinomatous meningitis
	CNS lymphoma
	Paraneoplastic
Psychiatric disorders	Acute psychosis
	Schizophrenia
Toxic-metabolic	Intoxication
	Thiamine deficiency from Wernicke encephalopathy

hypomania, Klüver-Bucy syndrome, and amnesia. All patients should have brain neuroimaging before lumbar puncture to assess for brain inflammation and to rule out a mass lesion. The lumbar puncture in HSV-1 encephalitis typically shows inflammatory and hemorrhagic CSF with lymphocytic pleocytosis. Patients should be empirically treated with CNS dosing of acyclovir until the HSV-1 polymerase chain reaction test is negative and an alternative etiology is discovered. Bacterial meningitis should also be considered but is less likely to present with florid psychiatric symptoms. However, empiric antibiotics should be instituted to broadly cover bacterial infections such as *Streptococcus pneumoniae*, *Neisseria meningitidis*, *Haemophilus influenzae*, and *Listeria monocytogenes* depending on the patient's age, demographics, and comorbidities until gram stain and culture results are obtained. Lumbar puncture for acute bacterial infection often shows turbid CSF with a neutrophilic predominance and low CSF glucose.

■ TREATMENT

If infectious and malignant etiologies of LE are reasonably excluded, empiric treatment for autoimmune LE should be seriously considered. If an autoimmune basis is highly suspected, empirical treatment is initiated because antibody testing results may not return for several weeks. Early immunosuppression is the mainstay of therapy in autoimmune LE. First-line immuno-modulatory medications include high-dose intravenous steroid methylprednisolone, 1,000 mg/day for 3–5 days; IVIg, 2 g/kg divided over 5 days; and five cycles of plasma exchange, often in combination. Second-line treatments frequently considered include intravenous rituximab or cyclophosphamide. If the eti-ology is autoimmune LE, seizures are more responsive to immu-notherapy than to conventional antiseizure drugs, with a low response rate of about 10%. Levetiracetam is commonly used in the hospital for seizure control; however, approximately 20% of patients develop psychiatric side effects with this medication (see Chapter 9, "Epilepsy and Limbic System Disorders"). Be-cause many patients with autoimmune LE present with florid psychiatric dysfunction, alternate antiseizure drugs may need to be considered.

■ ANTI-NMDAR ENCEPHALITIS

Anti-NMDAR encephalitis remains the most common and well-studied autoimmune LE, characterized by a combination of florid, new-onset psychiatric dysfunction; seizures; memory loss; decreased consciousness; movement disorder, including orofacial dyskinesias or dystonia; central hypoventilation; auto-nomic dysfunction; and speech/language disorder. Diagnosis can be made by identifying the characteristic clinical syndrome and be further confirmed by detection of serum or CSF IgG–specific antibodies against the GluN1 subunit of the NMDAR. This paraneoplastic antibody syndrome predominantly affects younger females and is associated with an ovarian teratoma in 50%. The disorder is treatable by removing the underlying ma-lignancy and administering immunotherapy, but patients often have a prolonged and severe course, typically weeks to months, and sometimes require intensive care. Prognosis is good in ap-proximately 80% of patients, especially those who receive early immunosuppressive treatment.

■ ANTI-LGI1 ENCEPHALITIS

The second most common LE is anti-LGI1 syndrome, typically associated with seizures and cognitive and memory dysfunc-tion. Patients are usually older than 40 years. The IgG antibody attacks the LGI1 glycoprotein, a subunit of the voltage-gated potassium complex that bridges the presynaptic K^+ channel to the postsynaptic AMPA receptor. A pathognomonic feature of LGI1 encephalitis is faciobrachial dystonic seizures, which occur in 50% of patients. These are brief, focal dystonic contractions of the face and arm that may occur many times per day either unilaterally or bilaterally. They can be mistaken for complex stereotypies or psychogenic nonepileptic events. Patients may also develop hyponatremia. Brain MRI can show typical changes of LE, and CSF is often normal. About 10% of cases are associated with an underlying tumor, most often thymoma. Patients with LGI1 encephalitis may respond to high-dosage steroids, 1 mg/kg/day up to 90 mg/day. They may also respond to other immunotherapies. Observational studies have shown that Na^+ channel blockers appear to be more effective than levetiracetam for seizure control; however, Na^+ channel blockers, such as carbamazepine and oxcarbazepine, may cause hyponatremia and rash. Patients with LGI1 encephalitis are predisposed to adverse effects, including rash on aromatic antiseizure drugs in 50%, hyponatremia, and psychiatric side effects.

■ SUMMARY

LE is a subacute inflammatory brain disorder characterized by new-onset subacute (<12 weeks) neuropsychiatric changes and CNS findings, such as seizures or a movement disorder. Limbic encephalitis has many etiologies, including infectious and noninfectious causes. The diagnostic workup should include lumbar puncture, serum and CSF antibody testing, brain MRI, and electroencephalography. Autoimmune LE, particularly neuronal cell surface antibody syndromes, should be recognized and treated early with immunotherapy for better outcomes. A search for an underlying malignancy is often warranted.

■ REFERENCES

Cabezudo-García P, Mena-Vázquez N, Villagrán-García M, Serrano-Castro PJ: Efficacy of antiepileptic drugs in autoimmune epilepsy: a systematic review. Seizure 59:72–76, 2018 29754014

Dalmau J: NMDA receptor encephalitis and other antibody-mediated disorders of the synapse: the 2016 Cotzias Lecture. Neurology 87(23):2471–2482, 2016 27920282

Dubey D, Samudra N, Gupta P, et al: Retrospective case series of the clinical features, management and outcomes of patients with autoimmune epilepsy. Seizure 29:143–147, 2015 26076858

Dubey D, Singh J, Britton JW, et al: Predictive models in the diagnosis and treatment of autoimmune epilepsy. Epilepsia 58(7):1181–1189, 2017 28555833

Gable MS, Sheriff H, Dalmau J, et al: The frequency of autoimmune N-methyl-D-aspartate receptor encephalitis surpasses that of individual viral etiologies in young individuals enrolled in the California Encephalitis Project. Clin Infect Dis 54(7):899–904, 2012 22281844

Graus F, Titulaer MJ, Balu R, et al: A clinical approach to diagnosis of autoimmune encephalitis. Lancet Neurol 15(4):391–404, 2016 26906964

Husari KS, Dubey D: Autoimmune Epilepsy. Neurotherapeutics 16(3):685–702, 2019 31240596

Lancaster E: The diagnosis and treatment of autoimmune encephalitis. J Clin Neurol 12(1):1–13, 2016 26754777

Nosadini M, Mohammad SS, Ramanathan S, et al: Immune therapy in autoimmune encephalitis: a systematic review. Expert Rev Neurother 15(12):1391–1419, 2015 26559389

Scheffer IE, Berkovic S, Capovilla G, et al: ILAE classification of the epilepsies: position paper of the ILAE Commission for Classification and Terminology. Epilepsia 58(4):512–521, 2017 28276062

Schmerler DA, Roller S, Espay AJ: Teaching video neuroimages: facio-brachial dystonic seizures: pathognomonic phenomenology. Neurology 86(6):e60–e61, 2016 26857958

Schmitt SE, Pargeon K, Frechette ES, et al: Extreme delta brush: a unique EEG pattern in adults with anti-NMDA receptor encephalitis. Neurology 79(11):1094–1100, 2012 22933737

Shin YW, Ahn SJ, Moon J, et al: Increased adverse events associated with antiepileptic drugs in anti-leucine-rich glioma-inactivated protein 1 encephalitis. Epilepsia 59(suppl 2):108–112, 2018 30159879

Vora NM, Holman RC, Mehal JM, et al: Burden of encephalitis-associated hospitalizations in the United States, 1998–2010. Neurology 82(5):443–451, 2014 24384647

Zong S, Hoffmann C, Mané-Damas M, et al: Neuronal surface autoantibodies in neuropsychiatric disorders: are there implications for depression? Front Immunol 8:752, 2017 28725222

21

HIV NEUROCOGNITIVE DISORDERS

Peter H. Marcus, Psy.D.
Lawrence M. McGlynn, M.D., M.S.

Combination antiretroviral therapy (cART) has transformed HIV/AIDS into a manageable condition. Measures of success include the CD4+ t-cell count and the viral load. The *CD4 count* is an indicator of immune competence. The *viral load* quantifies the amount of virus measured in a sample (typically blood but may also be measured in cerebrospinal fluid). An undetectable viral load is one of the goals of cART.

■ HIV IN THE BRAIN

HIV-infected mononuclear cells enter the CNS by crossing the blood-brain barrier shortly after the primary infection occurs. These cells then facilitate the replication of HIV inside the CNS, which leads to infection of other cells. Microglia and perivascular macrophages are the main target cells in the CNS for productive infection. These cells are then free to produce virions and viral proteins that can infect, activate, or injure other resident cells. Although HIV does not infect all cell types within the brain, most notably the neurons, the dramatic change in the normal CNS environment can lead to neuronal injury via multiple mechanisms induced by the presence of HIV, immune activation, and the release of neurotoxic cytokines and metabolites. Unchecked, HIV in the CNS can ultimately produce a range of cognitive and behavioral symptoms that becomes more severe as the immune system declines.

■ HIV-ASSOCIATED NEUROCOGNITIVE DISORDERS

HIV-associated neurocognitive disorders (HANDs) encompass three levels of impairment: 1) asymptomatic neurocognitive impairment (ANI), 2) mild neurocognitive disorder (MND), and 3) HIV-associated dementia (HAD) (Figure 21–1). ANI is defined by performance at least one standard deviation below the mean of demographically adjusted normative cognitive functioning scores involving at least two ability domains. The neuropsychological assessment must survey at least the following abilities: verbal/language, attention/working memory, memory (learning, recall), abstraction/executive function, speed of information processing, sensory-perceptual, and motor skills. If patients meet criteria for cognitive impairment, it must not be of sufficient severity to interfere with their everyday functioning to qualify for ANI. In addition, the cognitive impairment must not meet the criteria for delirium or dementia, and there cannot be evidence of another preexisting cause for the ANI. cART may improve ANI in some cases, so one can make the diagnosis of "ANI in remission."

The cognitive criteria for MND are equivalent to those for ANI. MND, however, requires that the cognitive impairment cause at least mild interference in the person's daily functioning. This can be self-reported (or observed by others) impairment in mental acuity or reduced inefficiency in work, homemaking, or social functioning. As in the diagnosis of ANI, the cognitive impairment must not meet criteria for delirium or dementia, and there can be no evidence of another preexisting cause for the MND. In cases in which improvement occurs, "MND in remission" is a valid diagnosis.

Diagnosis of HAD is also based on cognitive performance and functional impairment, but of a greater severity. The cognitive impairment must affect at least two domains and be two standard deviations below demographically corrected means. It must produce marked interference with day-to-day functioning. One cannot diagnose HAD during a period of delirium unless HAD was already established prior to the delirium. As with ANI and MND, there cannot be evidence of another preexisting cause for the presentation. An improvement in HAD can lead to a diagnosis of "HAD in remission."

Since the introduction of cART, the burden of HAD has decreased significantly to about 2%–3%. In total, however, HAND

Asymptomatic neurocognitive impairment	Mild neurocognitive disorder	HIV-associated dementia
• Cognitive functioning at least 1.0 SD below the mean involving at least two ability domains • No interference with everyday functioning	• Cognitive functioning at least 1.0 SD below the mean involving at least two ability domains • Mild interference with everyday functioning	• Cognitive functioning at least 2.0 SD below the mean involving at least two ability domains • Marked interference with everyday functioning

FIGURE 21–1. Categories of HIV-associated neurocognitive disorder

affects 25%–47% of individuals living with HIV today. In a cross-sectional study conducted in 1,555 patients positive for HIV, the CNS HIV Anti-Retroviral Therapy Effects Research study found that 52% met criteria for HAND, of which 33% had ANI, 12% MND, and 2% HAD.

The European AIDS Clinical Society (EACS) saw the need for a structured approach to assessing patients for HAND (Figure 21–2). Although other, more detailed algorithms are available, this model allows for a straightforward, concise approach while acknowledging the need for more comprehensive testing when indicated. Before screening patients for HAND, clinicians should determine whether confounding conditions are present. These conditions, including any disorder affecting the CNS or cognition, would need to be treated prior to administering neuropsychological testing. Some of these conditions, however, may not be identified until the differential diagnosis is addressed.

After the assessment for confounding conditions, cognitive screening tools are available if HAND is suspected. These include the Montreal Cognitive Assessment, HIV Dementia Scale, and International HIV Dementia Scale. Each has its strengths and limitations in screening for cognitive impairment in HIV/AIDS. The Mini-Mental State Examination, although broadly used in medical settings, is a more appropriate screen for cortical diseases, such as Alzheimer's dementia, but not necessarily for more subcortical disorders, such as HAND.

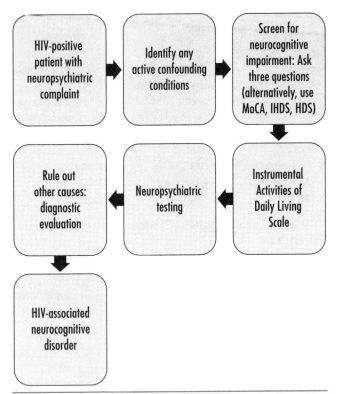

FIGURE 21-2. **A structured approach to assessing for neurocognitive impairment in HIV based on the European AIDS Clinical Society.**
HDS=HIV Dementia Scale; IHDS=International HIV Dementia Scale; MoCA=Montreal Cognitive Assessment.

Rather than endorsing any one of these screening tools, the EACS proposed an algorithm starting with three questions:

1. Do you experience frequent memory loss?
2. Do you feel that you are slower when reasoning, planning activities, or solving problems?
3. Do you have difficulties paying attention?

If patients answer "yes" to any of these questions, further evaluation is recommended. Because HAND requires evaluation of functional ability, the EACS recommends the Instrumental Activities of Daily Living (IADL) Scale by Lawton and Brody. Other functional assessment scales are also available. The IADL Scale produces scores of 1) no impairment, 2) mild impairment, or 3) severe impairment. If results from the three screening questions (or, optionally, screening questionnaire) and IADL Scale indicate some level of impairment, the next step is to administer formal neuropsychological testing to obtain a quantification of the impairment and thus determine whether the patients have ANI, MND, or HAD.

■ DIAGNOSTIC EVALUATION

The etiology for neuropsychiatric changes in HIV is complex, yet effective treatment has always depended on a comprehensive differential diagnosis. Even for seemingly simple presentations such as ANI, providers should consider multiple etiologies, especially in cases of poor adherence or otherwise low CD4 counts. Because diagnosis dictates treatment, multiple levels of testing may be required to fully rule in or out possible contributing factors (Tables 21–1 and 21–2).

■ TREATMENT OF HIV-ASSOCIATED NEUROCOGNITIVE DISORDERS

cART is the main backbone of treatment for HAND. Effective treatment has involved at least three medications, which are often combined into one pill. Most recently, a combination of two medications (dolutegravir-lamivudine) has shown efficacy as a stand-alone treatment. The goals of therapy include reducing the viral load, increasing the $CD4^+$ t-cell count, and preventing transmission of the virus to others. The individual components of cART, each of which targets a different phase of the HIV life cycle, fall into one of the following categories:

- Nonnucleoside reverse transcriptase inhibitors (inhibit reverse transcription, a necessary step in HIV replication)
- Nucleoside/nucleotide reverse transcriptase inhibitors (inhibit reverse transcription)
- Protease inhibitors (block the enzyme protease, responsible for producing mature virions)
- Integrase strand transfer inhibitors (inhibit viral enzyme integrase, responsible for integration of viral DNA into the DNA of the infected cell)

TABLE 21–1.	Differential diagnosis: HIV-related components to be aware of

HIV-associated neurocognitive disorders

Intrinsic involvement of the brain with HIV (encephalitis, viral escape*) or opportunistic infections or cancers

Mental status changes secondary to antiretroviral therapies (especially efavirenz)

Adverse side effects or toxicity of treatments for opportunistic infections, cancers, and other comorbidities

Drug–drug interactions (especially when ritonavir or cobicistat are used in combination antiretroviral therapy because both are potent metabolic inhibitors)

HIV-induced mood disorder: depression, mania, insomnia

Delirium*

Immune reconstitution inflammatory syndrome*

Methamphetamine-HIV compound effect (neurocognitive impairment, psychosis)*

*See sections that follow.

- Fusion/entry inhibitors (interfere with binding, fusion, and entry of HIV into the host cell)

Each class of treatment has unique profiles. Thus, it is essential to consider possible adverse events and drug–drug interactions for each component of cART when evaluating a patient who is being treated for HIV.

Adherence is essential because the goal is to minimize the presence of HIV in the CNS. cART needs to be able to penetrate the brain sufficiently without creating toxicity. If HIV is present in the CSF, the HIV genotype may ultimately be the guide to optimizing cART in order to reduce the brain's exposure to HIV and thus improve the likelihood of treating HAND.

A small prospective, double observer–blinded, open-label pilot randomized controlled trial demonstrated neurocognitive improvement when cART was augmented with the antiretroviral agent maraviroc in virally suppressed patients with HAND. A 24-week randomized, double-blind, placebo-controlled study examined the use of paroxetine and fluconazole in patients with HAND. Subjects in the paroxetine arm showed improved performance on a summary neuropsychological measure. Drugs used to treat non-HIV dementia include acetylcholinesterase inhibitors, angiotensin-converting enzyme inhibitors, and NMDA receptor antagonists. However, these have not shown significant clinical efficacy in the treatment of HAND.

TABLE 21–2. Tests and procedures
Medical evaluation with laboratory tests: complete blood count, chemistry screen (including liver and renal function tests), CD4+ t-cell count, viral load, urinalysis, chest radiography, electrocardiogram
Additional lab work: toxicology screen, therapeutic drug levels, thyroid function tests, vitamin B_{12} and B_6 levels, free or bioavailable testosterone
Evaluation for hepatitis C, syphilis
Neuroimaging (MRI preferable)
Lumbar puncture: examination of cerebrospinal fluid for evidence of infection, neoplasia, inflammation; presence of HIV

Cognitive rehabilitation is a treatment option for patients with HAND consisting of therapeutic, systematic activities oriented toward improvement in overall functioning.

■ SPECIALIZED COMPONENTS IN THE DIFFERENTIAL DIAGNOSIS SPECIFIC TO HIV

Delirium

Delirium in patients with HIV/AIDS may be superimposed on HAND. Patients with HAND are at increased risk of delirium when they are medically hospitalized. The etiology of delirium in patients with HIV/AIDS is often multifactorial. Treatment, as in those without HIV, involves identifying and treating the offending condition(s).

Immune Reconstitution Inflammatory Syndrome

Immune reconstitution inflammatory syndrome refers to the paradoxical worsening that often occurs within the first 4–8 weeks after starting cART. The reconstituted immune system creates a robust inflammatory response that worsens a known, underlying infection or unmasks a subclinical indolent infection. The most common CNS infections reported to be involved in this syndrome are HIV encephalitis, toxoplasmic encephalitis, cryptococcal meningitis, and progressive multifocal leukoencephalopathy (associated with John Cunningham viral infection). Risk factors include being naïve to cART and/or having an active or subclinical opportunistic infection, CD4+ t-cell count <50 cells/mm^3, elevated CD8+ cells, anemia, and a rapid decline in HIV viral load. Treatment of CNS immune reconstitution inflammatory syndrome involves optimizing the opportunistic infection treatment, but it may include corticosteroids when the diagnosis is certain and a viral etiology has been ruled out.

Viral Escape

There are cases in which patients with HIV may have an unde-tectable viral load in the periphery as measured by blood testing but a detectable viral load in the CNS, typically measured by examining the cerebrospinal fluid from a lumbar puncture. This phenomenon is referred to as *viral escape*. Symptomatic patients may present with neurological symptoms ranging from head-ache to coma. Viral escape may indicate suboptimal cART, poor adherence, drug–drug interactions reducing cART's CNS con-centration, or development of resistance to cART. Viral escape has been observed in approximately 10% of patients. Treatment targets the etiology and may include changing cARTs, adher-ence counseling, or changing interacting agents.

Methamphetamine Use

Combined HIV infection and methamphetamine use increases the likelihood of neuronal injury in the CNS. Effects include cognitive impairment and increased tendency toward impaired behavioral inhibition. Given methamphetamine's ability to in-crease dopamine to excessively high levels, it is not uncommon to observe paranoia, delusions, and hallucinations in individ-uals using methamphetamine. These symptoms may continue for extended periods after patients achieve abstinence. Beyond abstinence, treatment for neuropsychiatric disorders related to HIV and methamphetamine include the use of atypical neuro-leptics for psychosis (caution with metabolic syndrome); anti-depressants, including bupropion or mirtazapine; and ongoing addiction-focused therapy.

■ REFERENCES

Ances BM, Ellis RJ: Dementia and neurocognitive disorders due to HIV-1 infection. Semin Neurol 27(1):86–92, 2007 17226745
Antinori A, Arendt G, Becker JT, et al: Updated research nosology for HIV-associated neurocognitive disorders. Neurology 69(18):1789–1799, 2007 17914061
Atkinson JH, Grant I: Natural history of neuropsychiatric manifestations of HIV disease. Psychiatr Clin North Am 17(1):17–33, 1994 8190664
Breitbart W, Marotta R, Platt MM, et al: A double-blind trial of halo-peridol, chlorpromazine, and lorazepam in the treatment of delir-ium in hospitalized AIDS patients. Am J Psychiatry 153(2):231–237, 1996 8561204

Brew BJ, Chan P: Update on HIV dementia and HIV-associated neurocognitive disorders. Curr Neurol Neurosci Rep 14(8):468, 2014 24938216

Calcagno A, Di Perri G, Bonora S: Treating HIV infection in the central nervous system. Drugs 77(2):145–157, 2017 28070871

Carroll A, Brew B: HIV-associated neurocognitive disorders: recent advances in pathogenesis, biomarkers, and treatment. F1000 Res 6:312, 2017 28413625

Chan P, Brew BJ: HIV associated neurocognitive disorders in the modern antiviral treatment era: prevalence, characteristic, biomarkers, and effects of treatment. Curr HIV/AIDS Rep 11:317–324, 2014

Ciccarelli N: Considerations on nosology for HIV-associated neurocognitive disorders: it is time to update? Infection 48(1):37–42, 2020 31691905

Clifford DB, Ances BM: HIV-associated neurocognitive disorder. Lancet Infect Dis 13(11):976–986, 2013 24156898

DeVaughn S, Müller-Oehring EM, Markey B, et al: Aging with HIV-1 infection: motor functions, cognition, and attention—a comparison with Parkinson's disease. Neuropsychol Rev 25(4):424–438, 2015 26577508

Farhadian S, Patel P, Spudich S: Neurological complications of HIV infection. Curr Infect Dis Rep 19(12):50, 2017 29164407

Fernandez F, Tan J: Neuropsychiatric aspects of human immunodeficiency virus infection of the central nervous system, in Neuropsychiatry and Behavioral Sciences. Edited by Yudofsky SC, Hales RE. Washington, DC, American Psychiatric Publishing, 2008, pp 765–798

Ferrando SJ, Rabkin J, Rothenberg J: Psychiatric disorders and adjustment of HIV and AIDS patients during and after medical hospitalization. Psychosomatics 39:214–215, 1998

Gardner EM, McLees MP, Steiner JF, et al: The spectrum of engagement in HIV care and its relevance to test-and-treat strategies for prevention of HIV infection. Clin Infect Dis 52(6):793–800, 2011 21367734

Gates TM, Cysique LA, Siefried KJ, et al: Maraviroc-intensified combined antiretroviral therapy improves cognition in virally suppressed HIV-associated neurocognitive disorder. AIDS 30(4):591–600, 2016 26825032

Goodkin K, Miller EN, Cox C, et al: Effect of aging on neurocognitive function by stage of HIV infection: evidence from the Multicenter AIDS Cohort Study. Lancet HIV 4(9):e411–e422, 2017

Gorman AA, Foley JM, Ettenhofer ML, et al: Functional consequences of HIV-associated neuropsychological impairment. Neuropsychol Rev 19(2):186–203, 2009 19472057

Graf C: The Lawton instrumental activities of daily living scale. Am J Nurs 108(4):52–62, quiz 62–63, 2008 18367931

Haddow LJ, Floyd S, Copas A, Gilson RJ: A systematic review of the screening accuracy of the HIV Dementia Scale and International HIV Dementia Scale. PLoS ONE 8(4):e61826, 2013 23613945

Heaton RK, Clifford DB, Franklin DR Jr, et al: HIV-associated neurocognitive disorders persist in the era of potent antiretroviral therapy: CHARTER Study. Neurology 75(23):2087–2096, 2010 21135382

Heaton RK, Franklin DR, Ellis RJ, et al: HIV-associated neurocognitive disorders before and during the era of combination antiretroviral therapy: differences in rates, nature, and predictors. J Neurovirol 17(1):3–16, 2011 21174240

Henrich TJ, Hsue PY, VanBrocklin H: Seeing is believing: nuclear imaging of HIV persistence. Front Immunol 10:2077, 2019 31572355

Hoffmann C, Llibre JM: Neuropsychiatric adverse events with dolutegravir and other integrase strand transfer inhibitors. AIDS Rev 21(1):4–10, 2019 30899113

Hong S, Banks WA: Role of the immune system in HIV-associated neuroinflammation and neurocognitive implications. Brain Behav Immun 45:1–12, 2015 25449672

Legesse B, Babadi B, Forester B: Management of neuropsychiatric symptoms in neurocognitive disorders. Focus Am Psychiatr Publ 15(1):18–25, 2017 31975836

Letendre S, Iudicello J, Ances B, et al: HIV-associated neurocognitive disorders, in Comprehensive Textbook of AIDS Psychiatry. Edited by Cohen MA, Gorman JM, Letendre SL. New York, Oxford University Press, 2017, pp 175–203

Livelli A, Orofino GC, Calcagno A, et al: Evaluation of a cognitive rehabilitation protocol in HIV patients with associated neurocognitive disorders: efficacy and stability over time. Front Behav Neurosci 9:306, 2015 26635558

Makinson A, Dubois J, Eymard-Duvernay S, et al: Increased prevalence of neurocognitive impairment in aging people living with human immunodeficiency virus: the ANRS EP58 HAND 55-70 Study. Clin Infect Dis 70(12):2641–2648, 2020 31755936

Meintjes G, Scriven J, Marais S: Management of the immune reconstitution inflammatory syndrome. Curr HIV/AIDS Rep 9(3):238–250, 2012 22752438

Munjal S, Ferrando SJ, Freyberg Z: Neuropsychiatric aspects of infectious diseases: an update. Crit Care Clin 33(3):681–712, 2017 28601141

Norman LR, Basso M: An update of the review of neuropsychological consequences of HIV and substance abuse: a literature review and implications for treatment and future research. Curr Drug Abuse Rev 8(1):50–71, 2015 25751583

Purohit V, Rapaka R, Shurtleff D: Drugs of abuse, dopamine, and HIV-associated neurocognitive disorders/HIV-associated dementia. Mol Neurobiol 44(1):102–110, 2011 21717292

Sacktor N, Skolasky RL, Seaberg E, et al: Prevalence of HIV-associated neurocognitive disorders in the Multicenter AIDS Cohort Study. Neurology 86(4):334–340, 2016 26718568

Sacktor N, Skolasky RL, Moxley R, et al: Paroxetine and fluconazole therapy for HIV-associated neurocognitive impairment: results from a double-blind, placebo-controlled trial. J Neurovirol 24(1):16–27, 2018 29063516

Sanmarti M, Ibáñez L, Huertas S, et al: HIV-associated neurocognitive disorders. J Mol Psychiatry 2(1):2, 2014 25945248

Sathekge M, McFarren A, Dadachova E: Role of nuclear medicine in neuroHIV: PET, SPECT, and beyond. Nucl Med Commun 35(8):792–796, 2014 24781008

Singer EJ, Thames AD: Neurobehavioral manifestations of human immunodeficiency virus/AIDS: diagnosis and treatment. Neurol Clin 34(1):33–53, 2016 26613994

Singer EJ, Valdes-Sueiras M, Commins D, Levine A: Neurologic presentations of AIDS. Neurol Clin 28(1):253–275, 2010 19932385

Sinharay S, Hammoud DA: Brain PET imaging: value for understanding the pathophysiology of HIV-associated neurocognitive disorder (HAND). Curr HIV/AIDS Rep 16(1):66–75, 2019 30778853

Sonneville R, Ferrand H, Tubach F, et al: Neurological complications of HIV infection in critically ill patients: clinical features and outcomes. J Infect 62(4):301–308, 2011 21329724

Soontornniyomkij V, Kesby JP, Morgan EE, et al: Effects of HIV and methamphetamine on brain and behavior: evidence from human studies and animal models. J Neuroimmune Pharmacol 11(3):495–510, 2016 27484318

Spudich S: HIV and neurocognitive dysfunction. Curr HIV/AIDS Rep 10(3):235–243, 2013 23860944

Spudich S, González-Scarano F: HIV-1-related central nervous system disease: current issues in pathogenesis, diagnosis, and treatment. Cold Spring Harb Perspect Med 2(6):a007120, 2012 22675662

Subra C, Trautmann L: Role of T lymphocytes in HIV neuropathogenesis. Curr HIV/AIDS Rep 16(3):236–243, 2019 31062168

Sütterlin S, Vögele C, Gauggel S: Neuropsychiatric complications of efavirenz therapy: suggestions for a new research paradigm. J Neuropsychiatry Clin Neurosci 22(4):361–369, 2010 21037119

Tavazzi E, White MK, Khalili K: Progressive multifocal leukoencephalopathy: clinical and molecular aspects. Rev Med Virol 22(1):18–32, 2012 21936015

Underwood J, Winston A: Guidelines for evaluation and management of cognitive disorders in HIV-positive individuals. Curr HIV/AIDS Rep 13(5):235–240, 2016 27353598

Valcour VG: HIV, aging, and cognition: emerging issues. Top Antivir Med 21(3):119–123, 2013 23981600

Valcour V, Paul R, Chiao S, et al: Screening for cognitive impairment in human immunodeficiency virus. Clin Infect Dis 53(8):836–842, 2011 21921226

Valcour V, Sithinamsuwan P, Letendre S, Ances B: Pathogenesis of HIV in the central nervous system. Curr HIV/AIDS Rep 8(1):54–61, 2011 21191673

Watkins CC, Treisman GJ: Cognitive impairment in patients with AIDS: prevalence and severity. HIV AIDS (Auckl) 7:35–47, 2015 25678819

Wendelken LA, Valcour V: Impact of HIV and aging on neuropsychological function. J Neurovirol 18(4):256–263, 2012 22528478

Zipursky AR, Gogolishvili D, Rueda S, et al: Evaluation of brief screening tools for neurocognitive impairment in HIV/AIDS: a systematic review of the literature. AIDS 27(15):2385–2401, 2013 23751261

TREATMENTS IN NEUROPSYCHIATRY

John J. Barry, M.D.

All treatments in neurology and psychiatry exert their effects by altering brain function. This altered function is largely achieved by changes in neurotransmitters or their receptors, although in neurosurgical procedures, this alteration is effected by the placement of structural lesions or devices. Neurologists and psychiatrists use a similar spectrum of drugs.

■ BASIC CONCEPTS

The *bioavailability* of a drug is the proportion of an oral dose that reaches its site of action. Intravenous drugs are assumed to have 100% bioavailability. The *clearance* of a drug is the volume of plasma cleared of that drug in a unit of time. Some drugs, when given orally, are partially metabolized by the gut and liver; this is known as the *first-pass effect*. The *half-life* of a drug is the time taken for its concentration to fall by 50%. With *first-order* kinetics, there is a linear relationship between the dose taken and the serum drug levels. In *second-order* kinetics, this relationship is curvilinear. *Steady state* defines that circumstance in which the amount absorbed equals the amount eliminated, and plasma levels remain stable. Steady state is usually achieved after five half-lives of the administered drug.

Optimization of pharmacotherapy is aided by therapeutic drug monitoring (TDM). TDM is particularly useful in specific patient populations, such as the young and the geriatric populations. In addition, the lack of response to therapeutic drug dosing may be the result of noncompliance, drug–drug interactions, or other causes, and TDM may aid in clarifying causation. Idiosyncratic individual pharmacokinetics may result in a 20-fold variation in serum concentration. This may be the result of individual differences in absorption, metabolism, and excretion. Genetic factors may also be causative; when two active alleles on CYP450 are associated with elevated, reduced, or absent activity alleles, drug levels may change accordingly. Thus, these genetic polymorphisms may be important clinically. The utility of TDM has become clear; routine with the use of antiepileptic drugs, tricyclic antidepressants (TCAs), and mood stabilizers; and mandatory with administering lithium.

Therapeutic reference ranges are determined by the lower limit below which a drug response is no better than that for placebo and the upper limit at which tolerability declines or further improvement is unlikely. However, individual differences exist. Indications for TDM include compliance (50% of drugs issued for chronic disease are not taken) and relapse prevention. TDM is recommended for dosage titration of drugs such as lithium, carbamazepine, and valproic acid; antipsychotics such as clozapine; and depot formulations. It is less useful for selective serotonin reuptake inhibitors (SSRIs), antidementia medications, and antianxiety drugs for which clinical response and low toxicity can guide psychopharmacology. The timing of drug collection is also important and should occur after steady state is achieved, usually four to six elimination half-lives, and at a trough that represents the minimal effective drug concentration. With drugs for which effectiveness correlates more with maximal drug dosage, such as those with short half-lives, the maximum drug concentration might be more appropriate (e.g., antiparkinsonian drugs and methylphenidate).

Drugs that are active in the CNS affect unique receptors that control synaptic transmission. The neuron membrane is opened and closed by specific channels, of which there are two types: voltage-gated and ligand-gated. Receptors are either the ligand-gated type or metabotropic; both of these can bind to g-protein complexes. An excitatory neurotransmitter that affects an ionotropic receptor allows for increased permeability of the membrane, resulting in an excitatory postsynaptic potential. This is in contrast to an inhibitory postsynaptic potential that results from the opening of a chloride channel.

The cytochrome P450 system is a group of liver and intestinal enzymes that catalyze oxidation and influence the rate at which drugs are metabolized—and hence their resultant serum concentrations. These isoenzymes may be inhibited or induced by drugs, thus leading to pharmacokinetic interactions. The main enzymes are referred to by their family (number), subfamily (letter), and further specification (number). The isoenzymes most relevant for neuropsychiatry are CYP1A2, CYP2A6, CYP2B, CYP2D6, CYP3A4, CYP2E1, and CYP2C9. Of these, CYP3A4 accounts for 50% of drug metabolism. Genetic polymorphisms affecting the oxidative process may result in ultrarapid or poor metabolizers. Allelic variants are present for CYP2D6, CYP2C19, CYP2C9, and CYP2B6. A classification system for the main psychotropic agents is shown in Table 22–1.

■ ANTIDEPRESSANTS

Antidepressants are primarily useful in the treatment of depressive disorder. Their clinical effectiveness may revolve around improving monoamine deficiencies in neurotransmitter systems including serotonin, norepinephrine, and dopamine. Neurotrophic drugs, especially those that involve brain-derived neurotrophic factor and endocrine dysfunction, play significant roles as well. Categories of antidepressants are listed in Table 22–1.

Monoamine oxidase inhibitors (MAOIs) act by inhibiting the activity of both the A and B forms of monoamine oxidase (MAO), an enzyme widely distributed throughout the body. The substrates for MAO-A include norepinephrine and serotonin; the substrate for MAO-B is phenylalanine. Tyramine and dopamine are substrates for both but primarily reflect MAO-A and MAO-B, respectively.

Beyond their specificity for MAO, these drugs vary in the extent that they degrade the enzyme and thus must be regenerated on drug cessation. When they degrade it, they serve as an irreversible inhibitor. When they mask the enzyme but do not degrade it, they function as a reversible inhibitor. Phenelzine and tranylcypromine are irreversible inhibitors of MAO-A and release dopamine and norepinephrine. Tranylcypromine has an amphetamine-like stimulating effect, whereas phenelzine is more sedating than its counterparts. In contrast, moclobemide is a reversible inhibitor of MAO-A, and selegiline and rasagiline are selective and irreversible inhibitors of MAO-B. Selegiline can be administered transdermally in order to avoid significant effects on MAO in the gut and therefore has fewer dietary interactions. Selegiline is a selective MAO-B at low dosages and requires no dietary exclusions. Only at high dosages does it inhibit MAO-A and MAO-B and thus require dietary restrictions. Selegiline administered by patch, in low doses, avoids these restrictions.

TABLE 22–1. Classification system for psychotropic drugs

Antidepressants	5-HT$_2$ receptor antagonists
	Ketamine and esketamine
	Monoamine oxidase inhibitors (MAO-A, MAO-B)
	Selective serotonin reuptake inhibitors
	Serotonin-norepinephrine reuptake inhibitors
	Tetra- and unicyclic antidepressants
	Tricyclics
Antipsychotics (neuroleptics)	See Table 22–4
Cholinesterase inhibitors (see Chapter 10)	Donepezil
	Galantamine
	Rivastigmine
Hypnotic, antianxiety, and sedative drugs	Barbiturates
	Benzodiazepines
	Buspirone
	Melatonin receptor agonists
	Orexin receptor agonists
Mood-stabilizing drugs	Lithium
	Others*
Psychostimulants	Dextroamphetamine
	Dextroamphetamine/Amphetamine
	Lisdexamfetamine
	Methylphenidate
	Modafinil/armodafinil
Other psychotropics	Analgesics
	β-Blockers
	Dopaminergic agents
	Narcotics

*Other mood-stabilizing drugs include anticonvulsants, valproic acid, and carbamazepine and lamotrigine.

The "cheese reaction" is due to an interaction between the inhibition of peripheral MAO activity and the ingestion of certain primary amines. Irreversible inhibition of MAO-A blocks the metabolism of tyramine and may result in a pressor effect catalyzing a severe hypertensive episode. This reaction limits the ingestion of certain foods and is one reason these drugs are not widely used. However, with the newer selective drugs (e.g., moclobemide, which is reversible but is not approved in the United States), this reaction is much less likely to occur.

TABLE 22–2. Disorders most likely to respond to monoamine oxidase (MAO) inhibitors

MAO-A inhibitors	MAO-B inhibitors
Agoraphobia and social phobias	Parkinson's disease
Atypical depression	
Melancholic depression	
Phobic anxiety with depersonalization	
Somatic anxiety	

The disorders most likely to respond to MAOIs in clinical practice are listed in Table 22–2.

Although this is controversial, selegiline may play a neuroprotective role in Parkinson's disease because of its ability to reduce the generation of free radicals. It also may be neuroprotective against the parkinsonian effects of the neurotoxin mPTP (1-methyl-4-phenyl 1–1,2,3,6 tetrahydropyridine). Both selegiline and the newer MAO-B blocker rasagiline may be neuroprotective and antiapoptotic. Dopamine neurons may be especially vulnerable to oxidative stress through reactions catalyzed by MAO; however, their utility may be secondary to their increase in dopamine and not a direct neuroprotective effect. In clinical studies, rasagiline had a possible disease-modifying effect at low dosages of 1 mg/day, but it was not effective at higher dosages of 2 mg/day. Neither drug has demonstrated unequivocal positive clinical effects. Further study is indicated. This is discussed further in Chapter 12, "Movement Disorders."

Safinamide is a reversible MAOI-B inhibitor that is used in the treatment of Parkinson's disease. It was approved by the FDA in 2017 (see Chapter 12).

Two types of drug toxicity may result from use of MAOIs. The first is interactions from their combined use with SSRIs, which results in serotonin syndrome and sympathomimetic responses from tyramine or other amines. Second, they can cause serotonin syndrome secondary to an interaction with some opioids, especially meperidine. Fentanyl, methadone, tramadol, and tapentadol are not recommended for similar reasons. MAOIs can also cause orthostatic hypotension, weight gain, insomnia, and anorgasmia.

When switching from an SSRI or TCA to an MAOI, taper the non-MAOI for a period of 2–4 weeks and then discontinue the antidepressant for 2 weeks (5 weeks for fluoxetine) before starting the MAOI. To switch from an MAOI to an SSRI or TCA, the same taper is recommended, followed by a 2-week wash-out period to allow for enzyme regeneration.

Tricyclic Antidepressants

TCAs are traditionally thought to inhibit monoamine reuptake from the synaptic cleft. Drugs such as imipramine and amitriptyline are metabolized into desipramine and nortriptyline, respectively. In the former case, imipramine affects serotonin and norepinephrine, in contrast to desipramine, which is more selective for norepinephrine. Clomipramine is much more selective for serotonin. Anticholinergic effects are common, especially with imipramine, amitriptyline, and clomipramine. TCAs may also have cardiotoxicity. Discontinuation syndrome may occur with abrupt withdrawal, especially with clomipramine. Several TCAs have antihistaminic properties, and some are commonly used for pain control, such as amitriptyline. Nortriptyline has a therapeutic window, with an increase in dosage leading to less clinical efficacy for depression.

Serotonin Augmenting Agents

Molecular targets separate the remaining antidepressants. The SSRIs are selective for serotonin and have clinical utility not only for major depressive disorder but also for OCD, premenstrual dysphoric disorder, and anxiety disorders. They have fewer side effects than the TCAs and are safer in overdose. These drugs include fluoxetine, sertraline, citalopram and its (S) enantiomer escitalopram, fluvoxamine, and paroxetine. They are generally well tolerated except for sexual dysfunction (seen in 30%–40% of those treated with SSRIs) and risk of serotonin syndrome, especially when combined with MAOIs.

The latest generation of antidepressant medications has been developed to be even more specific for various receptors. These include the serotonin-norepinephrine reuptake inhibitors (SNRIs), which consist of venlafaxine, its metabolite desvenlafaxine, and duloxetine and are often used for major depressive disorder and for pain control, fibromyalgia, and neuropathies. Milnacipran and levomilnacipran also fall into this category. These medications bind serotonin and norepinephrine transporters.

Trazodone and nefazodone are 5-HT_2 receptor inhibitors. In the past, they were often used for treatment of major depressive disorder, but they are now often used to control anxiety and used off-label as hypnotics. Because of its hepatotoxicity, nefazodone was given a black box warning by the FDA.

Vortioxetine is a new antidepressant that has antagonist activity at a variety of serotonin receptors, agonist activity at the 5-HT_{1A} receptor, and partial agonist activity at 5-HT_{1B}. It is utilized for the treatment of major depressive disorder and is particularly useful for treating the cognitive complaints associated with depressive disorders.

Tetracyclic and Unicyclic Antidepressants

Bupropion is an antidepressant with a unicyclic aminoketone structure. It is an indirect norepinephrine agonist that has some dopaminergic properties. Bupropion is used as an antidepressant with activating properties, as an anoriexant in combination with naltrexone, and as an aid to stop smoking. Seizures are a particularly problematic side effect in patients with bulimia and potentially in patients with a history of head injuries. Please refer to Chapters 9 ("Limbic System Disorders") and 16 ("Head Injury and Its Sequelae").

Mirtazapine is a noradrenergic and specific serotonergic antidepressant. It increases noradrenergic and serotonergic transmission via blockade of α_2 receptors but also blocks 5-HT_2 and 5-HT_3 receptors, accentuating serotonin activity by stimulating the 5-HT_1 receptor. Its antihistaminergic effect causes sedation, and the drug may also cause weight gain. It is only infrequently associated with sexual side effects.

Vilazodone binds to the serotonin transporter and 5-HT_{1A} but binds weakly to the transporter for norepinephrine and dopamine.

Novel Antidepressants

Ketamine and its enantiomer esketamine present a new class of antidepressant that appears to work by a different mechanism. Ketamine blocks the glutamate NMDA receptor and may have other targets that might be responsible for its antidepressant activity, such as receptor subtypes, increased brain-derived neurotrophic factor, and monoamine and opiate effects. Up to 60% of patients with treatment-refractory depression may have a positive response to the drug, which can last for 3–7 days.

The side effects of ketamine may be problematic. These include the development of dissociation and elevations in blood pressure. Ketamine can also be abused, and its antidepressant effects may be blocked by naltrexone. In addition, patients may develop uropathy, psychosis, and cognitive difficulties. Esketamine has been found comparably effective with ketamine and been given an FDA "breakthrough therapy" designation. However, concerns about its long-term use remain to be clarified.

Diagnostic Evaluation for Bipolar Depression

Regardless of the CNS disorder, it is imperative to determine the correct diagnosis when evaluating patients with depression. Is the affective disorder a cyclic bipolar or a unipolar depression? Depression appearing as part of bipolar disorder often does not respond to antidepressants and requires mood-stabilizing medication. Screening instruments have poor sensitivity and specificity. In addition to these patients having a response similar to placebo, their use of antidepressants may induce a manic episode. Venlafaxine and the TCAs are more prone to this side effect. Treatment entails the use of a mood stabilizer (discussed later) such as lithium, a second-generation atypical neuroleptic agent, or an anticonvulsant with antimanic properties. If an antidepressant is used, the recommendation is to also include a mood-stabilizing agent.

Diagnosing a bipolar depression is often difficult, but the following clinical history and symptoms may alert clinicians to that probability:

- Earlier onset of illness (i.e., as adolescent or young adult)
- Psychosis
- Presence of other comorbid psychiatric conditions
- Multiple episodes of major depression
- Family history of bipolar disorder
- Antidepressant treatment resistance

When in doubt, refer patients for further evaluation.

Side Effects

The side effects of the non-MAOI antidepressants are shown in Table 22–3. The nausea, weight reduction, and tremor reported with the SSRIs probably reflect their serotonin agonist activity.

One of the most problematic side effect concerns is the induction of seizure activity by antidepressant medications, especially in patients with epilepsy. This side effect is discussed fully in Chapter 9, "Epilepsy and Limbic System Disorders."

TABLE 22–3. Side effects of non–monoamine oxidase inhibitor antidepressants

Agitation, aggression	Impaired cognition
Anorgasmia, impotence	Myopathy
Ataxia	Nausea, vomiting, gastrointestinal upset
Blurred vision	Neuropathy
Cholestatic jaundice	Palpitations
Constipation	Paralytic ileus
Convulsions	Postural hypotension
Delirium	Rash
Depersonalization	Sedation
Dry mouth	Sweating, fever
Dyskinesias	Transient hypomania
Electrocardiographic changes	Tremor
	Urinary retention
Galactorrhea	Weight gain
Glaucoma	

Drug Interactions

Enzyme-inducing agents may decrease the serum levels of antidepressant substrates. Induction of the 2D6 isoenzyme by carbamazepine, phenytoin, and phenobarbital can decrease the serum levels of TCAs. The reverse can take place with fluoxetine and paroxetine. These drug interactions can be important clinically; this is discussed further later in the chapter.

Some SSRIs inhibit the metabolism of selected drugs, including tricyclic antidepressants, carbamazepine, and haloperidol. The primary isoenzymes involved are CYP2D6, CYP1A2, and CYP3A4.

The primary use of antidepressants is in managing depression. However, they are also utilized to treat chronic pain syndromes and migraine, panic disorder, OCD, and narcolepsy (clomipramine can be used for cataplexy).

■ ANTIPSYCHOTICS (NEUROLEPTICS)

Agents

Neuroleptics are drugs that produce extrapyramidal reactions (EPRs) when used clinically. They are commonly categorized as either conventional—that is, typical or first-generation antipsychotics—or as the newer "atypical" antipsychotics that produce less severe EPRs. Clozapine was the first medication in this category and the template for the introduction of a series of atypical agents (see Table 22–4 for select typical and atypical agents). Newer antipsychotics include asenapine, cariprazine, brexpiprazole, iloperidone, paliperidone, and sertindole. It should be noted that haloperidol, fluphenazine, chlorpromazine, droperidol, aripiprazole, olanzapine, paliperidone, risperidone, and ziprasidone come as injectable medications.

Pharmacokinetics

Most antipsychotics are dosed to provide 60%–80% dopamine (D_2) occupancy. There are five important dopaminergic pathways. The most relevant to the development of psychosis are the mesolimbic-mesocortical and nigrostriatal pathways. The distinguishing features of neuroleptics are their antipsychotic effects and blockade of dopamine receptors. The atypical neuroleptics act preferentially on dopamine receptors outside the dorsal striatum, which gives them a different side effect profile compared with typical antipsychotics. Some atypicals occupy lower levels of D_2 receptors and bind preferentially to limbic as opposed to striatal receptors. The atypical antipsychotics also have greater affinity for blocking cortical 5-HT_{2A} receptors, an effect thought to be important in their action, especially against the negative symptoms of schizophrenia. The antipsychotics also have a range of effects on the 5-HT (especially 5-HT_{2A} and 5-HT_{2C}), α-adrenergic, histaminic, and cholinergic receptors.

Side Effects

Extrapyramidal Reactions

The standard antipsychotic agents evoke EPRs (see Chapter 12, "Movement Disorders"). The most common EPRs are the acute, agitated restlessness of akathisia and the loss of spontaneous movement in akinesia. Akathisia occurs with clozapine at a rate of 6%, in contrast to haloperidol in which it occurs in 30% of patients. Atypical antipsychotics, especially clozapine, are thought less likely to lead to extrapyramidal complications. Clozapine has been the most studied of this class and has been reported to produce improvement in some movement disorders (e.g., dystonias, dyskinesias, tremor).

TABLE 22–4. Select antipsychotics*

	Potency	EPR	Sedation	Weight gain	Seizures	Prolactin	Tardive dyskinesia	OH	QTc changes
Aripiprazole	High	Low	Low	Low	Low	Low	Med	Low	Med
Chlorpromazine	Low	Med	High	Med	Med-high	Med	High	High	High
Clozapine	Med	Low	Low	High	High	Low	Low	High	Med
Haloperidol	High	High	Low	Low	Low	High	High	Low	High
Lurasidone	Med	Med	Low	Low	Low	Low	Med	Low	Low
Olanzapine	High	Low	Med	High	Low	Med	Med	Low	Med
Risperidone	High	Low	Low	Low	Low	High	Med	Med	Med
Quetiapine	Low	Low	Med	Med	Low	Low	Med	Low-med	Med
Thiothixene	High	Med	Med	Low	Low	High	High	Med	Low
Ziprasidone	Med	Low	Low	Low	Low	Mod	Med	Low	Med

EPR=extrapyramidal reaction; OH=orthostatic hypotension.

*Values from *Clinical Handbook of Psychotropic Drugs* are relative (i.e., higher, moderate, and lower), whereas values from *Basic and Clinical Pharmacology* are absolutes (i.e, low, medium, high). All values have been changed to absolutes.

Source. Adapted from DeBattista C: "Antipsychotic Agents and Lithium," in *Basic and Clinical Pharmacology*, 14th Edition. Edited by Katzung BG. New York, McGraw-Hill Education, 2015, pp. 511–531, and Procyshyn RM, Bezchlibnyk-Butler KZ, Jeffries JJ (eds): *Clinical Handbook of Psychotropic Drugs*. Boston, MA, Hogrefe, 2015.

Tardive Dyskinesia

Tardive dyskinesia (TD), possibly due to dopaminergic super-sensitivity in the caudate/putamen, manifests as choreoathetoid movements. It is observed most commonly with the typical antipsychotics, with a frequency of 20%–40%. Early recognition is important, followed by reducing or discontinuing the offending agent and switching to an atypical antipsychotic as well as discontinuing central anticholinergics, especially antiparkinsonian drugs and TCAs. GABAergic medications may also be helpful. After discontinuing or switching the antipsychotic, vesicular monoamine transporter type-2 (VMAT2) inhibitors such as tetrabenazine, deutetrabenazine, and valbenazine are the treatments of choice but may be associated with the induction of depression.

Cardiac

Because some antipsychotic medications have been shown to increase the QT interval on the electrocardiogram, caution is required, particularly in elderly patients and those with cardiac disease, in order to avoid torsades de pointes. An electrocardiographic investigation should be performed before an antipsychotic is prescribed. Newer antipsychotic agents may affect the QT interval, especially ziprasidone and quetiapine, but the actual induction of arrhythmias is suspect. Other potential side effects include seizure induction (see Chapter 9), endocrine effects (i.e., prolactin elevation), and induction of metabolic syndrome.

Neuroleptic Malignant Syndrome

Neuroleptic malignant syndrome, possibly secondary to a rapid blockade or to postsynaptic dopamine receptors, may be manifested by muscle rigidity, elevated creatine kinase levels, autonomic instability, and fever. Treatment is with dopamine agonists such as bromocriptine and muscle relaxants, coupled with discontinuation of the offending agent.

Agranulocytosis

Agranulocytosis may be seen in 1%–2% of patients secondary to clozapine use and requires caution. The incidence is higher in weeks 6–18 of use. Protocols for patient monitoring are provided by the FDA.

Indications

TDM for some antipsychotics may be useful to ensure adherence, to prevent relapse, and for safe use in elderly patients. It is also helpful with the use of drugs such as clozapine, for which there is an association with serum concentration and seizure induction, and when switching from an oral to a depot form of an antipsychotic. The main use of neuroleptics is to treat psychotic disorders, particularly schizophrenia and schizoaffective disorder, mania, and psychosis in neurological disorders. They are also used in the management of delirium (see Chapter 10, "Delirium"), Gilles de la Tourette's syndrome and Huntington's chorea (see Chapter 12), and borderline personality disorder. Antipsychotic agents aripiprazole, brexpiprazole, cariprazine, olanzapine (often combined with fluoxetine), risperidone, and ziprasidone are also used in the treatment of bipolar and unipolar depression as augmenters and as single agents. Lurasidone can be used for depression in bipolar affective disorder as well.

Atypical antipsychotics are also used to control agitation in patients with Alzheimer's disease but have been associated with increased mortality (see Chapter 13, "Cerebrovascular Disease–Stroke"). Intramuscular ziprasidone, olanzapine, and aripiprazole have also been used to treat agitation in other disorders and have a decreased incidence of EPRs compared with haloperidol. The hallucinations associated with Lewy body dementia can be treated with quetiapine or clozapine with less fear of motor deterioration (see Chapters 11 and 12). Psychosis associated with Parkinson's disease can present a problem for treatment; see Chapter 12 for further discussion. Pimavanserin was approved in 2016 for treatment of psychosis associated with Parkinson's disease. It has no dopaminergic antagonist properties and is a serotonin inverse agonist at the 5-HT$_{2A}$ receptor, with less potency at 5-HT$_{2C}$. Pimavanserin is also being evaluated for the treatment of dementia-related psychosis (see Chapter 11), with one negative study in 2018; more data are needed.

■ SEDATIVE-HYPNOTICS

Indications

Sedative agents produce anxiolytic effects, whereas hypnotics produce drowsiness and onset of sleep. Barbiturates are rarely used as first-line treatment because of their linear kinetic side effects, especially CNS depression. Alternative medications are as

TABLE 22–5.	Pharmacological differences among benzodiazepines*	
Long-acting (tranquilizers, antiepileptics)	**Intermediate-acting (hypnotics, tranquilizers)**	**Short-acting (hypnotics)**
Chlordiazepoxide	Alprazolam	Midazolam
Clobazam	Flunitrazepam	Triazolam
Clonazepam	Lorazepam	
Clorazepate	Nitrazepam	
Diazepam	Oxazepam	
Flurazepam	Temazepam	

*Main uses are indicated in parentheses.

effective but without concomitant side effects. Barbiturates have been used in the past as anticonvulsants, especially for treatment of status epilepticus. They may be associated with hyperactivity and ADHD in children and with depression in adults and can cause respiratory depression leading to death in overdose.

Benzodiazepines

Benzodiazepines differ in their duration of action (Table 22–5). Several are used to control epilepsy, most often in patients with status epilepticus. The primary benzodiazepines utilized in the oral therapy of epilepsy are clobazam, clonazepam, and lorazepam. Benzodiazepines are also utilized as hypnotics agents, to treat spasticity and myoclonus, and to induce preoperative amnesia, especially lorazepam and midazolam. Clonazepam has been given in large doses to patients with acute mania.

Pharmacokinetics

Benzodiazepines have a common structure but a spectrum of activity that ranges from full agonist to antagonist to inverse agonist effects. Because of their various neurotransmitter actions, the benzodiazepines have tranquilizing, muscle-relaxant, anticonvulsant, and amnestic properties (producing memory impairment; see Chapter 8, "Memory and Its Disorders"). They act at the benzodiazepine–GABA receptor. Because anxiolytics are fast acting, treatment efficacy can be guided by clinical observation, and TDM is not as useful.

Side Effects

Side effects of benzodiazepines include seizures and a return of acute anxiety on rapid withdrawal, concentration and memory impairment, ataxia, and fetal hypotonia. The inverse agonists are both proconvulsant and anxiogenic. Flumazenil is a competitive benzodiazepine antagonist with no effect on barbiturates or alcohol.

Other Agents

Buspirone is an azaspirodecanedione, nonbenzodiazepine anxiolytic that is a partial 5-HT_{1A} agonist and may have affinity for CNS D_2 receptors. It does not show cross-tolerance with the benzodiazepines and has fewer sedative, hypnotic, and amnestic effects. It has no anticonvulsant effects. Its main disadvantage is its delayed onset of action, which may be up to 2–4 weeks.

Newer hypnotics developed include those that are GABA agonists, which also influence the benzodiazepine site; these include zaleplon, zolpidem, and zopiclone. Additional hypnotics include the melatonin receptor agonists ramelteon and tasimelteon and the orexin antagonists suvorexant (approved by FDA) and almorexant. The metabolism of benzodiazepines is hepatic, especially via CYP2C19 and CYP3A4. Only oxazepam and lorazepam have no active metabolites (they are conjugated in the liver), thus making these two benzodiazepines especially useful in patients with hepatic disease.

■ MOOD-STABILIZING DRUGS

The mood stabilizers were originally focused on the treatment and prevention of mania. However, their present utility refers to the acute intervention and prevention of mania and bipolar depression.

Lithium

Lithium is utilized to stabilize mood. Its exact mode of action is unclear. It is used in a number of cyclical conditions, such as bipolar disorder, recurrent affective disorder, cluster headache, migraine, and paroxysmal aggression. Lithium is associated with a reduction in suicide risk in patients with unipolar and bipolar affective disorders.

Lithium has several neuropsychiatric side effects; the most frequent and disabling are cognitive impairment (>10%), muscle weakness (>30%), tremor (>30%; responsive to β-blockers), gastrointestinal upset (>30%), hypothyroidism (30%), and polyuria and polydipsia (>30%). These side effects can be avoided to some extent by monitoring serum lithium levels; treatment with lithium is a main indication for the routine monitoring of serum levels of psychotropic drugs. Severe intoxication may lead to delirium and subsequent encephalopathy. Severe CNS side effects are occasionally seen with lithium levels below the given upper limits of tolerance. Following patients' thyroid and renal function at least every 6 months is also recommended.

Other Agents

Several anticonvulsants are utilized as mood-stabilizing agents or to treat acute mania, including carbamazepine and valproic acid. Lamotrigine is FDA-approved for preventing recurrence of bipolar depression; however, gabapentin, oxcarbazepine, and topiramate are not FDA approved for this purpose. The typical antipsychotic agent chlorpromazine and the atypical agents aripiprazole, quetiapine, olanzapine, risperidone, cariprazine, and ziprasidone are FDA-approved for the treatment of acute mania. The combination of olanzapine plus fluoxetine and the individual use of quetiapine, lurasidone, and cariprazine are all FDA-approved for the treatment of depression appearing in bipolar affective disorder. See discussion earlier in this chapter.

■ ANTICONVULSANT DRUGS

It has become fashionable to refer to anticonvulsants as antiepileptic drugs. Although they do have antiseizure activity, these drugs also have a range of other effects, including important psychotropic actions. Carbamazepine and valproate have antimanic and mood-stabilizing properties; carbamazepine is also used to treat trigeminal neuralgia, paroxysmal aggressive disorders, and schizophrenia. Gabapentin and pregabalin can be used for pain control.

Table 22–6 lists of older and newer antiepileptic drugs introduced after 1993. Their clinical applications—that is, the type of epilepsy that responds to each drug—are also listed. Therapeutic drug levels and common side effects are also included. Additionally, antiepileptics may have significant positive and

TABLE 22–6. Some clinical properties of select anticonvulsant drugs

Drug	Recommended serum level, μg/mL	Indications and side effects
Older agents		
Carbamazepine	4–12	Focal-aware and -impaired and focal to bilateral tonic-clonic seizures
		May exacerbate some types of generalized epilepsies, including myoclonic and absence seizures
		May cause rash and leukopenia, hyponatremia, and Stevens-Johnson syndrome, especially in those with the HLA-B1502 allele, particularly patients of Asian ethnicity
		Hypersensitivity incidence increased fivefold in the presence of the HLA-A 3101 allele
Clobazam	0.03–0.30	Approved for the treatment of Lennox-Gastaut syndrome but also used for focal seizure in other countries
		Modulator of GABA-A receptor
		Dosage-dependent side effects and withdrawal symptoms with abrupt discontinuation
Clonazepam	19–70	Long-acting benzodiazepine used in generalized absence, atonic, and myoclonic seizures and Lennox-Gastaut syndrome
		Has sedative effects, possible paradoxical response and tolerance
Ethosuximide	40–100	Generalized absence seizures
		May cause gastrointestinal complaints, headache, and sedation

TABLE 22–6. Some clinical properties of select anticonvulsant drugs *(continued)*

Drug	Recommended serum level, µg/mL	Indications and side effects
Phenobarbital	15–40	Focal-aware and -impaired, generalized tonic-clonic, and myoclonic seizures
		Depression and cognitive impairment are common; may worsen generalized absence seizures and infantile spasms; serious rash occurs rarely
Phenytoin	10–20	Focal-aware and -impaired and generalized tonic-clonic seizures, status epilepticus
		May cause ataxia, nystagmus, confusion, bone demineralization, agranulocytosis, and rarely Stevens-Johnson syndrome
Primidone	8–12	Focal-aware and -impaired and generalized tonic-clonic and partial seizures
		Side effects similar to those of phenobarbital
Valproate	40–100	Generalized absence, myoclonic, and atonic to bilateral generalized seizures; migraine prophylaxis
		May cause tremor, hyperammonemia, gastrointestinal effects, hypocarnitinemia, decreased bone mineral density, thrombocytopenia.
		Use in first trimester may be associated with neural tube defects, cardiovascular digital and orofacial abnormalities, and cognitive impairments; hepatotoxicity and pancreatitis may also occur
Newer agents (since 1993)		
Felbamate	30–60	Focal-aware and -impaired seizures and Lennox-Gastaut syndrome
		Associated with aplastic anemia and severe hepatitis, thus used only for refractory epilepsy

TABLE 22-6. Some clinical properties of select anticonvulsant drugs (*continued*)

Drug	Recommended serum level, µg/mL	Indications and side effects
Gabapentin	12–21	Focal-aware and -impaired seizures, anxiety, and neuropathic pain control
		May cause somnolence; may cause aggressive behavior and irritability in children and worsen absence and myoclonic seizures
Lacosamide	10–20	Focal-aware and -impaired seizures
		May increase PR interval; dizziness, somnolence, depression, and nausea may occur
Lamotrigine	3–15	Focal-aware and -impaired, generalized tonic/clonic, absence, and other generalized seizures; Lennox-Gastaut syndrome; bipolar affective disorder
		Serious rash seen in 0.08%–0.3% of adults and higher in children, risk decreased with slow titration; arrhythmias
Levetiracetam	12–46	Focal-aware and -impaired, generalized tonic-clonic, and myoclonic seizures
		May cause depression, agitation, irritability
Oxcarbazepine	5–35	Use is the same as carbamazepine but better tolerated. Effects similar to those of carbamazepine except more hyponatremia and less induction of hepatic enzymes
Perampanel	0.05–0.4	AMPA noncompetitive receptor blocker; focal-aware and -impaired, focal to bilateral, and generalized tonic-clonic seizures
		May cause somnolence, aggression, irritability
Pregabalin	2.8–8.2	Focal-aware and -impaired seizures, pain syndromes, anxiety
		Effects similar to those of gabapentin

TABLE 22–6. Some clinical properties of select anticonvulsant drugs (continued)

Drug	Recommended serum level, µg/mL	Indications and side effects
Rufinamide	9–40	Focal-aware and -impaired seizures and Lennox-Gastaut syndrome
Tiagabine	0.02–0.2	May cause somnolence, gastrointestinal complaints, depression Focal-aware and -impaired seizures May cause nervousness, depression, cognitive effects, rarely psychosis
Topiramate	5–20	Focal-aware and -impaired and generalized tonic-clonic seizures, Lennox-Gastaut syndrome, migraine prophylaxis May cause weight loss, depression, psychosis, and dosage-dependent cognitive, expressive language, and memory impairment
Vigabatrin	0.8–36	Focal-aware and -impaired seizures and infantile spasms May cause visual field defects, irreversible retinal dysfunction, memory and cognition impairment, psychosis, depression, or mania; may increase seizure activity
Zonisamide	10–40	Focal-aware and -impaired, generalized tonic/clonic, and myoclonic seizures May cause cognitive impairment, behavioral irritability, paranoia, depression, psychosis, weight loss, renal stones, rarely skin rash/Stevens-Johnson syndrome

Source. Adapted from Porter RJ, Rogawski MA: "Antiseizure Drugs," in *Basic and Clinical Pharmacology*, 14th Edition. Edited by Katzung BG. New York, McGraw-Hill, 2015, pp. 409–439; and Patsalos PN, Bourgeois BFD: *The Epilepsy Prescriber's Guide to Antiepileptic Drugs*, 2nd Edition. Cambridge, UK, Cambridge University Press, 2014.

negative psychiatric side effects. Psychosis that develops as a side effect of a newly administered antiepileptic may be secondary to the phenomenon of forced normalization, as reviewed in Chapter 9.

Recommended anticonvulsant serum levels, indications for use, and major toxicities are listed Table 22–6. A new classification scheme from the International League Against Epilepsy is outlined in Chapter 9. Recommendations from both references have been changed to reflect this new classification.

Newer drugs added to the list include cannabidiol, stiripentol, cenobamate, eslicarbazepine, and ezogabapine, which has been removed from the market because of toxicity. Brivaracetam was added to the list in 2019. It is a derivative of levetiracetam with perhaps better tolerability.

Pharmacokinetics

Serum-level monitoring is especially important for phenytoin. This drug has nonlinear pharmacokinetics and interacts with several other drugs (Table 22–7) via the liver's cytochrome P450 system. Carbamazepine induces its own hepatic metabolism, with serum levels falling despite a constant dosage in the first weeks of therapy. It is also associated with increased risk of Stevens-Johnson syndrome in patients with the HLA-B1502 allele, which is 10 times more frequent in persons of Asian ethnicity.

Carbamazepine, phenytoin, primidone, and phenobarbital are all hepatic enzyme–inducing drugs and are associated with osteoporosis. With the exception of felbamate, newer-generation antiepileptic drugs seem relatively devoid of significant interactions with other anticonvulsants. Lamotrigine metabolism is inhibited by valproate (see Table 22–6); slow dosage titration and avoidance of abrupt discontinuation are indicated.

Carbamazepine, phenytoin, primidone, lamotrigine, oxcarbazepine, eslicarbazepine, and phenobarbital are the most allergenic and the most prone to risk for Stevens-Johnson syndrome and rash.

Gabapentin and pregabalin do not act through effects on GABA but by attachment to $\alpha_2\delta$ and by effects on voltage-gated calcium channels. They are widely utilized in the management of chronic pain and have few side effects. Lamotrigine acts on voltage-dependent sodium channels, has a wide spectrum of activity against seizures, and may have an antidepressant effect; rashes are its main side effect. As antiepileptic drugs, lamotrigine, levetiracetam, lacosamide, felbamate, and brivaracetam are

TABLE 22-7. Significant anticonvulsant interactions

Interaction	Drugs
Causes hepatic enzyme induction	Carbamazepine*, phenobarbital, phenytoin, primidone
Has levels reduced by enzyme-inducing drugs	Anticonvulsants Other drugs: e.g., warfarin, antidepressants, antipsychotics, cyclosporine, modafinil, protease inhibitors, methylphenidate, corticosteroids, propranolol, and benzodiazepines
Reduces steroid oral contraceptive efficacy	Topiramate, felbamate, oxcarbazepine, phenobarbital, carbamazepine, phenytoin
Has most antiepileptic vs. antiepileptic interactions (N)	Felbamate (15), lamotrigine (17), oxcarbazepine (14), rufinamide (13)
Inhibits hepatic enzyme	Valproate increases phenobarbital and primidone levels by 30%–50%, lamotrigine levels by up to 200%; Drug–drug interaction results in a high incidence of Stevens-Johnson syndrome
Induces anticonvulsant toxicity	Isoniazid, dicoumarol, disulfiram, erythromycin, chloramphenicol

*Carbamazepine reduces the serum concentration of phenytoin, and vice versa.

neurocognitively better tolerated. Levetiracetam binds synaptic vesicle 2A and may block release of glutamate; it is frequently associated with the advent of depression and agitation.

Oxcarbazepine is a prodrug and is rapidly transformed to the monohydroxy derivative after ingestion. Metabolized by reduction independent of the P450 system, oxcarbazepine has no liver enzyme–inducing properties and is without autoinduction. However, like carbamazepine, it interferes with the metabolism of oral contraceptives. With both carbamazepine and oxcarbazepine, therefore, high-estrogen compounds are recommended. Oxcarbazepine is associated with hyponatremia, as is carbamazepine but less frequently.

Tiagabine inhibits the reuptake of GABA from the synaptic cleft into glial cells and neurons. It can precipitate seizures and has been associated with onset of nonconvulsive status epilepticus. Topiramate has several actions, including inhibiting glutamate and enhancing GABA activity, and is a carbonic anhydrase inhibitor. A small number of patients taking topiramate develop renal stones, which are usually passed spontaneously. Other side effects include depression and speech disturbance, which can occur if the dosage is increased too rapidly.

■ APATHY

Apathy in neurocognitive disorders is discussed in Chapters 11, 12, 13, 15 ("White Matter Diseases"), and 18 ("Autism Spectrum Disorder").

■ PSEUDOBULBAR AFFECT

Pseudobulbar affect is reviewed in Chapters 3 ("Neuropsychiatric Symptoms and Syndromes"), 15 ("White Matter Diseases"), and 16 ("Head Injury and Its Sequelae").

■ COGNITIVE ENHANCERS

Cognitive enhancers are discussed in Chapter 11.

■ REFERENCES

Abou-Khalil BW: Update on antiepileptic drugs 2019. Am Acad Neurol 25(2, Epilepsy):508–536, 2019

Alper K, Schwartz KA, Kolts RL, Khan A: Seizure incidence in psychopharmacological clinical trials: an analysis of Food and Drug Administration (FDA) summary basis of approval reports. Biol Psychiatry 62(4):345–354, 2007 17223086

Ballard C, Banister C, Khan Z, et al: Evaluation of the safety, tolerability, and efficacy of pimavanserin versus placebo in patients with Alzheimer's disease psychosis: a phase 2, randomized, placebo-controlled, double-blind study. Lancet Neurol 17:213–222, 2018

Barry JJ, Lembke A, Huynh N: Affective disorders in epilepsy, in Psychiatric Issues in Epilepsy: A Practical Guide to Diagnosis and Treatment. Edited by Ettinger A, Kanner AM. Philadelphia, PA, Lippincott Williams and Wilkins, 2001, pp 45–72

Berman K, Brodaty H, Withall A, Seeher K: Pharmacologic treatment of apathy in dementia. Am J Geriatr Psychiatry 20(2):104–122, 2012 21841459

Chong TTJ, Husain M: The role of dopamine in the pathophysiology and treatment of apathy. Prog Brain Res 229:389–426, 2016 27926449

358

Correia MA: Drug biotransformation, in Basic and Clinical Pharmacology, 14th Edition. Edited by Katzung BG. New York, McGraw Hill Education, 2018, pp 56-73

Cummings JL, Devanand DP, Stahl SM: Dementia related psychosis and the potential role for pimavanserin. CNS Spectr 2020 32811586 Epub ahead of print

de Toffol B, Trimble M, Hesdorffer DC, et al: Pharmacotherapy in patients with epilepsy and psychosis. Epilepsy Behav 88:54–60, 2018 30241054

DeBattista C: Antidepressant agents, in Basic and Clinical Pharmacology, 14th edition. Edited by Katzung BG. New York, McGraw-Hill Education, 2015, pp 532–552

DeBattista C: Antipsychotic agents and lithium, in Basic and Clinical Pharmacology, 14th edition Edited by Katzung BG. New York, McGraw-Hill Education, 2015, pp 511–531

Hiemke C, Bergemann N, Clement HW, et al: Consensus guidelines for therapeutic drug monitoring in neuropsychopharmacology: update 2017. Pharmacopsychiatry 51:9–62, 2018

Iqbal SZ, Mathew SJ. Ketamine for depression clinical issues. Adv Pharmacol 89:131–162, 2020 32616205

Mitchell PB: Therapeutic drug monitoring of psychotropic medications. Br J Clin Pharmacol 49(4):303–312, 2000 10759685

Molero P, Ramos-Quiroga JA, Martin-Santos R, et al: Antidepressant efficacy and tolerability of ketamine and esketamine: a critical review. CNS Drugs 32:411–420, 2018

Mula M: The clinical spectrum of bipolar symptoms in epilepsy: a critical reappraisal. Postgrad Med 122(4):17–23, 2010 20675967

Patsalos PN: Drug interactions with the newer antiepileptic drugs (AEDs), part 1: pharmacokinetic and pharmacodynamic interactions between AEDs. Clin Pharmacokinet 52:927–966, 2013

Patsalos PN: Drug interactions with the newer antiepileptic drugs (AEDs), part 2: pharmacokinetic and pharmacodynamic interactions between AEDs. Clin Pharmacokinet 52:1045–1061, 2013

Patsalos PN, Bourgeois BFD: The Epilepsy Prescriber's Guide to Antiepileptic Drugs, 2nd Edition. Cambridge, UK, Cambridge University Press, 2014

Perucca E: New anticonvulsants, in Seizures, Affective Disorders and Anticonvulsant Drugs. Edited by Trimble MR, Schmitz B. Guildford, UK, Clarius, 2002

Porter RJ, Rogawski MA: Antiseizure drugs, in Basic and Clinical Pharmacology, 14th edition. Edited by Katzung BG. New York, McGraw-Hill Education, 2015, pp 409–439

Procyshyn RM, Bezchlibnyk-Butler KZ, Jeffries JJ (eds): Clinical Handbook of Psychotropic Drugs 2015. Boston, MA, Hogrefe, 2015

Rosenberg PB, Lanctôt KL, Drye LT, et al: Safety and efficacy of methylphenidate for apathy in Alzheimer's disease: a randomized, placebo-controlled trial. J Clin Psychiatry 74(8):810–816, 2013 24021498

Schatzberg A, DeBattista C: Schatzberg's Manual of Clinical Psychopharmacology. Washington, DC, American Psychiatric Association
Publishing, 2019

Spiegel DR, Warren A, Takakura W, Servidio L: Disorders of diminished motivation: what they are and how to treat them. Current
Psychiatry 17(1):11–19, 2018

Stahl SM: Stahl's Essential Psychopharmacology. Cambridge, UK,
Cambridge University Press, 2013

Starkstein SE, Pahissa J: Apathy following traumatic brain injury. Psychiatr Clin North Am 37(1):103–112, 2014 24529426

Steinhoff BJ, Staack AM: Levetiracetam and brivaracetam: a review of
evidence from clinical trials and clinical experience. Ther Adv Neurol Disord 12:1756286419873518, 2019 31523280

Szoko E, Tabit T, Riederer P, et al: Pharmacological aspects of the neuroprotective effects of irreversible MAO-B inhibitors, selegiline and
rasagiline, in Parkinson's disease. J Neural Transm (Vienna)
125(11):1735–1749, 2018 29417334

Walsh M-T, Dinan TG: Selective serotonin reuptake inhibitors and violence: a review of the available evidence. Acta Psychiatr Scand
104(2):84–91, 2001 11473500

INTERVENTIONAL PSYCHIATRY

John P. Coetzee, Ph.D.
Ian H. Kratter, M.D., Ph.D.
Mahendra T. Bhati, M.D.
Nolan Williams, M.D.

Interventional psychiatry is a growing subspecialty that uses neurotechnologies to identify the dysfunctional brain circuitry underlying neuropsychiatric disorders and applies neuromodulatory techniques to alter that circuitry therapeutically. Most studies have focused on neuromodulation for treatment-resistant depression (TRD), and this indication is the primary focus here, although we also highlight other indications. Depending on the modality chosen, direct modification of neural activity in discrete brain areas or systems may have a number of potential advantages over more traditional treatments of neuropsychiatric disorders. For example, focal modulation of a dysfunctional circuit may speed onset of therapeutic benefit while decreasing risk of adverse effects. This, in turn, may ultimately make such a treatment more cost-effective, especially when compared with the cost of untreated or ineffectively treated neuropsychiatric illness.

Neuromodulatory treatments can be divided into two broad categories: noninvasive and invasive. Noninvasive techniques, including transcranial magnetic stimulation (TMS), theta-burst stimulation (TBS; a high frequency form of patterned TMS), and electroconvulsive therapy (ECT), have a potentially broader clinical application than invasive techniques, given the significantly lower risks and costs associated with them. Invasive treatments such as ablative surgeries, deep brain stimulation (DBS), and vagus nerve stimulation (VNS) are typically reserved for the most severe cases because of the inherently greater risks involved. These approaches are discussed later in the chapter. Additional modalities under active study include transcranial direct-current stimulation, epidural cortical stimulation, magnetic seizure therapy, and focal electrically administered seizure therapy; however, these modalities are not discussed further here given their purely investigational status.

When choosing a treatment for a particular patient, clinicians should consider the indication, treatment history, severity of symptoms, patient's ability to adhere to treatment, and likely efficacy in addition to the potential side effects, risks, and cost of treatment. In general, noninvasive approaches should be tried first. The effectiveness, tolerability, and precision of these techniques will likely continue to improve, resulting in more widespread adoption of neuromodulation therapies.

■ NONINVASIVE INTERVENTIONS

Transcranial Magnetic Stimulation

In TMS, a coil placed near the scalp generates a pulsed magnetic field that safely passes through intervening skin and bone and induces an electrical current in the brain region below. The nature and intensity of the stimulation is dependent on the shape and placement of the coil, the frequency of pulsation, and the intensity of the magnetic field. Repetitive TMS (rTMS) induces long-term changes in neuronal excitability, allowing dysfunctional brain circuits to be modulated in a more durable manner.

rTMS targeting the left dorsolateral prefrontal cortex, an area shown to be hypoactive in patients with depression, was approved by the FDA in 2008 for TRD. Multiple studies have demonstrated rTMS to be more effective than sham but not as effective as ECT. A typical treatment course is a 37.5-minute stimulation session daily, 5 days per week, for 4–6 weeks; maintenance rTMS may improve response durability for some patients. rTMS has proven to be quite safe and well-tolerated. Headache and scalp pain are the most common adverse effects. Earplugs are advised for comfort and safety; although the sound produced by rTMS can be loud enough to produce hearing loss, studies have found that in practice the changes in hearing produced by rTMS are transient in nature, with only rare exceptions. The most serious adverse event is a seizure, which occurs at a rate of <0.1% and usually in patients receiving a dose of rTMS that exceeds guidelines or those concurrently taking drugs that lower the seizure threshold.

rTMS for TRD comes with several advantages compared with ECT. rTMS does not require induction of a seizure and, importantly, does not have cognitive risks like those associated with ECT. Finally, rTMS does not carry the significant cultural stigma of ECT. Despite these advantages, the efficacy of rTMS is inferior to that of ECT (see "Efficacy").

rTMS is useful for other conditions as well. In 2018, "deep" rTMS targeting the medial prefrontal cortex was approved by the FDA for treatment of OCD. The orbitofrontal cortex and the presupplementary motor area are additional potential therapeutic targets for OCD under active study. rTMS continues to be studied as a possible treatment for a diverse range of neuropsychiatric disorders such as Tourette's syndrome, Parkinson's disease, bipolar disorder, anxiety disorders, substance use disorders, schizophrenia, chronic pain, and more.

Theta Burst Stimulation

TBS is a patterned form of rTMS that makes use of theta rhythms similar to those produced intrinsically by the human hippocampus to promote neuronal plasticity. TBS is more efficient than conventional rTMS, thereby allowing a considerable shortening in the duration of each treatment session. A large, randomized trial of patients with TRD in 2018 demonstrated that a course of TBS to the left dorsolateral prefrontal cortex lasting 3 minutes per treatment but otherwise equivalent in terms of frequency and number of treatments is non-inferior to a course of standard rTMS (37.5 minutes per treatment). This trial led to FDA approval of TBS for treatment of TRD that year. The safety profile of TBS is at least as good as that of rTMS (as described earlier). Given its improved efficiency, TBS is one of the most promising forms of noninvasive therapies for the near future, and innovative forms of the treatment are actively being developed.

Electroconvulsive Therapy

ECT is the oldest noninvasive treatment for TRD and remains the gold standard for efficacy (see "Efficacy" section). It is especially valuable for the most severe cases of depression, such as those involving catatonia or psychosis. It also can be effective for bipolar disorder, schizophrenia, catatonia of other etiologies, and neuroleptic malignant syndrome. During an ECT session, an electric current is applied to the scalp to induce a seizure. Typically, a series of 9–12 seizures are induced over several weeks, with 2–3 occurring each week. Treatments are given with the patient under general anesthesia and the influence of a paralyzing drug.

Patients who have benefited from ECT continue to be at risk for relapse. As such, they should continue to be treated with antidepressant medications or maintenance ECT. The optimal approach to maintaining remission after a successful course of ECT remains uncertain. Although serious complications, such as status epilepticus, are rare, several transient adverse events are common with ECT, including nausea, headaches, muscle aches, and arrhythmias. The side effects that have played the largest role in limiting the application of ECT, however, are cognitive in nature, including acute cognitive impairment typically lasting minutes to hours and retrograde or anterograde amnesia. The risk of lasting cognitive impairment is increased in geriatric populations, with bilateral electrode placement, and with longer courses of treatment. Unfortunately, ECT continues to be associated with stigma due to its past administration without anesthesia and its depictions in popular culture and media.

ECT can be safely administered in patients with coexisting neuropsychiatric illnesses, including epilepsy, Parkinson's disease, and dementia. If there is clinical concern regarding active lesion(s) in patients with multiple sclerosis, then a brain MRI with contrast may be considered prior to ECT, although no clear evidence has shown that such lesions increase the risk for post-ECT delirium or cognitive impairment. See Table 23–1 for special considerations in specific neuropsychiatric populations.

Effic.acy

Both rTMS and ECT are effective treatments for TRD, although ECT has demonstrably superior rates of remission. *Remission* is defined as the presence of few or no symptoms, usually indicated by a score below a specific threshold on a standardized measure of depression, and is generally considered to be a more reliable outcome comparison in such studies than treatment response, which only requires a 50% reduction in symptoms. Open-label studies of ECT for TRD have found remission rates of 48% for patients with a prior pharmacotherapy failure (although rates can range as high as 90%, depending on various factors, including the level of treatment resistance, the presence of comorbid medical and psychiatric conditions, and the type of ECT stimulation conducted), compared with remission rates of 27% for standard rTMS and 32% for intermittent TBS. In randomized controlled trials, remission rates for standard rTMS fall even further, to 16%. Similarly, a randomized controlled trial that directly compared ECT with rTMS found remission rates of 59% and 17%, respectively. Although ECT is more effective than rTMS, it is not as well tolerated as rTMS and is associated with greater risks, as described earlier.

TABLE 23–1. Neuropsychiatric illnesses and electroconvulsive therapy (ECT)

	Pros of ECT	Cons of ECT
Dementia	May transiently help with apathy and agitation	May worsen cognitive impairment.
Epilepsy	Raises seizure threshold and has an anticonvulsant effect	Anticonvulsants interfere with it and may need to be reduced or discontinued
Multiple sclerosis	May help with related mood symptoms (both depression and mania)	May increase risk of delirium and cognitive impairment.
Parkinson's disease	May help improve motor and mood symptoms	May contribute to cognitive impairment.
Stroke	May help with stroke-related depression	May result in cardiovascular alterations, increasing risk of stroke, and may contribute to cognitive impairment.

■ INVASIVE INTERVENTIONS

Ablative Surgery

Surgical treatments for psychiatric disorders also suffer from stigma, primarily stemming from the field's troubled history. The popularity of the prefrontal leucotomy (commonly known as the frontal lobotomy) during the early to mid-20th century perhaps most famously (and tragically) illustrates both the ethical concerns and the risks inherent in this kind of treatment. However, increased understanding of the neural circuitry associated with particular pathological mental states, combined with significant improvements in stereotactic neurosurgical targeting, has led to a cautious reemergence of focal ablation therapies for intractable psychiatric conditions. Ongoing advancements in targeting based on functional neuroimaging and tractography and the development of newer modalities, such as gamma knife radiosurgery or magnetic resonance–guided focused ultrasound, that avoid the need for craniotomy in some cases have led to further refinements in these treatments.

Anterior cingulotomy for TRD or OCD is the most studied of these treatments. Bilateral lesions of the dorsal anterior cingulate gyrus are intended to disrupt fibers connecting the anterior cingulate to the orbitofrontal cortex and subcortical limbic structures. The procedure has a good record of safety, and while

366

no randomized trials have been completed, reduction in symptoms is usually in the 30%–60% range. Other ablative procedures for TRD and OCD include anterior capsulotomy targeting the anterior limb of the internal capsule; subcaudate tractotomy targeting the substantia innominata (specifically thalamocortical white matter tracts inferior to the anterior striatum); and limbic leucotomy, which combines cingulotomy with subcaudate tractotomy. Despite recent advances, these surgical approaches are irreversible and are generally associated with greater risk than noninvasive approaches. Accordingly, they are reserved for use in only the most severe cases when other treatments have failed. Compared with DBS, ablative procedures offer the benefits of requiring neither clinic visits for programming nor eventual battery replacement.

Deep Brain Stimulation

DBS differs in several important ways from its surgical predecessors. Unlike ablative or disconnective surgeries, DBS is reversible and adjustable, meaning that sham studies can more easily be conducted and that devices can be reprogrammed to change the intensity or pattern of stimulation and even the specific location of stimulus delivery (by changing which contact[s] on the lead are active). Although the chronic introduction of electrodes into subcortical brain structures for clinical purposes has been practiced in one form or another since at least the 1950s, DBS in its modern form was developed in the 1980s for the treatment of intractable motor disorders (e.g., Parkinson's disease, tremor, dystonia), for which it has been a life-changing treatment. This dramatic success led neurosurgeons to explore the possibility of replacing destructive interventions for other disorders with DBS as well, applying it successfully for TRD, epilepsy, Tourette's syndrome, OCD, obesity, and cluster headache, among others. DBS currently has FDA approval in the United States for the treatment of Parkinson's disease, essential tremor, and dystonia, and in 2009 it received FDA approval for treatment-resistant OCD under a humanitarian device exemption.

Regarding TRD, various potential targets have been tested, and there is at least preliminary evidence for both the efficacy and safety of DBS in the subgenual anterior cingulate cortex (ACC), the ventral capsule/ventral striatum, the nucleus accumbens, the lateral habenula, the inferior thalamic peduncle, the medial forebrain bundle, the bed nucleus of the stria terminalis, and the ventral anterior limb of the internal capsule. Although the ideal target for treatment of TRD with DBS is still unknown, the evidence for the subgenual ACC (i.e., Brodmann area 25) may be the strongest, with at least 16 studies displaying the safety of DBS in this area, along with high rates of response and remission. By contrast, the published studies supporting the efficacy of other DBS targets for TRD are somewhat smaller in number. Stimulation of this area can result in immediate antidysphoric effects. The reduction in depressive symptoms with DBS also appears durable, with relief in one study persisting at 1 year and in another lasting several years. The efficacy of stimulating the subgenual ACC may be enhanced by individualized target identification utilizing connectomic analysis, although this has only been explored in a small pilot study. However, a large multicenter controlled trial for the purpose of gaining FDA approval of DBS for TRD failed to find a statistically significant difference between the groups. Future DBS trials may benefit from allowing time for stimulation optimization, which is an influential factor in the effectiveness of DBS.

Because DBS entails brain surgery as well as longitudinal follow-up for programming and battery replacement, it comes with significant risks and requires a multidisciplinary management team. Risks of the surgery include infection, persistent pain or discomfort, and hemorrhage. The potential psychiatric side effects of stimulation depend on the stimulation target and settings but generally include worsening of mood, anxiety, sleep disturbance, (hypo)mania, agitation, or suicidal ideation or attempt, although it is often difficult to determine whether these are related to the intervention or to the underlying illness itself. Nonpsychiatric side effects of DBS may include paresthesias, headache, a pulling sensation at the surgical sites, or other nonspecific somatic symptoms. Some of these side effects are transient or can be mitigated with programming changes.

Vagus Nerve Stimulation

VNS is primarily used as a treatment for intractable epilepsy, and chronic stimulation has been found to have antidepressant effects. Although the efferent fibers of the vagus nerve primarily originate in the medulla oblongata and descend to modulate the heart and other internal viscera, the antiseizure and antidepressant benefits of VNS are associated with stimulation to the ascending afferent vagal fibers, which innervate various structures including the cingulate gyrus and frontal areas. The stimulating leads are usually wrapped around the left vagus nerve (less cardiac innervation than the right) at the carotid sheath by a trained surgeon, and the procedure is lower risk compared with other invasive interventions. An interventional psychiatrist is responsible for managing the stimulation parameters. The possibility of transcutaneous VNS at the auricular branch of the afferent vagus nerve currently is being explored.

VNS can alter regional cerebral blood flow in several regions, including the amygdala and subgenual ACC. Stimulation of the vagus nerve also reduces inflammatory responses, which are thought to be involved in the pathogenesis of depression. Regarding efficacy, a large, controlled trial found no detectable effect of VNS for TRD, but the duration of the study may have been too short to detect an effect. A subsequent open-label trial found an improvement of 0.45 points per month on the Hamilton Rating Scale for Depression, and it was on this basis that the FDA approved VNS in 2005 for the adjunctive long-term treatment of chronic or recurrent depression in patients 18 years of age or older who are experiencing a major depressive episode without adequate response to four or more adequate antidepressant treatments. Despite this approval, most insurers (including the Centers for Medicare and Medicaid Services) did not find the evidence sufficiently strong to justify reimbursement. However, a recent, long-term observational study provided evidence that the effects of VNS are durable, with a significantly higher response and remission rate compared with treatment as usual after 5 years. A more definitive randomized clinical trial is currently under way to determine efficacy.

VNS complications come in two categories: those related to surgery and those related to stimulation. The most common surgical problems are infection (3%–6%), vocal cord paresis (1%), and lower facial weakness (1%). The most common complications related to stimulation include (but are not limited to) voice alteration, cough, paresthesia, dyspnea, headache, and pain. The latter complications are more common, with as many as 62% of patients experiencing voice changes while the device is actively stimulating. However, stimulation issues tend to decline over time, with the proportion of patients experiencing voice problems dropping to 18.7% after 5 years.

■ REFERENCES

Bergfeld IO, Mantione M, Hoogendoorn MLC, et al: Deep brain stimulation of the ventral anterior limb of the internal capsule for treatment-resistant depression: a randomized clinical trial. JAMA Psychiatry 73(5):456–464, 2016 27049915

Blumberger DM, Vila-Rodriguez F, Thorpe KE, et al: Effectiveness of theta burst versus high-frequency repetitive transcranial magnetic stimulation in patients with depression (THREE-D): a randomised non-inferiority trial. Lancet 391(10131):1683–1692, 2018 29726344

Chen JJ, Zhao LB, Liu YY, et al: Comparative efficacy and acceptability of electroconvulsive therapy versus repetitive transcranial magnetic stimulation for major depression: a systematic review and multiple-treatments meta-analysis. Behav Brain Res 320:30–36, 2017 27876667

Cusin C, Dougherty DD: Somatic therapies for treatment-resistant depression: ECT, TMS, VNS, DBS. Biol Mood Anxiety Disord 2(1):14, 2012 22901565

Dougherty DD: Deep brain stimulation: clinical applications. Psychiatr Clin North Am 41(3):385–394, 2018 30098652

Eranti S, Mogg A, Pluck G, et al: A randomized, controlled trial with 6-month follow-up of repetitive transcranial magnetic stimulation and electroconvulsive therapy for severe depression. Am J Psychiatry 164(1):73–81, 2007 17202547

George MS, Lisanby SH, Avery D, et al: Daily left prefrontal transcranial magnetic stimulation therapy for major depressive disorder: a sham-controlled randomized trial. Arch Gen Psychiatry 67(5):507–516, 2010 20439832

Heijnen WT, Birkenhäger TK, Wierdsma AI, van den Broek WW: Antidepressant pharmacotherapy failure and response to subsequent electroconvulsive therapy: a meta-analysis. J Clin Psychopharmacol 30(5):616–619, 2010 20814336

Holtzheimer PE, Husain MM, Lisanby SH, et al: Subcallosal cingulate deep brain stimulation for treatment-resistant depression: a multisite, randomised, sham-controlled trial. Lancet Psychiatry 4(11):839–849, 2017 28988904

Krames ES, Hunter Peckham P, Rezai A, Aboelsaad F: What is neuromodulation?, in Neuromodulation. Edited by Krames ES, Peckham PH, Rezai AR. San Diego, CA, Academic Press, 2009, pp 3–8

Krystal AD, Coffey CE: Neuropsychiatric considerations in the use of electroconvulsive therapy. J Neuropsychiatry Clin Neurosci 9(2):283–292, 1997 9144111

Lam RW, Chan P, Wilkins-Ho M, Yatham LN: Repetitive transcranial magnetic stimulation for treatment-resistant depression: a systematic review and metaanalysis. Can J Psychiatry 53(9):621–631, 2008 18801225

Lisanby SH: Electroconvulsive therapy for depression. N Engl J Med 357(19):1939–1945, 2007 17989386

Milev RV, Giacobbe P, Kennedy SH, et al: Canadian Network for Mood and Anxiety Treatments (CANMAT) 2016 clinical guidelines for the management of adults with major depressive disorder: section 4. neurostimulation treatments. Can J Psychiatry 61(9):561–575, 2016 27486154

O'Reardon JP, Solvason HB, Janicak PG, et al: Efficacy and safety of transcranial magnetic stimulation in the acute treatment of major depression: a multisite randomized controlled trial. Biol Psychiatry 62(11):1208–1216, 2007 17573044

Petrides G, Fink M, Husain MM, et al: ECT remission rates in psychotic versus nonpsychotic depressed patients: a report from CORE. J ECT 17(4):244–253, 2001 11731725

Rosa MA, Lisanby SH: Somatic treatments for mood disorders. Neuropsychopharmacology 37(1):102–116, 2012 21976043

Rush AJ, Sackeim HA, Marangell LB, et al: Effects of 12 months of vagus nerve stimulation in treatment-resistant depression: a naturalistic study. Biol Psychiatry 58(5):355–363, 2005 16139581

Sehatzadeh S, Daskalakis ZJ, Yap B, et al: Unilateral and bilateral repetitive transcranial magnetic stimulation for treatment-resistant depression: a meta-analysis of randomized controlled trials over 2 decades. J Psychiatry Neurosci 44(3):151–163, 2019 30720259

INDEX

*Page numbers printed in **boldface** type refer to tables or figures.*

378